theclinics.com

HEART FAILURE CLINICS

Noninvasive Imaging of Heart Failure

GUEST EDITORS
Vasken Dilsizian, MD
Mario J. Garcia, MD
David Bello, MD

CONSULTING EDITORS
Jagat Narula, MD, PhD
James B. Young, MD

April 2006 • Volume 2 • Number 2

SAUNDERS

An Imprint of Elsevier, Inc.
PHILADELPHIA LONDON TORONTO MONTREAL SYDNEY TOKYO

W.B. SAUNDERS COMPANY
A Division of Elsevier Inc.

1600 John F. Kennedy Boulevard • Suite 1800 • Philadelphia, Pennsylvania 19103-2899

http://www.theclinics.com

HEART FAILURE CLINICS
April 2006
Editor: Karen Sorensen

Volume 2, Number 2
ISSN 1551-7136
ISBN 1-4160-3508-7

Heart Failure Clinics (ISSN 1551-7136) is published quarterly by W.B. Saunders, 360 Park Avenue South, New York, NY 10010-1710. Months of publication are January, April, July, and October. Business and editorial offices: 1600 John F. Kennedy Boulevard, Suite 1800, Philadelphia, PA 19103-2899. Accounting and circulation offices: 6277 Sea Harbor Drive, Orlando, FL 32887-4800. Periodicals postage paid at New York, NY and additional mailing offices. Subscription prices are USD 145 per year for US individuals, USD 245 per year for US institutions, USD 50 per year for US students and residents, USD 175 per year for Canadian individuals, USD 275 per year for Canadian institutions, USD 175 per year for international individuals, USD 275 per year for international institutions and USD 60 per year for foreign students/residents. To receive student and resident rate, orders must be accompanied by name of affiliated institution, date of term, and the *signature* of program/residency coordinator on institution letterhead. Orders will be billed at individual rate until proof of status is received. Foreign air speed delivery is included in all *Clinics* subscription prices. All prices are subject to change without notice. POSTMASTER: Send address changes to *Heart Failure Clinics*, Elsevier Periodicals Customer Service, 6277 Sea Harbor Drive, Orlando, FL 32887-4800. **Customer Service: 1-800-654-2452 (US). From outside of the US, call (+1) 407-345-4000.**

Printed in the United States of America.

Cover artwork courtesy of Umberto M. Jezek.

CONSULTING EDITORS

JAGAT NARULA, MD, PhD, Professor, Medicine; Chief, Division of Cardiology; and Associate Dean, University of California Irvine School of Medicine, Irvine, California

JAMES B. YOUNG, MD, Chairman and Professor, Department of Medicine, Lerner College of Medicine; and George and Linda Kaufman Chair, Cleveland Clinic Foundation, Case Western Reserve University, Cleveland, Ohio

GUEST EDITORS

VASKEN DILSIZIAN, MD, Professor, Department of Medicine and Radiology, University of Maryland School of Medicine; Director of Cardiovascular Nuclear Medicine and Cardiac Positron Emission Tomography, University of Maryland Medical Center, Baltimore, Maryland

MARIO J. GARCIA, MD, Director, Cardiac Imaging; and Professor of Medicine, Cleveland Clinic Lerner College of Medicine, Cleveland, Ohio

DAVID BELLO, MD, Mid-Florida Cardiology, Orlando Regional Hospital, Orlando, Florida; Division of Cardiology, Department of Medicine, University of California–Irvine, Irvine, California

CONTRIBUTORS

THEODORE P. ABRAHAM, MD, Associate Professor, Division of Cardiology, Johns Hopkins University, Baltimore, Maryland

JAMES A. ARRIGHI, MD, Associate Professor, Department of Medicine and Diagnostic Imaging, Brown Medical School; and Director, Nuclear Cardiology, Rhode Island Hospital, Providence, Rhode Island

JEROEN J. BAX, MD, PhD, Department of Cardiology, Leiden University Medical Center, Leiden, The Netherlands

DAVID BELLO, MD, Mid-Florida Cardiology, Orlando Regional Hospital, Orlando, Florida; Division of Cardiology, Department of Medicine, University of California–Irvine, Irvine, California

VASKEN DILSIZIAN, MD, Professor, Department of Medicine and Radiology, University of Maryland School of Medicine; Director of Cardiovascular Nuclear Medicine and Cardiac Positron Emission Tomography, University of Maryland Medical Center, Baltimore, Maryland

WILLIAM C. ECKELMAN, PhD, Molecular Tracer, LLC, Bethesda, Maryland

ABDOU ELHENDY, MD, PhD, Thorax Center, Erasmus Medical Center, Rotterdam, The Netherlands

STEVEN J. FOWLER, MD, Division of Cardiology, University of California at Irvine, Orange, California

MARIO J. GARCIA, MD, Director, Cardiac Imaging; and Professor of Medicine, Cleveland Clinic Lerner College of Medicine, Cleveland, Ohio

SWAMINATHA V. GURUDEVAN, MD, Division of Cardiology, University of California at Irvine, Orange, California

TAKAHIRO HIGUCHI, MD, PhD, Nuklearmedizinische Klinik und Poliklinik, Klinikum rechts der Isar der Technische Universität München, München, Germany

DAVID A. KASS, MD, Abraham and Virginia Weiss Professor of Cardiology and Professor of Biomedical Engineering, Johns Hopkins University, Baltimore, Maryland

ALBERT C. LARDO, PhD, Assistant Professor of Medicine, Radiology and Biomedical Engineering, Johns Hopkins University, Baltimore, Maryland

MANDEEP R. MEHRA, MD, FACC, FACP, Herbert Berger Professor of Medicine; and Head of Cardiology, University of Maryland School of Medicine, Baltimore, Maryland

JAGAT NARULA, MD, PhD, Professor, Medicine; Chief, Division of Cardiology; and Associate Dean, University of California Irvine School of Medicine, Irvine, California

DON POLDERMANS, MD, PhD, Thorax Center, Erasmus Medical Center, Rotterdam, The Netherlands

AIDAN R. RANEY, BA, Department of Medicine, Division of Cardiology, University of California, Irvine, California

ARTHUR J.H.A. SCHOLTE, MD, Department of Cardiology, Leiden University Medical Center, Leiden, The Netherlands

JOANNE D. SCHUIJF, MSc, Department of Cardiology, Leiden University Medical Center, Leiden, The Netherlands

MARKUS SCHWAIGER, MD, Nuklearmedizinische Klinik und Poliklinik, Klinikum rechts der Isar der Technischen Universität München, München, Germany

JAMSHID SHIRANI, MD, Department of Cardiology, Geisinger Medical Center, Danville, Pennsylvania

ERIC M. THORN, MD, Clinical Fellow, Division of Cardiology, University of Maryland School of Medicine, Baltimore, Maryland

ERNST E. van der WALL, MD, PhD, Department of Cardiology, Leiden University Medical Center, Leiden, The Netherlands

JAMES B. YOUNG, MD, Chairman and Professor, Department of Medicine, Lerner College of Medicine; and George and Linda Kaufman Chair, Cleveland Clinic Foundation, Case Western Reserve University, Cleveland, Ohio

CONTENTS

FORTHCOMING ISSUES

July 2006

Natriuretic Peptides
John Burnett, MD, Roger Mills, MD, and
W.H. Wilson Tang, MD, *Guest Editors*

October 2006

Valvular Disease and Heart Failure
Blasé Anthony Carabello, MD, *Guest Editor*

January 2007

Advances in Pre- and Post-Transplant Management
Mandeep R. Mehra, MD, *Guest Editor*

RECENT ISSUES

January 2006

Diabetic-Hypertensive Pre–Heart Failure Patient
David S.H. Bell, MB, *Guest Editor*

October 2005

Myocarditis
G. William Dec, MD, *Guest Editor*

July 2005

Pathogenesis of Heart Failure
Roger J. Hajjar, MD, and
Federica del Monte, MD, PhD, *Guest Editors*

ELSEVIER
SAUNDERS

Heart Failure Clin 2 (2006) ix – x

HEART
FAILURE
CLINICS

Editorial

Imaging Heart Failure: Premonition to Prevention in Predisposed. . .

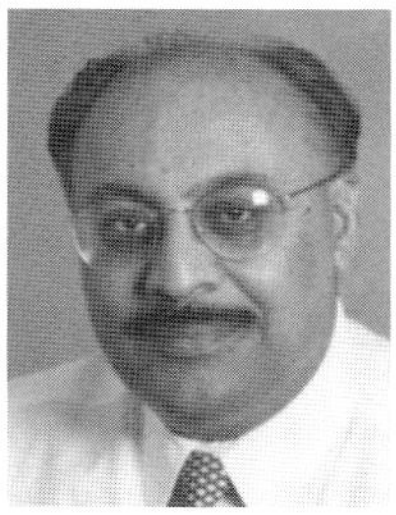
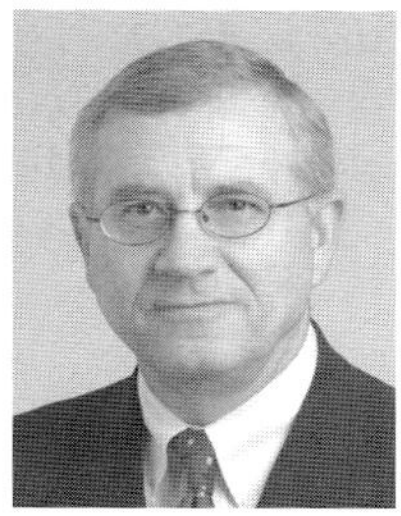

Jagat Narula, MD, PhD   James B. Young, MD
Consulting Editors

The short story "The Minority Report" by Philip Dick and its subsequent cinematic translation by director Steven Spielberg portray the metaphysical concept of predicting and preventing a murder that is supposed to occur 50 years later. Three elite "pre-cogs" provide imagery of the future time, mode, and place of the crime, and the "pre-crime" unit acts on the premonition by arresting the "potential" criminal. The pre-cogs do not always agree about the future, and the "minority report" refers to their dissenting opinion, which must be crystallized to establish the certainty that is necessary for the program's validity. Summarily, because a crime has not occurred, the foreknowledge is likely to change the future!

The paradigm of medical management (and prevention) of some diseases may evolve similarly if we focus on strategies that identify the likelihood of development of infirmity. The recent ACC-AHA guidelines—in addition to the commonly accepted group of patients who have manifest heart failure (HF) that includes symptomatic patients who have ventricular dysfunction (stage C) and those who have advanced HF (stage D)—include all subjects who are susceptible to the development of HF (stage A) and those who have asymptomatic ventricular dysfunction (stage B) within the broader category of HF. Much energetic, and, at times, contentious discussion occurred when the "staging" concept was proposed. How could someone have "heart failure" if there are no symptoms or physical findings to suggest fluid retention and congestion, despite the presence of systolic or diastolic dysfunction on echocardiography? More contentious was the concept of "pre"-heart failure, whereby patients were asymptomatic and had no evidence of structural heart disease. Surely a type of futuristic murder. It is believed that in addition to the 5 million patients who have manifest HF (stages C–D) in the United States, 75 million subjects may be at risk for developing HF (stages A–B). The mortality that is attributed to HF surpasses that for all cancers and HIV-related deaths combined, and the economic burden of the management of stages C–D HF is enormous. Therefore, emphasis on the diagnosis and management of stages C–D HF alone is grossly inadequate. It is necessary to develop diagnostic schemes and treatment strategies to prevent the progression of stages A–B "heart failure" to stages C–D manifest and symptomatic HF. Ultimately, such strategies will require genotypic characterization of the susceptibility to HF and the development of novel imaging techniques for phenotypic characterization before morphologic alterations become apparent.

1551-7136/06/$ – see front matter
doi:10.1016/j.hfc.2006.05.001

The study of HF provides a prime setting for the introduction of new and innovative imaging strategies designed that identify new targets and provide relevant clinical information concerning pathophysiology and patient outcome. Although the assessment of perfusion and ventricular function have provided important insights, they are insufficient to address key issues of remodeling, including the ability to reverse this process, identify arrhythmogenic substrate, and determine the potential for myocyte death or recovery. Future imaging strategies could be developed based on new biologic insights into the failing myocardium that were acquired from in vitro studies and studies in genetically altered small animal models. These strategies would focus on myocytic, interstitial, and neuronal cardiac compartments. The potential imaging targets include altered myocyte surface proteins, receptors, or channels; interstitial and matrical collagen synthesis and dissolution; and the efficiency of presynaptic neurons in concentrating adrenergic mediators. Novel imaging strategies also will probe cytokine activation, local myocardial neurohumoral upregulation, mediators of inflammation, and metabolic perturbations in the failing myocytes; provide better definition of cell death mechanisms; and characterize the expression of fetal genes in failing myocytes. Additionally, because the future therapy of HF is likely to include novel biologic strategies, such as gene therapy and stem cell transplantation, effective imaging approaches to follow these therapeutic options also will be necessary. This issue of *Heart Failure Clinics*, edited so ably by Dilsizian, Garcia, and Bello, brings established, evolving, and futuristic imaging techniques together. The issue culminates with a stimulating proposal that the imaging of the renin–angiotensin axis in the myocardium will predict remodeling and allow for the recognition of gullible amongst the predisposed. As is obvious in the ensuing issue, it has become mandatory that we adopt a preventive ideology and invest in finding imaging pre-cogs to contain the impending global HF epidemic. If a murder can be prevented 50 years before it is committed, why can we not develop strategies for the prevention of HF only 6 to 12 months in the future? The future of preventing heart failure is the imaging future! These techniques are the "pre-cogs" of our specialty.

Jagat Narula, MD, PhD
Professor, Medicine
Chief, Division of Cardiology
Associate Dean
University of California Irvine
School of Medicine
101 The City Drive
Building 53, Mail Route 81
Irvine, CA 92868-4080, USA
E-mail address: narula@uci.edu

James B. Young, MD
Chairman, Department of Medicine
Professor, Medicine
Lerner College of Medicine
Case Western Reserve University
Cleveland Clinic Foundation
9500 Euclid Avenue
Desk T-13
Cleveland, OH 44195, USA
E-mail address: youngj@ccf.org

ELSEVIER
SAUNDERS

Heart Failure Clin 2 (2006) xi – xii

HEART
FAILURE
CLINICS

Preface

Noninvasive Imaging of Heart Failure

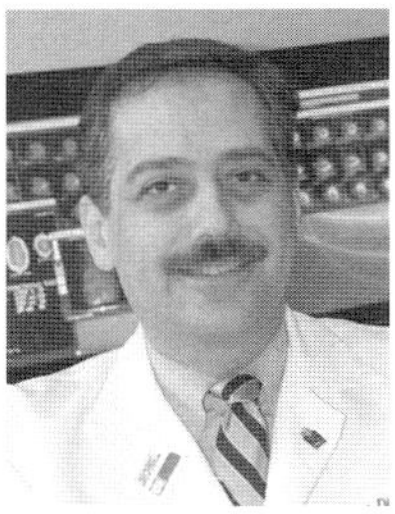

Vasken Dilsizian, MD

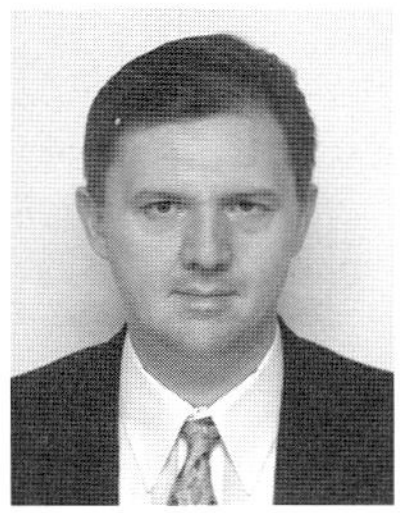

Mario J. Garcia, MD

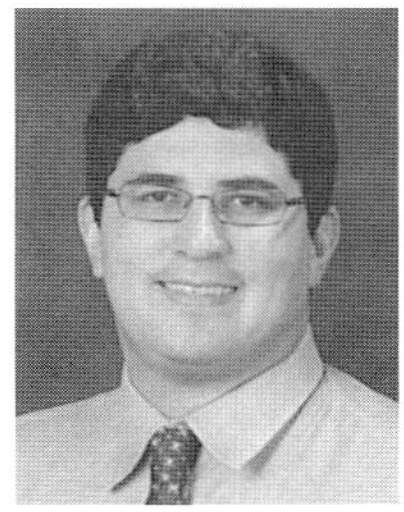

David Bello, MD

Guest Editors

Despite remarkable advances in our understanding and clinical management of patients who have heart failure, the prevalence of the disease and the resultant death rates have almost tripled in the past three decades. Left ventricular dysfunction is the final stage of most primary cardiovascular diseases; the more severe the left ventricular dysfunction and clinical failure, the worse the prognosis. After the initial injury to the myocardium, left ventricular dysfunction may continue to dilate and decompensate, either through direct loss of myocardial tissue (necrosis or apoptosis) or altered hemodynamic processes. Such left ventricular remodeling can progress even in the absence of clinical signs and symptoms of heart failure. Conversely, patients with symptoms of heart failure can present with abnormalities in diastolic function in the absence of systolic left ventricular dysfunction. Hence, noninvasive techniques that can identify patients with systolic as well as diastolic left ventricular dysfunction early in the disease process may favorably alter patient outcome.

This issue of the *Heart Failure Clinics* includes a comprehensive review of current and novel clinical applications of cardiac imaging in heart failure. World-renowned experts in molecular and nuclear imaging, echocardiography, and cardiac magnetic resonance have reviewed the role of imaging from the basic molecular level to the most advanced clinical applications. Cardiac imaging has facilitated the development of new drugs and devices by providing end points that may be used to determine clinical effectiveness and safety in small-scale animal and human clinical trials. Measurements of left ventricular mass, volume, and function are now accepted as clinical end points, reducing the need for large-scale clinical trials that rely primarily on clinical events. Differentiation of dysfunctional but viable myocardium (stunned or hibernating) from nonviable myocardium have resulted in more appropriate use of health care resources in patients with end-stage heart failure. Information provided by such imaging techniques are used to guide clinicians to intervene early and undertake appropriate preventative measures in the evolution and progression of left ventricular remodeling and heart failure.

Current noninvasive approaches in the diagnosis and management of heart failure include evaluation of regional perfusion, function, and metabolism with nuclear techniques, and assessment of valvular structure, myocardial perfusion and function with echocardiographic and cardiac magnetic resonance techniques. These noninvasive imaging studies allow the differentiation between ischemic, hypertrophic, restrictive, and dilated cardiomyopathies, as well as pericardial constriction in patients presenting with new onset of heart failure symptoms. Hemodynamic status of these patients can be evaluated both at rest and during exercise. Advanced Doppler echocardiographic techniques for the assessment of myocardial dyssynchrony are now emerging as the most accurate modalities for predicting response to cardiac resyn-

1551-7136/06/$ – see front matter
doi:10.1016/j.hfc.2006.05.004

chronization therapy. With the advent of hybrid SPECT and PET/CT systems, complimentary information on coronary artery anatomy and physiology can be realized immediately, at the same imaging session. In patients with ischemic, dilated, and hypertrophic cardiomyopathies, the finding of diminished quantitative flow reserve measurement by PET (reflecting microvascular dysfunction) is associated with unfavorable outcome over the ensuing years. The ability to image the shift in cardiac metabolism from fatty acids to glucose with PET in the setting of reduced blood flow has become the cornerstone of the decision-making process to appropriately select patients with systolic dysfunction for revascularization, transplantation, or medical therapy. The potential use of quantitative assessment of myocardial fibrosis with cardiac magnetic resonance (delayed contrast enhancement) and the assessment of beta-adrenergic receptor density with I^{131}-meta-iodobenzylguanidine single photon emission CT as markers of prognosis and risk of sudden death are currently under investigation. Such indices that forecast poor outcomes may be used to monitor response to standard and novel therapeutic interventions. More recently, CT angiography has been introduced as a reliable method for detecting coronary artery disease noninvasively. These and other emerging techniques and applications are extensively reviewed in this issue.

As we face the growing pandemic of heart failure, the value of cardiac imaging will continue to expand. The topics reviewed in this issue of the *Heart Failure Clinics* are not only relevant to cardiac imaging specialists, but also to all medical and surgical specialists managing patients who have heart failure.

Vasken Dilsizian, MD
Professor
Department of Medicine and Radiology
University of Maryland School of Medicine
Director
Cardiovascular Nuclear Medicine and
Cardiac Positron Emission Tomography
University of Maryland Medical Center
Gudelsky Building, Room N2W78
22 South Greene Street
Baltimore, MD 21201, USA
E-mail address: vdilsizian@umm.edu

Mario J. Garcia, MD
Cleveland Clinic Foundation
9500 Euclid Avenue, F-15
Cleveland, OH 44195, USA
E-mail address: garciam@ccf.org

David Bello, MD
Mid-Florida Cardiology
Orlando Regional Hospital
Orlando, FL 32806, USA
E-mail address: davidcraf@aol.com

ELSEVIER
SAUNDERS

Heart Failure Clin 2 (2006) 107 – 115

HEART
FAILURE
CLINICS

Imaging Patients with Heart Failure: Expectations of the Clinician

James B. Young, MD[a,b,*]

[a]Cleveland Clinic Foundation, Cleveland, OH, USA
[b]Lerner College of Medicine of Case Western Reserve University, Cleveland, OH, USA

Obviously the clinical evaluation of a patient who is known to have, or suspected of having, heart failure is extraordinarily important. All of the world's major societies with guidelines for diagnosing and managing patients who have heart failure have emphasized the importance of a complete evaluation [1–4]. Diagnostic tools are essential to help the skilled clinician define the illness and manage these individuals to achieve optimal outcomes. A variety of tests assist with the clinical evaluation of patients during the initial presentation as well as at long-term follow-up points. Specifically, the clinician is challenged when choosing from the wide spectrum of noninvasive imaging techniques that is available to assist with the task. The clinician's expectations that the results of these tests will be helpful should be high, because individualized care of patients who have heart failure is critically important and is based largely on results that emerge from imaging evaluations. The complete evaluation of an individual who has heart failure demands synthesizing and integrating clinical data that are obtained during history taking and physical examination as well as studying ancillary laboratory test results, physiologic performance, and imaging modalities. Although no one test should be used to diagnose heart failure, determine prognosis, or guide therapy and interventions, imaging procedures dominate these decisions. Therefore, the completeness of an examination and its accuracy, with skilled reporting of results that is done quickly and efficiently is essential to the clinician. It is extraordinarily important for individuals who provide noninvasive cardiovascular imaging services to know and anticipate what the clinician needs to manage his patient best.

Goals of a noninvasive evaluation of a patient who has heart failure

Box 1 summarizes the important goals that a clinician should have when caring for a patient who is suspected of having or is diagnosed with heart failure. The clinician expects that the information that is provided from noninvasive imaging evaluations will assist in achieving these goals. First and foremost, will the imaging data confirm the diagnosis of heart failure? Patient and symptoms and physical examination data can be misleading, and it often falls to a noninvasive imaging test to confirm a heart failure diagnosis. Noninvasive imaging information often gives a specific diagnosis in addition to determining if cardiac dysfunction and failure is present. Fairly, the clinician is going to ask what the problem is. Is aortic stenosis present? Is mitral regurgitation complicating a dilated cardiomyopathy? Are there multiple problems present? Is significant aortic stenosis noted in a patient who has a dilated left ventricle and regional wall motion abnormalities that might suggest coronary artery disease?

Clinicians also expect to receive information from noninvasive imaging that defines the severity of the

* Division of Medicine, Cleveland Clinic Foundation, 9500 Euclid Avenue, T13, Cleveland, OH 44195.
E-mail address: youngj@ccf.org

1551-7136/06/$ – see front matter
doi:10.1016/j.hfc.2006.05.003

Box 1. Goals of a noninvasive imaging evaluation of a patient who has heart failure

Diagnosis

Does the patient have heart failure?
What is the specific diagnosis?
Are there multiple problems?

Prognosis

How severe is the problem?
What are likely to be long-term difficulties?
Can a prognosis be determined?

Therapeutic discussion

Medical therapy versus percutaneous interventions versus surgical therapy?
What additional diagnostic procedures are required to make therapeutic decisions?

problem and assists with prognosis. Patients, particularly, want to know how bad the ailment is and what to expect in the future. Prognosticating in patients who have heart failure is a challenge that is fraught with hazard and inconsistency, but is helped when the clinician focuses on readily available information that often is provided by noninvasive imaging. Specifically, left ventricular ejection fraction, chamber dimensions, valve abnormalities, and pericardial effusions give guidance with respect to therapeutic intervention possibilities and related prognosis.

The clinician also expects information that helps to determine the need and wisdom of further diagnostic testing that assists with therapeutic decisions. For example, a patient with a newly diagnosed congestive heart failure syndrome and severely dilated left ventricle in a setting of atherosclerosis risk factors probably should go directly to coronary angiography (of one sort or another) to determine if coronary artery disease is present, irrespective of the symptom complex at initial presentation. More specific examples of how noninvasive imaging can direct therapeutic decisions relate to the ability of echocardiography to quantify valvular stenosis and insufficiency and give a complete picture of multiple cardiac lesions that can be present. For example, echocardiography is essential in helping to determine the wisdom of aortic valve replacement in patients who have aortic stenosis and low ejection fraction, but low gradients across the valve.

Specific noninvasive imaging modalities: expectations

Box 2 lists the generally available noninvasive imaging modalities a clinician might select during the evaluation of patients who are suspected of having heart failure. Chest radiography and basic echocardiography (usually two-dimensional and Doppler studies) are recommended in everyone. Special circumstances dictate the use of the other modalities, such as positron emission tomography (PET) or gadolinium-enhanced MRI, to determine if myocardial viability that might respond to surgical intervention exists in a patient who has ischemic cardiomyopathy. Rapidly emerging CT angiographic technology is capturing our imagination with crisp noninvasive coronary lumen characterization. Expectations of the clinician will be that the imaging specialist helps guide choice of study and then provide cogent and accurate interpretation of the studies without over interpretation.

Box 2. Noninvasive imaging modalities

Chest radiography
Echocardiography
- M-mode
- Two-dimensional
- Three-dimensional
- Pulsed Doppler
- Continuous wave Doppler
- Tissue Doppler
- Stress studies

Nuclear scintigraphic imaging
- Single photon emission CT (Thallium-201)

Positron emission tomography
- Fluorine-19 deoxyglucose viability

MRI
- Gadolinium studies

CT
- Noncontrast-enhanced imaging
- Contrast-enhanced CT angiography

Chest radiography

Because of the plethora and sophistication of newer noninvasive imaging modalities, one of the earliest, chest radiography, has been marginalized despite its potential value. Chest radiography can provide important information and the clinician who is evaluating a patient who has heart failure always should obtain one, and expect an expert and complete study commentary. Critical review of this simple and inexpensive test can demonstrate important findings. The clinician should expect a chest radiograph interpretation to include measured cardiothoracic ratio because this has been demonstrated to be an independent predictor of survival. There is a poor correlation between cardiothoracic ratio and left ventricular ejection fraction, however, and the clinician cannot expect this observation to translate into a direct measurement of systolic function. Nonetheless, cardiothoracic ratio can increase in patients who have substantive left ventricular hypertrophy, severe diastolic dysfunction, and normal ejection fraction. Congestive states that manifest as plural effusions or pulmonary parenchymal congestion should be commented upon. Furthermore, the presence of pulmonary infiltrates that suggest an inflammatory or infectious process are important in the overall management of the patient, particularly when there is the suggestion of comorbidities. Congestive heart failure is known to worsen in the presence of pulmonary infection, and sometimes pneumonia is misdiagnosed as congestive heart failure and vice versa. Also important is the suggestion that chronic obstructive pulmonary disease may be present, and, of course, interstitial processes that are seen on chest radiographs are not always due to pulmonary edema. The suggestion of interstitial fibrosis becomes important and the interpreting physician must comment on this if appropriate. Valuable, too, is commentary on the presence or absence of findings that are compatible with calcification in the great vessels or heart itself, as well as abnormalities in the mediastinum or with the great vessels. Finally, compulsively performed calculation of heart volumes by chest radiography that is coupled to certain electrocardiographic findings (specifically low voltage in the limb leads and Q-wave formation in the inferior and precordial leads) can give valuable insight into left ventricular systolic performance. This has become a lost art but could be extremely cost effective and valuable during long-term follow-up of patients in certain circumstances. The expectations of a clinician regarding patients who undergo chest radiography for evaluation of heart failure are high, and, unfortunately, most radiology reports fall short.

Echocardiography

Box 3 focuses on echocardiography and the information that a clinician would like to see provided. Most of our attention is spent on this modality because it is, arguably, the most widely performed noninvasive imaging examination in patients who have heart failure, and it is recommended uniformly in all guidelines regarding the care of these individuals. Study performance and reports must be detailed and complete with many calculated and qualitative observations noted. Many types of echocardiographic imaging studies are done, which range from transthoracic, two- and three-dimensional study, to transesophageal evaluation and the more subtle and esoteric pulsed, continuous wave, and tissue Doppler examinations. The clinician expects a report of the specific type of study, and it is reasonable to know the system used, the technician who performed the study, and the interpreting physician, because variability does exist in many of the subjectively analyzed components of an echocardiogram. Quality of the study should be commented upon because data can be influenced highly by technical issues, such as obesity and severe obstructive pulmonary disease. Therefore, it is reasonable for the clinician to know the degree of certainty that the echocardiographic interpretation carries. A report of inferior quality might drive the clinician to another noninvasive imaging modality to quantify better an important parameter, such as ejection fraction or wall motion abnormality.

Other information that is valuable to the clinician includes basic demographic data, although this usually is readily at hand, and some clinical information regarding the purpose of the study. It is important for the clinician to know the patient's heart rhythm during the echocardiographic study, as well as what the heart rate and blood pressure are. These should be components of any echocardiographic report. Obviously echocardiography has the ability to provide multidimensional information on the patient. Arguably, left ventricular ejection fraction is the most important piece of information, because this has been viewed as the most common index of the degree of left ventricular systolic dysfunction and is a powerful prognosticating observation; however, it often does not correlate strongly with exercise tolerance or the degree of a patient's disability. Because the ejection fraction is the ratio of stroke volume to end diastolic volume, precise measurements of end systolic and end diastolic dimensions are expected and must be made. This must be linked to commentary about the quality of a study, because precise determination of these measurements is problematic if images are

Box 3. Expectations of a clinician: echocardiography information on reports

- *Type of study*
  - Transthoracic
  - Two-dimensional/three-dimensional
  - Doppler/Tissue Doppler
  - Stress for ischemic evaluation
  - Pulse wave Doppler
  - Evaluating physician
  - Technicians
  - Machine
- *Quality of study*
- *Basic information*
  - Patient age, sex, date of study
  - Clinical information
    - Height
    - Weight
    - Body mass index/body surface area
    - Heart rate
    - Blood pressure
    - Rhythm
  - Reason for study
- *Measurements*
  - Aorta (at valve leaflets)
  - Left atrium (diameter and systolic area)
  - Left ventricle: end diastole
  - Left ventricle: end systole
  - Interventricular septum
  - Posterior wall thickness
  - End diastolic volume
  - End systolic volume
  - Shortening fraction
  - Ejection fraction
- *Specific findings*
- *Left ventricle*
  - Left ventricular size
  - Left ventricular systolic function
    - Qualitative commentary only if ejection fraction cannot be calculated
  - Left ventricular diastolic function
    - Normal
    - Stage 1 dysfunction
    - Stage 2 dysfunction (''pseudonormal'')
    - Stage 3 dysfunction
  - Wall motion abnormalities
    - Normal wall motion
    - Hypokinesis
    - Akinesis
    - Dyskinesis
    - Left ventricular aneurysm
    - Location of wall motion abnormalities
    - Presence of ''thrombus''
      - Adherent, layered, mural
      - Mobile or flopping
- *Right ventricle*
  - Qualitative estimate of size
  - Qualitative estimate of systolic function
  - Identification of device presence (pacer leads, Swan-Ganz catheter)
- *Left atrium/pulmonary veins*
  - Commentary on size
- *Right atrium/inferior vena cava/superior vena cava*
  - Commentary on size
  - Inferior vena cava inspiratory collapse
- *Mitral valve*
  - Structural commentary
  - Degree of stenosis/insufficiency
  - Quantification of mitral regurgitation
  - Calcification of annulus
  - ''Forward'' pressure gradient across mitral valve
- *Tricuspid valve*
  - Structure commentary
  - Degree of stenosis/insufficiency
  - Quantification of tricuspid regurgitation
    - Doppler-derived regurgitant velocity
    - Estimated right ventricular systolic pressure
- *Pulmonic valve*
  - Qualitative commentary on structure
  - Estimation of degree of insufficiency
- *Aortic valve/left ventricular outflow tract*
  - Tricuspid or bicuspid valve
  - Presence of calcification / thickening
  - Orifice area
  - Left ventricular outflow tract characteristics and size

Mean and peak pressure gradient across aortic valve
Aortic root
Supravalvular dimensions
Pulmonary arteries
Doppler left atrium inflow pattern
Interatrial and ventricular septa
Paradoxic motion
Aneurysmal
Patent foramen ovale
Pericardium
Presence of effusion
Size of effusions
Signs of ''tamponade''
Pericardial thickening
Special considerations
Congenital abnormalities
Unusual left ventricular muscle findings
Sinusoidal patterns
Scintillations suggesting amyloid
Congenital cardiac structural abnormalities
Specific commentary
Relevance to acute heart failure
Relevance to chronic heart failure
Relevance to congenital heart disease
Relevance to various hypertrophic cardiomyopathies

hazy. The clinician should know if that is the case and what formula was used to calculate the ejection fraction. A normal left ventricular ejection fraction should be more than 50%, but this can vary depending on loading conditions, heart rate, medications taken, and other clinical variables. Furthermore, the error of measurement is related to wide variability of the measurement of ventricular dimensions and volumes that are performed often by visual estimation rather than mathematical derivation (eg, biplane "Simpson" rule method).

Other measurements that the clinician expects his echocardiographer to provide include the aortic orifice size measured at the valve leaflets with an explanation of the technique used. Intraventricular wall thickness in systole and diastole and posterior wall thickness also are critical to give the clinician insight into ventricular hypertrophy. Particularly important during measurement of ventricular wall thickness are the identification of asymmetric septal hypertrophy and obstruction to the left ventricular outflow tract that are created by intraventricular septal and mitral valve abnormalities in hypertrophic cardiomyopathy. Complementing the importance of determining systolic dysfunction with an ejection fraction is an observation regarding diastolic filling patterns and dysfunction. Clinicians are becoming aware of the fact that many patients present with typical heart failure symptoms but "preserved" or mostly normal left ventricular systolic function, because their ejection fraction is in the range of 50% and greater. These individuals often are said to have "diastolic heart failure" or heart failure with "preserved left ventricular systolic function." Treating these patients is different than treating those who have systolic ventricular dysfunction and the prognosis may be better. Echocardiographic data can be extremely important in diagnosing this elusive problem. Therefore, the echocardiographic report should include information regarding transmitral inflow velocity as determined by Doppler interrogation. Stages 1, 2, and 3 "diastolic dysfunction" refer to the perturbation of mitral inflow. Because the E-wave on a mitral inflow filling Doppler pattern corresponds to early filling and the a-wave reflects atrial contraction, a normal E/a ratio is greater than 1.6. A ratio of less than 1 is seen commonly in patients who have hypertension, left ventricular hypertrophy, and coronary artery disease; this reflects Doppler echocardiographic evidence of diastolic dysfunction.

Measurement of ventricular chamber size is the next most important characteristic (after the determination of ejection fraction) when evaluating a patient who has heart failure. Left and right ventricular dimensions should be determined. Because they bear some relationship to body surface area, absolute measurements and an index that is related to body surface should be reported. This should be reported in every case because patients who have known heart failure and systolic left ventricular dysfunction and a dilated left ventricle have a poor prognosis. Conversely, small left ventricular chamber cavities are noted often in individuals who have severe diastolic dysfunction, "preserved" ejection fraction, and hypertrophic cardiomyopathy.

Sometimes right ventricular chamber dimension is ignored but commentary regarding its size and function gives insight into pulmonary hypertension and volume or pressure overload on the right side of the heart. Left atrial dimension is extremely important because this often relates to the presence or risk for development of atrial fibrillation. One becomes vitally interested in this observation, particularly when considering procedures (eg, percutaneous pulmonary vein isolation) to treat atrial fibrillation.

Wall motion abnormalities give insight into the possible presence of ischemic heart disease; however, it should be emphasized that patients who have idiopathic dilated congestive cardiomyopathy and normal coronary arteries can present with wall motion abnormalities. To characterize wall motion best with echocardiography, the ventricle is divided into 16 segments and a score can be provided for each that is determined by classifying movement during systole as normal, akinetic, hypokinetic, or frankly dyskinetic.

In addition to abnormal left ventricular wall thickness, thinning of the left ventricular wall also can be noted on echocardiography, and commentary should be made if this is present. Generally, this observation represents ventricular scarring from coronary artery disease and myocardial infarction and might prompt consideration of further imaging studies to determine if surgical intervention is warranted.

Infiltrative cardiomyopathy, such as amyloid heart disease, leads to increased wall thickness with no, for the most part, accompanying left ventricular voltage increase on the electrocardiogram. Often, amyloid deposition produces a scintillating pattern in the seemingly hypertrophied left ventricular muscle, but this is not a consistent feature and is highly subjective in its analysis. Generally, patients who have infiltrative cardiomyopathies have normal-sized left ventricles with thick-walled muscle chambers, moderately reduced systolic function, and a dilated left atrium. The ejection fraction decreases in the latter stages of infiltrative cardiomyopathy. The echocardiographic report should contain information that will push the clinician to suspect an infiltrative myopathic process so that plans can be made for further diagnostic studies.

Valvular function

Echocardiography can be extraordinarily valuable for identifying and quantifying valvular disease. Generally, patients who have dilated cardiomyopathy develop mitral regurgitation as the left ventricle increases in size and the mitral valve annulus becomes distorted by papillary muscle dysfunction and chamber realignment. Arguably, the mitral valve becomes the major focus in patients who have heart failure, and the clinician expects commentary regarding intrinsic pathology of the valve versus anatomic distortion that is due to left ventricular dilation. This should be coupled to a qualitative estimate of the degree of mitral regurgitation that is based on Doppler interrogation of the valve and left atrium. Also important is the degree of tricuspid insufficiency that follows the pulmonary hypertension that develops in patients who have heart failure. Differentiating between mitral and tricuspid regurgitation that are due to primary valvular abnormalities and "functional" regurgitation is important because primary abnormalities are addressed surgically more often. Nonetheless, mitral valve repair may become an important therapeutic strategy in select patients who have heart failure with dilated ventricles and normal valves, but substantive valvular insufficiency.

Aortic stenosis and regurgitation also are seen commonly in patients who have heart failure, and frequently are the cause of left ventricular dysfunction and congestive heart failure. Clinicians realize that quantifying the severity of aortic stenosis is difficult in the face of depressed left ventricular systolic function because patients can have critical aortic stenosis but only a moderate aortic valve gradient. It is important that the interpreting echocardiographer assist the clinician in determining the orifice size of the aortic valve to help with decisions regarding surgery. Additional tests, if appropriate, should be recommended to clarify this issue. Often, a dobutamine stress echocardiogram that is designed to improve myocardial systolic function reveals that a significantly stenotic aortic valve is present in the setting of left ventricular systolic dysfunction.

Decisions also have to be made about the impact of aortic insufficiency on ventricular dysfunction and heart failure. Aortic insufficiency is well known to have a long and protracted course whereby individuals are asymptomatic despite severe aortic regurgitation. The rate of progression to symptoms or significant left ventricular systolic dysfunction is about 5% per year. When left ventricular systolic function is depressed, patients usually develop congestive states or significant exercise limitation that warrants surgery within 12 to 24 months. When patients have normal left ventricular systolic dysfunction, no symptoms, and severe grade 3 to 4+ aortic regurgitation careful echocardiographic follow-up should be done at approximately 6-month intervals. When patients who have left ventricular dilation (end diastolic dimension >70 mm and systolic dimension >50 mm) develop an ejection fraction of less than 50% aortic valve surgery (repair or replacement) should ensue, irrespective of symptomatic status. This decision-making process emphasizes the importance of the echocardiographer communicating these values to the attending clinician.

Other echocardiographic observations that should be reported to the clinician include the presence of valvular vegetations, intracardiac thrombus, lesions that could mean tumor, the presence of prosthetic valve associated with stenosis or regurgitation, the presence of a patent foramen ovale, or findings of volume and pressure overload in the right ventricle. Obviously, transesophageal echocardiography is better for evaluating certain situations, such as valvular vegetation and intracardiac thrombi (particularly that in the left atrial appendage).

Another extraordinarily important use of echocardiography by the clinician is dobutamine stress echocardiography to detect ischemia and infer "viable" myocardium. This technique is less sensitive than are radionuclide scintigraphic studies, PET, or MRI, which are more expensive and less available. Nonetheless, clinicians rely heavily on an echocardiographer's skill at determining this important finding. It has been pointed out that the test of choice for myocardial viability is dependent on the individual's expertise, and that is why reports should contain information regarding who interpreted the study.

Nuclear scintigraphic imaging

Arguably, some aspects of nuclear scintigraphic imaging are much less subjective than is qualitative echocardiographic assessment. Many clinicians desire a precise determination of ejection fraction and when gated left ventricular radionuclide images are obtained a more precise quantification of ejection fraction is possible. Despite the prognostic power of an ejection fraction, however, quantification to this degree may not be necessary or advantageous. In patients who have heart failure, the most important use of scintigraphic imaging is to determine the presence of myocardial ischemia and hibernation, or the presence of "viable" myocardium. Thallium-201 is the most commonly used imaging agent during single photon emission CT. In this setting the radioisotope usually is acquired by a viable myocardial cell and typical protocols use stress-redistribution-reinjection or rest-redistribution techniques to detect abnormalities. The clinician expects the interpreting physician to describe precisely which protocol was used. This technique allows determination of regional thallium-201 uptake in a quantitative rather than a qualitative fashion. Thallium-201 uptake of more than 50% of normal in regions of left ventricular "scar" have been useful in predicting functional recovery after coronary revascularization. The myocardial segments with the highest probability of recovery are those that show rest-redistribution of the isotope. Areas lacking thallium uptake at rest, at stress, and at reinjection generally do not respond to revascularization and are said to be "nonviable." Alternative radioisotopes for the assessment of viability include technetium-99 sestamibi.

Positron emission tomography

Many investigators believe that PET is the best technique for determining myocardial viability when coupled with fluorine-19 deoxyglucose (FDG). FDG is a glucose analog that becomes trapped within the myocardial cells when phosphorylated. FDG uptake identifies hibernating or "stunned" myocardium that is created by viable myocytes that are nonfunctional. Chronically reduced coronary blood flow may cause myocardial contractile elements to move into this "hibernation" state to allow for survival in settings of relative chronic ischemia. Myocardial stunning refers to persistent postischemic dysfunction following a short-term, low blood flow insult, despite subsequent return of normal or improved myocardial blood flow. Stunned and hibernating myocardium include features of positive response to inotropic stimulation and conservation of glucose metabolism. When PET studies are done, it is important to report areas that appear "ischemic" and "viable." Because of PET scanning's high predictive value (often said to be >80% for detection of ischemia) and the ability to couple a viability study to this determination, it has become the noninvasive imaging study of preference for many heart failure clinicians. Rubidium gives the clinician an assessment of regional coronary blood flow and dipyridamole usually is the provocative agent that is administered to facilitate the diagnosis of ischemia. If there are regional reductions in coronary blood flow determined by rubidium imaging, coupled to a matched proportional decrease in glucose metabolism as determined by FDG administration, nonviability is said to be present and revascularization of these areas are unlikely to result in improved clinical myocardial performance. Conversely, diminished regional blood flow that is associated with increased FDG activity suggests a "flow/viability mismatch" that might respond to revascularization of one sort or another in patients who have left ventricular systolic dysfunction and chronic coronary artery disease. The clinician expects precise description of techniques that were used to characterize "ischemia," "scar," and "viability," which will help the clinician to guide therapy.

MRI

MRI is becoming an additional and sensitive tool to identify potentially reversible myocardial dysfunction in patients who have ischemic cardiomyopathy.

A gadolinium-based agent can be administered intravenously and produces MRI image enhancement in the presence of myocardial scar. This allows precise measurement of segmental wall thickening and gives an index of contractility that can be scored in a manner similar to stress echocardiographic evaluation. Global left ventricular ejection fraction can be determined precisely and myocardial perfusion also measured as with PET scanning. MRI also can be valuable in characterizing left ventricular geometry for patients who undergo left ventricular reconstructive surgery, such as the Dor procedure. In contrast to radionuclide scintigraphic studies and dobutamine stress echocardiography, which have reduced predictive accuracy when severe left ventricular dysfunction is present, MRI has a greater ability to determine viable myocardial segments in patients with the lowest global left ventricular ejection fraction. Also important is the fact that gadolinium is an inert substance and is not nephrotoxic. Furthermore, gadolinium-enhanced MRI studies do not require the administration of agents to provoke ischemia, and some investigators believe that this approach is safer in patients who have severe coronary disease and active myocardial ischemia or angina pectoris. Clinicians expect, with these studies, determination of an ejection fraction, characterization of left ventricular geometry, and precise localization and quantification of viable and nonviable myocardial territories. This is important because a reduction in the hyperenhancement by contrast-enhanced MRI early after myocardial infarction, for example, is associated with a subsequent improvement in contractile performance. Characterization of viability, then, will drive a clinician's decisions regarding percutaneous intervention or surgical coronary revascularization, particularly coupled to surgical left ventricular remodeling procedures. The clinician relies heavily on an interpretation of the gadolinium-enhanced MRI study for clinical care direction.

CT

Cardiac CT evaluation can be noncontrast- or contrast-enhanced imaging and the resolution of the study becomes extraordinarily important. Noncontrast-enhanced imaging provides an assessment of coronary artery calcification that has led to the development of coronary calcification "scores" that can be helpful in gaining insight into the presence or absence of coronary artery disease and, possibly, ischemic heart disease. Determination of the significance of obstructive lesions, however, is not possible by simply identifying the presence of coronary calcification. Conversely, higher resolution CT angiography has been an exciting new development that is characterized well elsewhere in this issue. MRI and CT studies give additional information much like echocardiography. Constrictive pericarditis, pericardial effusions, and restrictive myocardial relaxation patterns can be identified nicely and it is essential to report these observations. Furthermore, great vessel imaging can be much more extensive with MRI and CT studies than with echocardiography. Finally, cardiac thrombus, particularly thrombus in the left atrial appendage, can be demonstrated nicely by these techniques and, particularly, cardiac CT.

When one compares cardiac CT with MRI, advantages include better spatial resolution, better detection of vessel calcification, better detection of acute hematoma formation, and better evaluation of the

Box 4. Expectations of a clinician: peeves

- Delays in report development
- Failure to call referring clinician when
  - Life-threatening findings present (cardiac tamponade for example)
  - Unanticipated findings noted (findings suggesting amyloidosis for example)
  - Problems observed during study (severe ischemia during stress study for example)
- Narrative reports based on qualitative study reviews
- Absence of measurements listed in Box 3, despite having a quality study that allows for their determination and calculation
- Specific peeves
  - No calculated left ventricular ejection fraction
  - No measured left ventricular dimensions
  - No calculated right ventricular systolic pressure when Doppler tricuspid regurgitation of any degree reported
  - No commentary regarding valve integrity
  - No assessment of left ventricular hypertrophy

lungs, mediastinum, and abdomen. Furthermore, MRI imaging includes confounding factors (eg, inability of getting some patients into the magnetic field) and contraindications (eg, presence of a pacemaker or defibrillator), something of increasing importance. Certainly the future of imaging of patients who have heart failure is bright for MRI and CT scan development.

Peeves of a heart failure clinician

Box 4 summarizes some of the author's peeves when trying to use the reports that are generated by his imaging colleagues. Of course, these rarely are noted at my present institution! Problematic are narrative reports that are based solely on qualitative study. The absence of measurements (when they can be done) listed in Box 3 is particularly irksome and suggests inattention to detail, lack of a passion for excellence, and, perhaps, laziness. Delays in getting reports out, and failure to call the clinician directly with life-threatening findings (eg, pericardial tamponade and valvular vegetations) or when unanticipated observations are made (eg, ventricular patterns suggesting amyloidosis) are major peeves. More specific peeves include the imaging specialist providing no calculated left ventricular ejection fraction, not measuring left ventricular internal chamber dimensions, not estimating right ventricular systolic pressure when Doppler detected tricuspid insufficiency is present, providing no information regarding valve integrity, and not assessing left ventricular hypertrophy.

Summary

Evaluating and treating patients who have heart failure is a demanding task that should integrate clinical skills with the proper choice of ancillary tools to help diagnose and determine the prognosis for individual patients. Furthermore, noninvasive imaging techniques have become critical in determining additional evaluation and therapies. The clinician relies heavily on the imaging expert to transmit information that is complete, accurate, and relevant to the patient who has heart failure. Heart failure specialists will be helped tremendously by their imaging colleagues if compulsive and complete reports are generated that avoid simple narrative descriptions of qualitative assessments and provide the discussed information.

References

[1] Hunt SA, Abraham WT, Chin MH, et al. ACC/AHA 2005 guidelines for the diagnosis and management of chronic heart failure in the adult. J Am Coll Cardiol 2005;46:1116–43.

[2] Nieminen MS, Bohm M, Cowie MR, et al. European Society of Cardiology guidelines on the diagnosis and treatment of acute heart failure. Eur Heart J 2005;26: 384–416.

[3] Adams Jr KF, Lindenfeld J, Arnold JMO. Heart Failure Society of America 2006 comprehensive heart failure practice guideline. J Card Fail 2006;12:10–38.

[4] Arnold JMO, Liu P, Demers C, et al. Canadian Cardiovascular Society consensus conference recommendations on heart failure 2006: diagnosis and management. Can J Cardiol 2006;22:23–45.

ELSEVIER
SAUNDERS

Heart Failure Clin 2 (2006) 117 – 127

HEART
FAILURE
CLINICS

Imaging Markers of Adverse Remodeling: from Organ to Organelle

Eric M. Thorn, MD, Mandeep R. Mehra, MD*

University of Maryland School of Medicine, Baltimore, MD, USA

Adverse ventricular remodeling is believed to play a causative role in heart failure progression and has a strong association with poor prognosis [1,2]. The identification of quantifiable markers of remodeling has been instrumental in the understanding of the natural history of heart failure progression and has proved useful for the clinical diagnosis of heart failure, the prediction of clinical outcomes, the assessment of a therapeutic response, and the evaluation of treatment effect within clinical trials. The structural and functional changes that typify adverse ventricular remodeling are part of a complex cascade of events (Fig. 1). The process begins with an "index event" that adversely affects the myocardial pump [3] and leads to initially compensatory local and systemic responses. These responses result in alterations in the genomic expression patterns of cardiac cells that underlie the remodeling process [4]. The resulting diverse phenotypic changes include myocyte hypertrophy, myocyte necrosis and apoptosis, myocyte regeneration, and nonmyocyte changes, including alterations in the balance and configuration of structural proteins such as collagen and elastin [5]. These phenotypic shifts, on a molecular and cellular level, result in macro-alterations in cardiac histopathology that is reflected in overall cardiac size, shape, and function. The assessment of adverse remodeling has been limited largely to the measurement of the large-scale structural and functional changes, but the increasing recognition of new potential markers is emerging (Box 1). This article reviews the traditional and emerging markers of remodeling and the non-invasive imaging techniques used to measure them.

Traditional markers of cardiac structure and function: the organ

As adverse remodeling progresses, eccentric hypertrophy and ventricular dilation develop, with associated change in geometry and decline in the ejection fraction [6]. Of these structural and functional changes, left ventricular ejection fraction has the most widespread use in clinical practice. However, ejection fraction and left ventricular volumes are limited by their dependence on the prevailing hemodynamic conditions and state of iontropy and lusitropy [7]. Left ventricular mass is theoretically load-independent. Unfortunately, mass is also a limited measure of adverse remodeling because it does not express geometric changes. The geometric changes in left ventricular shape that occur with adverse remodeling are not quantified easily. Lamas and colleagues [8] have defined a sphericity index, determined by dividing the left ventricular end diastolic volume by the volume of a sphere having a diameter equal to the ventricular long-axis dimension. Their group found that the sphericity index predicted progression to heart failure and decreased exercise capacity and that the index was lower in patients treated with captopril [8]. However, the sphericity index is a simplification of the shape change that occurs with remodeling, and as with left ventricular mass, the calculation of a sphericity index is dependent on volume measurement. Thus, although anatomic measurements can be

* Corresponding author. Division of Cardiology, University of Maryland School of Medicine, 22 South Greene Street, Room S3B06, Baltimore, MD 21201.

E-mail address: mmehra@medicine.umaryland.edu (M.R. Mehra).

1551-7136/06/$ – see front matter
doi:10.1016/j.hfc.2006.01.002

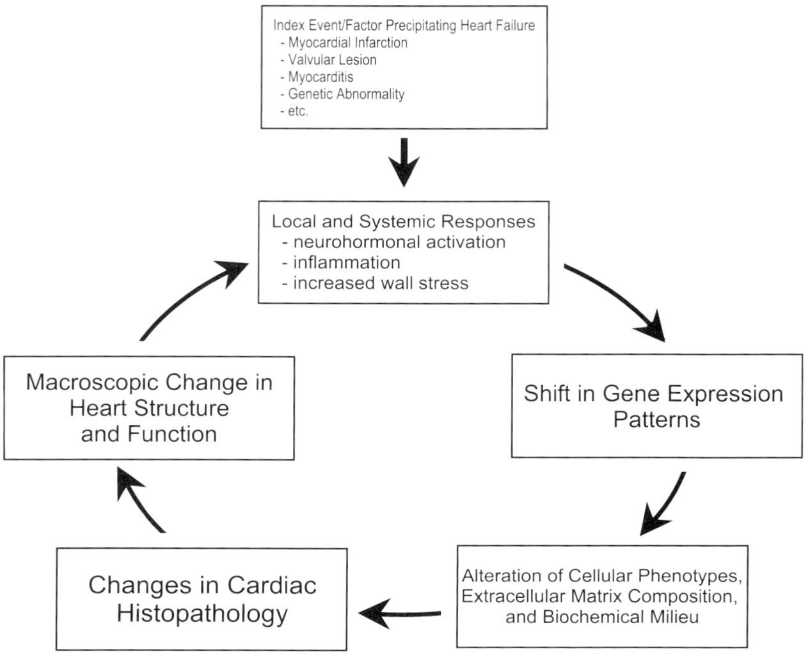

Fig. 1. Cascade of events that make up the adverse remodeling process in heart failure.

used to quantify a complex underlying remodeling process, one must use multiple markers in conjunction, recognizing that each marker measures a single facet of remodeling and that each has limitations (Table 1).

The modalities of two-dimensional transthoracic echocardiography (TTE), gated SPECT, and cardiac MRI (CMR) have been the standard means of imaging adverse remodeling. All modes have been used for (1) predicting clinical outcomes in individual patients; (2) identifying the presence of remodeling as a target for therapy; and (3) using markers of remodeling as surrogates for response to therapy in both the clinical setting and in clinical trials. Each modality has its own set of strengths and limitations for achieving these goals (Table 2).

Echocardiography

The primary advantages of TTE are its widespread use, portability, and relatively low cost. The limitations of TTE stem from the necessity of converting linear measurements or two-dimensional areas into three-dimensional volumes. This conversion is calculated using equations that make assumptions about the left ventricular geometry and uniformity of function. This limitation can be overcome to some degree by the use of the modified Simpson's rule, in which the left ventricle is divided into multiple cylinders that are then summed. However, one limitation is traded for another because the calculations of volume and mass in echocardiography require accurate identification of the endocardial cavity interface. The modified Simpson's method is limited by the necessity of using apical viewing windows from which endocardial borders are less readily identified [9]. As a result of its limitations, TTE has been found to underestimate left ventricular volumes [10]. TTE has been validated for the estimation of left ventricular mass [11]; however, both two-dimensional and M-mode echocardiographic calculations of left ventricular mass require the estimation of ventricular volumes and the volume of an outer epicardial "shell" [9]. Given the geometric assumptions required for estimating these volumes, the potential for error is high, limiting the accuracy and reproducibility [12,13]. TTE systematically overestimates mass compared with CMR [14,15]. This discrepancy is even more significant in patients who have left ventricular hypertrophy or ventricular dilation [16].

Gated SPECT

Unlike TTE, gated SPECT is a three-dimensional, dynamic, tomographic imaging modality. These char-

Box 1. Established and emerging markers of adverse remodeling accessible to noninvasive imaging

I. Structural and functional markers

A. Left ventricular end-systolic and end-diastolic volume
B. Left ventricular ejection fraction
C. Left ventricular mass
D. Sphericity index

II. Histopathologic markers

A. Late gadolinium enhancement (cardiac MRI)
B. Perfusable tissue index (PET)

III. Cellular and molecular markers

A. Apoptosis imaging
B. Matrix metalloproteinase (MMP) imaging
C. Stem-cell tracking

IV. Tissue neurohormonal markers

A. Sympathetic innervation
B. Tissue renin-angiotensin-aldosterone system activity

acteristics allow for the calculation of left ventricular volumes and ejection fraction, without resorting to geometric assumptions. The measurement of left ventricular volumes and ejection fraction by gated SPECT has been compared with CMR, with correlation coefficients generally greater than 0.8 [17]. Furthermore, the reproducibility of serial measurements of resting ventricular volumes and ejection fraction generally is good when the radionuclide dose is adequate [18–20]. The use of gated SPECT for the measurement of left ventricular mass is less well validated. An early report was disappointing, demonstrating only moderate correlation with TTE [21]. In this study, differences between left ventricular mass estimates were dependent on the use of systolic, diastolic, or summed images. More recently, two reports have found gated SPECT mass determinations to correlate well with TTE estimates of mass, using a proprietary software package called Quantitative-Gated SPECT or QGS (Ceders-Sinai Hospital, New York, New York) [22,23]. QGS automatically detects endocardial and epicardial borders using radioactivity counts and count gradients, thereby minimizing the problem of background radiation and changes in count recovery throughout the cardiac cycle.

Cardiac MRI

CMR is a true three-dimensional tomographic modality with high spatial resolution. It allows for the accurate reconstruction of the ventricle without the need for geometric assumptions [24,25]. Because of these advantages, CMR has become the reference standard for the measurement of structural and functional markers of adverse remodeling. Studies comparing left ventricular volumes with mass as measured by CMR for values obtained from cadaveric hearts have found correlation coefficients of 0.99 [24,26]. Furthermore, CMR is highly reproducible, making it particularly well suited for measuring the progression and regression of adverse remodeling. Studies of patients who have heart failure have shown intraobserver, interobserver, and test–retest variabili-

Table 1
Characteristics and limitations of structural and functional markers of adverse remodeling

Marker	Parameter measured	Limitations of marker
Left ventricular end-systolic and end-diastolic volumes	Ventricular dilation and cell slippage	Dependent on loading conditions and ionotropic/lusitropic state
Ejection fraction	Pumping ability	Not an accurate measure of contractile function as it is dependent on both dilation and stroke volume Calculated from volume measurements, thus also dependent on loading conditions and ionotropic/lusitropic state
Left ventricular mass	Combined myocyte and nonmyocyte mass	Does not differentiate concentric from eccentric hypertrophy May be influenced by loading conditions (likely due to technical differences in volume measurements)
Left ventricular geometry and sphericity index	Deviation from ideal ellipsoid ventricular shape	Shape changes can by extremely complex and are difficult to express as a discreet, quantifiable value

Table 2
Pros and cons of noninvasive imaging modalities for assessment of structural and functional markers of adverse remodeling

Imaging modality	Pros	Cons
TTE	Widely available Inexpensive and portable	Calculations require the use of geometric assumptions to convert linear measurements or two-dimensional areas into volumes Endocardial borders can be difficult to define Patient characteristics frequently limit available acoustic windows Image acquisition is operator dependent Intra- and interobserver variability and test-retest reliability are significantly greater than that of SPECT or CMR Overestimates left ventricular mass Underestimates left ventricular volumes
Gated SPECT	Widely available No geometric assumptions required Image acquisition is relatively independent of patient and operator characteristics Measurement of ejection fraction is highly reproducible	Requires regular heart rhythm and controlled heart rate Underestimates systolic volumes in patients with small hearts Reported normal values for ejection fraction are lower than those reported for other imaging modalities Accuracy and reproducibility for estimation of left ventricular mass is not well validated Requires exposure to ionizing radiation
Cardiac MRI	Image acquisition is relatively independent of patient and operator characteristics No geometric assumptions required Reference standard for measurement of volumes, ejection fraction, and mass	Limited availability of cardiac scanners and skilled readers Requires regular heart rhythm Not feasible in patients with claustrophobia or implanted metal devices (eg, pacemakers, defibrillators, etc.)
2-D TTE with tissue harmonic imaging and intravenous ultrasonic contrast	Inexpensive and portable Imaging acquisition is relatively independent of patient characteristics Intra- and interobserver variability and test-retest reliability similar to that of CMR	Calculations require the use of geometric assumptions to convert linear measurements or two-dimensional areas into volumes Image acquisition is operator dependent Not well validated for measurement of left ventricular mass
Real-time 3-D TTE	Inexpensive and portable Imaging acquisition is relatively independent of patient characteristics No geometric assumptions required Intra- and interobserver variability and test-retest reliability similar to CMR	Limited availability and expertise in use Requires regular heart rhythm

ties for left ventricular mass, volumes, and ejection fraction in the range of 2% to 8% [27,28]. More recently, the development of steady-state free precession CMR techniques has shortened acquisition times and improved blood–myocardium contrast, which further improve reproducibility and accuracy [29,30]. Because of this high reproducibility, Bellenger and colleagues [28] have calculated that the sample sizes of heart failure patients that are necessary to detect a 10-mL change in end-diastolic or end-systolic volume, a 3% change in ejection fraction, or a 10-g change in mass (with a power of 90% and *P* value of .05) would be 12, 10, 15, and 9 subjects, respectively. Myerson and colleagues [31] came to a similar conclusion, estimating that sample sizes for studies using CMR to measure left ventricular mass as an endpoint would need to be only one-sixth of the size needed by studies using TTE. Thus, CMR is a very useful tool for measuring markers of adverse remodeling as surrogate endpoints in clinical trials, making the performance of such trials more practical and likely less expensive.

Tissue harmonic imaging and ultrasonic contrast imaging

The new echocardiographic techniques of tissue harmonic imaging [32] and intravenous ultrasonic contrast imaging [33,34] greatly enhance the definition of endomyocardial borders. Harmonic imaging involves the transmission of ultrasound at one frequency and receiving the backscattered signals at double the transmitted frequency. Ultrasound contrast agents used to enhance left ventricular imaging consist of protein- or lipid-coated microspheres (1–8 μm in diameter) that resonate when excited by ultrasound, thus generating strongly echo-dense harmonic energy that contrasts sharply with the myocardium. The use of tissue harmonics and ultrasonic contrast has been shown to greatly increase the accuracy and reproducibility of two-dimensional TTE for the measurement of left ventricular volumes and ejection fraction [35–37]. Beyond improving accuracy and reproducibility, harmonic imaging and ultrasonic contrast allow for accurate imaging of patients who have poor acoustic windows [38]. Furthermore, the use of echocardiographic contrast has been demonstrated to allow for accurate automated endocardial border detection, thus streamlining the process of measurement [39].

Real-time three-dimensional echocardiography

Multiple studies have reported a very strong correlation of three-dimensional echo with CMR and contrast ventriculography for the measurement of left ventricular volumes, ejection fraction, and mass [40–47]. However, until recently, three-dimensional echocardiography has required time-consuming and technically demanding image acquisition and post-processing. These circumstances have changed with the introduction of real-time three-dimensional echocardiography (RT3DE). Second-generation RT3DE uses a matrix-array transducer with almost 3000 elements and a wide 93° × 80°-pyramidal ultrasound-sampling volume. These properties result in high spatial and temporal resolution, with coverage of a larger area of interest. Studies comparing RT3DE with CMR for the measurement of left ventricular volumes and ejection fraction show a high degree of correlation and no underestimation of volume by RT3DE [48–50]. In all of these studies, the inter- and intraobserver variability for RT3DE was low, much better than that seen with two-dimensional TTE [48–50]. RT3DE also has been validated for the measurement of left ventricular mass, with similarly low inter- and intraobserver variability [50–52].

Emerging markers of adverse remodeling: the organelle

Although noninvasive measurement of structural and functional markers of remodeling has proven to have great clinical and research value, the use of these markers for the assessment of adverse remodeling is limited. First, the structural changes are influenced by alterations in loading conditions, inotropy, and lusitropy. This lack of specificity limits the use of current noninvasive imaging techniques for measuring the progression or reversal of remodeling. Second, the measurement of structural and functional markers can identify only the result of an adverse remodeling process after it has already produced marked deleterious alterations to the ventricle. Third, the only way to determine the rate of progression of adverse remodeling using structural and functional markers is through serial measurement. Any single measurement does not tell the degree to which underlying genetic and molecular processes are active. Recently, however, a number of newer markers of adverse remodeling have been described that have the potential to overcome these shortcomings by allowing measurement of the heretofore less accessible aspects of the adverse remodeling process.

Histopathologic markers of adverse remodeling: imaging of fibrosis

Alterations in the extracellular matrix with concomitant changes in myocardial fibrosis are an integral part of adverse remodeling [53]. Two recently described markers of increased myocardial fibrosis have been described: late gadolinium enhancement (LGE) on CMR and the perfusable tissue index measured using PET. LGE is a relatively new CMR technique that was described initially for the detection of myocardial viability in ischemic cardiomyopathy [54] and the quantification of infarct size and transmural extent after myocardial infarction [55]. It is believed that the delayed enhancement is caused by the increased volume of distribution and slower washout kinetics of the gadolinium in regions of myocardial fibrosis. Although sensitivity and specificity of LGE for the quantification of fibrosis have not been reported, the extent of LGE has been shown to be inversely correlated with the degree of improvement in adverse remodeling as evidenced by declines in left ventricular volumes and improvements in ejection fraction in heart failure patients treated with β-blockers [56]. Similar to LGE, a perfusable tissue index was described initially as a PET technique for identifying myocardial viability [57]. The perfusable tissue index is a ratio of perfusable tissue fraction versus anatomic tissue fraction as measured using $H_2O^{15}O$ and $C^{15}O$ PET, respectively. This ratio is diminished in areas of myocardial fibrosis. Knaapen and colleagues [58] have recently demonstrated that, in comparison to controls, patients who have idiopathic dilated cardiomyopathy have decreased perfusable tissue indexes with increased heterogeneity across wall segments. This finding suggests that perfusable tissue index may be a valuable marker for myocardial fibrosis in adverse remodeling.

Cellular and molecular markers of adverse remodeling

Molecular imaging is a new, multidisciplinary field that encompasses the noninvasive imaging of targeted macromolecules and biologic processes in living organisms [59]. The principle underlying molecular imaging is the use of targeted, molecularly specific probes that use a reporter component to create contrast with tissue that is detected by various imaging modalities. Detection modalities that have been used for cardiac molecular imaging include CMR, SPECT or PET, and optical imaging. Recent reports have identified a number of novel markers of ventricular remodeling that can be detected and quantified by these techniques (Fig. 2).

Imaging of apoptosis

A prominent feature of adverse ventricular remodeling is the loss of cardiac myocytes through necrosis and apoptosis [60,61]. Although the precise role of apoptosis in remodeling has been difficult to define, there is evidence that the rate of apoptosis tracks with the progression and regression of remodeling [62,63], making it an attractive target for molecular imaging. Phosphatidylserine is a phospholipid that is normally confined to the inner leaflet of the cell membrane. During apoptosis, phosphatidylserine is externalized [64] and is bound by the phospholipid-binding protein annexin V. Molecular imaging techniques have exploited this phenomenon, using labeled annexin V as a targeted probe.

Molecular imaging of apoptosis was first reported in humans by Hofstra and colleagues using techne-

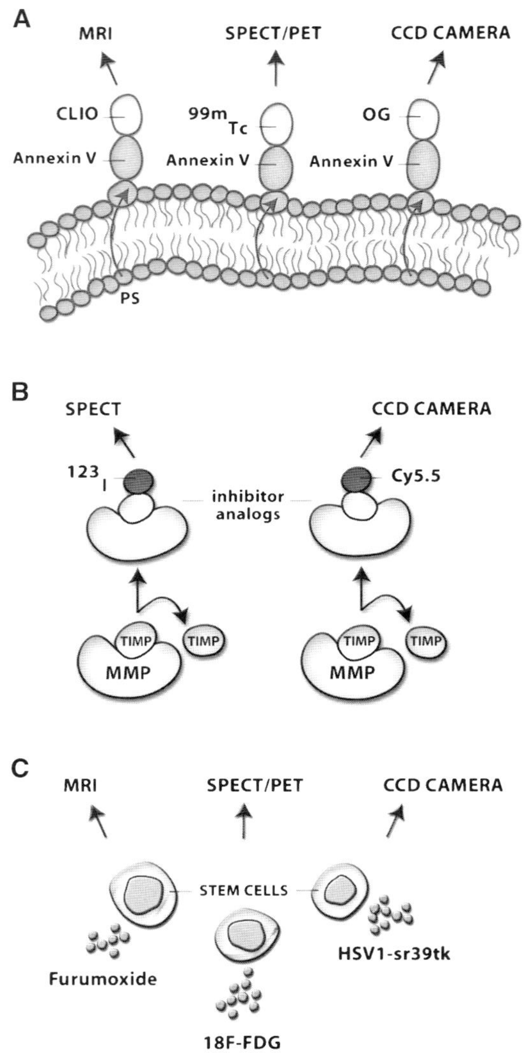

Fig. 2. Molecular imaging of adverse remodeling. (*A*) Apoptosis imaging. Phosphatidylserine (PS), normally found on the inner leaflet of cell membranes, is translocated to the external leaflets of apoptotic cells. It is bound there by engineered annexin V, labeled with a reporter that can be detected by MRI, SPECT, PET, or a CCD camera. (*B*) MMP imaging. Synthetic TIMP analogs labeled with reporters can be detected by SPECT–PET or a CCD camera. (*C*) Stem cell imaging. Stem cells used for therapy can be labeled before injection with reporters that can be detected by MRI, SPECT–PET or a CCD camera. CLIO, cross-linked iron oxide; Ferumoxide, ferumoxide injectable solution; OG, Oregon Green fluorescent probe.

tium Tc 99m (^{99m}Tc)-labeled annexin V detected by SPECT [65]. Seven patients were injected 2 hours after undergoing percutaneous transluminal coronary angioplasty. Six of the patients demonstrated detectable activity of the probe in the infarct zone at an average of 3 to 4 hours after injection. The localization of annexin V as detected by SPECT corresponded to SPECT perfusion defects found 6 to 8 weeks later, demonstrating the potential for early identification of cell death using apoptosis imaging. A similar ^{99m}Tc-labeled annexin V probe was used by Narula and colleagues [66] to noninvasively detect the presence or absence of biopsy grade 2 or greater heart transplantation rejection. Another approach that holds great promise for clinical value is the use of superparamagnetic iron oxide nanoparticles as a reporter for MRI imaging of apoptosis. MRI molecular imaging has the advantages of not requiring time for probe washout from the blood pool and the ability to provide anatomic colocalization with very good spatial resolution. Although MRI molecular imaging is not yet described in humans, Sosnovik and colleagues [67] have shown the feasibility of this approach by demonstrating selective localization of an annexin V–cross-linked iron oxide–targeted probe to hypocontractile myocardium after myocardial infarction in mice. Also described is the use of the fluorescent probe, Oregon Green, to optically image myocardial apoptosis in mice through a charged-coupled device (CCD) camera [68]. However, the limited depth of penetration and nontomographic nature of optical imaging techniques currently limit their clinical value.

Imaging of matrix metalloproteinases

The orderly degradation and repair of the extracellular matrix are dependent on the balance between MMPs and tissue inhibitors of MMPs (TIMP), and a shift toward one or the other can result in adverse remodeling [53]. Molecular imaging strategies take advantage of the MMP–TIMP interaction, using probes that bind to the TIMP binding site without inhibiting MMP function. Molecular imaging of MMP activation and inhibition in a live animal was first shown by Bremer and colleagues [69] using an activatable probe consisting of an engineered peptide substrate of MMP-2. On cleavage of this peptide, a linked near infrared (NIR) fluorochrome, Cy5.5, emits a signal detectable by a CCD camera. The cleavage of multiple probes by a single MMP molecule amplifies this NIR signal many times over. The same investigators have now used a similar strategy to image the expression of MMP-2 and MMP-9 in mice after myocardial infarction [70]. Using multiple probe injections, the investigators were able not only to localize MMP expression but also able to quantify it and track the levels over time. In similar experiments, Su and colleagues [71] have demonstrated the ability to image MMP activation after myocardial infarction in mice by SPECT, using a ^{99m}Tc-labeled MMP targeted radiotracer. In addition, they used hybrid SPECT–x-ray computed tomographic imaging to achieve precise spatial localization.

Imaging stem cells

The traditional view of myocytes as terminally differentiated cells that do not proliferate and are not replaced has been challenged recently [72,73]. Additionally, recent clinical investigations have demonstrated that intracoronary stem cell transplantation after myocardial infarction can improve ventricular ejection fraction and decrease left ventricular volumes, potentially by preventing or reversing adverse remodeling [74,75]. To date, it has not been possible to image stem cells or myocyte proliferation in vivo in human or animal models. However, noninvasive in vivo imaging of transplanted stem cells is possible by labeling with targeted probes before transplantation.

Kraitchman and colleagues [76] have recently demonstrated the use of superparamagnetic iron nanoparticles to label stem cells before injection into infarcted pig myocardium. Using a 1.5-T MRI scanner, investigators were able to track both the location and size of the stem cell population. Over a period of 3 weeks, the signal decreased in intensity while increasing in the overall area involved, suggesting that there was stem cell division or migration, or both. A similar study by Hill and colleagues [77] had comparable results. These studies highlight the strengths of molecular imaging with MRI: the fact that imaging protocols were very similar to those currently used in clinical practice and the ability of MRI to spatially colocalize stem cells with myocardial infarction.

Other groups have used the technique of radionuclide labeling of stem cells for noninvasively tracking the fate of stem cells after transplantation into myocardium. Aicher and colleagues [78] tagged endothelial progenitor cells with indium-111 (^{111}In)-oxine, a radiolabel well known for its use in leukocyte tagging for the imaging of localized inflammation. After injecting ^{111}In-oxine into mice after induced myocardial infarction, the investigators were able to identify increased radiotracer localized to the myocardium for up to 96 hours after injection. Unfortunately, this approach is limited by the short half-life of the ^{111}In radiotracer (2.8 days), which limits detection to 5 to 7 days, and by the poor spatial resolution of this isotope. Hoffmann and colleagues recently demonstrated the value of PET in the first report of the use of labeled stem cell transplantation in human subjects after experiencing myocardial infarction [79]. They labeled harvested bone marrow cells with 2-fluorine-18-fluoro-2-deoxy-D-glucose (^{18}F-FDG) and performed three-dimensional PET imaging within 50 to 75 minutes after injection. This approach proved fruitful for the exploration of differences in stem cell localization between three different harvesting–transplantation protocols.

A limitation of both SPECT–PET and MRI for the molecular imaging of transplanted stem cells is the inability to perform serial imaging. Nuclear techniques suffer from progressive radioactive decay. MRI techniques suffer from a diffusion of the original ferrous contrast particles and uncertainty as to whether late imaging truly represents living stem cells. Wu and colleagues [80] attempted to address these shortcomings using a reporter gene approach that theoretically would allow serial imaging through multiple administrations of a substrate. The investigators transfected embryonic rat cardiomyoblasts with an adenoviral vector containing a constitutively expressed herpes simplexvirus (HSV)-1 thymidine kinase derivative (HSV-1-sr39tk) or firefly luciferase. HSV-1-sr39tk can phosphorylate thymidine analog probes, trapping the probes intracellularly, thus amplifying any attached radionuclide signal. Firefly luciferase is an enzyme that cleaves luciferin, a light-emitting molecule. After the transplantation of the transfected myoblasts into mouse myocardium, investigators were able to localize them by both CCD camera and micro-PET. In this case, there was significant signal reduction after 1 to 4 days. However, reporter gene technology promises the opportunity for serial imaging of living cells through the serial administration of the requisite substrate.

Tissue neurohormonal markers of adverse remodeling

The neurohormonal signals that mediate and perpetuate adverse remodeling arise initially as compensatory reactions to an index insult to myocardial function. Once the adverse remodeling process is underway, it amplifies these neurohormonal signals further, resulting ultimately in clinical decompensation. This central role in the perpetuation of adverse remodeling and the progression of heart failure makes the neurohormonal systems attractive as markers of remodeling. SPECT and PET have been used for over a decade to measure presynaptic sympathetic innervation and catecholamine reuptake in heart failure [81,82]. Work is also ongoing on developing ligands for postsynaptic adrenergic receptors. In comparison, noninvasive imaging of the renin-angiotensin system remains in the experimental stages. Dilsizian and colleagues [83] have synthesized an ^{18}F-labeled lisinopril analog and demonstrated specific binding to angiotensin-converting enzyme in explanted myocardium. This preliminary work holds promise for the development of PET imaging of the renin-angiotensin system in vivo.

Summary

To date, noninvasive imaging of remodeling has been limited primarily to the measurement of structural and functional changes observed on an organ level. TTE, CMR, and gated SPECT have all been effective clinical tools for the measurement of these markers of adverse remodeling (ie, left ventricular volumes, ejection fraction, mass, and sphericity index). However, these markers do not give a complete picture of the adverse remodeling process, providing no information about preclinical remodeling or the rate of progression of remodeling. The development of new markers of adverse remodeling representing changes on a histopathologic, cellular, molecular, and neurohormonal level offers to provide a much fuller representation of the underlying process. Particularly exciting are a number of emerging molecular imaging techniques incorporating the use of targeted and activatable molecular probes with the modalities of CMR, SPECT, PET, and optical imaging. The imaging of apoptosis, MMP activity, and transplanted stem cell localization demonstrates how molecular imaging will allow identification and measurement of the underlying processes of remodeling rather than the end results.

Acknowledgments

The authors thank Anh Bui for artistic assistance.

References

[1] White HD, Norris RM, Brown MA, et al. Left ventricular end-systolic volume as the major determinant of survival after recovery from myocardial infarction. Circulation 1987;76:44–51.

[2] Vasan RS, Larson MG, Benjamin EJ, et al. Left ventricular dilatation and the risk of congestive heart failure in people without myocardial infarction. N Engl J Med 1997;336:1350–5.

[3] Mann DL. Basic mechanisms of left ventricular remodeling: the contribution of wall stress. J Card Fail 2004;10:S202–6.

[4] McKinsey TA, Olson EN. Toward transcriptional therapies for the failing heart: chemical screens to modulate genes. J Clin Invest 2005;115:538–46.

[5] Anand IS, Florea VG. Alterations in ventricular structure: role of left ventricular remodeling. In: Mann DL, editor. Heart failure: a companion to Braunwald's heart disease. 1st edition. Philadelphia: WB Saunders; 2004. p. 229–45.

[6] Cohn JN, Ferrari R, Sharpe N for the International Forum on Cardiac Remodeling. Cardiac remodeling–concepts and clinical implications: a consensus paper from an international forum on cardiac remodeling. J Am Coll Cardiol 2000;35:569–82.

[7] Katz AM. Organ Physiology: the failing heart as a weakend pump. In: Heart failure. Philadelphia: Lippincott Williams & Wilkins; 2000. p. 40–50.

[8] Lamas GA, Vaughan DE, Parisi AF, et al. Effects of left ventricular shape and captopril therapy on exercise capacity after anterior wall acute myocardial infarction. Am J Cardiol 1989;63:1167–73.

[9] Gottdiener JS, Bednarz J, Devereux R, et al. American Society of Echocardiography recommendations for use of echocardiography in clinical trials. J Am Soc Echocardiogr 2004;17:1086–119.

[10] Erbel R, Schweizer P, Lambertz H, et al. Echoventriculography–a simultaneous analysis of two-dimensional echocardiography and cineventriculography. Circulation 1983;67:205–15.

[11] Devereux RB, Alonso DR, Lutas EM, et al. Echocardiographic assessment of left ventricular hypertrophy: comparison to necropsy findings. Am J Cardiol 1986; 57:450–8.

[12] Gottdiener JS, Livengood SV, Meyer PS, et al. Should echocardiography be performed to assess effects of antihypertensive therapy? test-retest reliability of echocardiography for measurement of left ventricular mass and function. J Am Coll Cardiol 1995;25:424–30.

[13] Myerson SG, Montgomery HE, World MJ, et al. Left ventricular mass: reliability of M-mode and 2-dimensional echocardiographic formulas. Hypertension 2002;40:673–8.

[14] Bottini PB, Carr AA, Prisant LM, et al. Magnetic resonance imaging compared to echocardiography to assess left ventricular mass in the hypertensive patient. Am J Hypertens 1995;8:221–8.

[15] Missouris CG, Forbat SM, Singer DR, et al. Echocardiography overestimates left ventricular mass: a comparative study with magnetic resonance imaging in patients with hypertension. J Hypertens 1996;14: 1005–10.

[16] Stewart GA, Foster J, Cowan M, et al. Echocardiography overestimates left ventricular mass in hemodialysis patients relative to magnetic resonance imaging. Kidney Int 1999;56:2248–53.

[17] Sciagra R, Leoncini M. Gated single-photon emission computed tomography: the present-day "one-stop-shop" for cardiac imaging. Q J Nucl Med Mol Imaging 2005;49:19–29.

[18] Verberne HJ, Dijkgraaf MG, Somsen GA, et al. Stress-related variations in left ventricular function as assessed with gated myocardial perfusion SPECT. J Nucl Cardiol 2003;10:456–63.

[19] De Winter O, De Bondt P, Van De WC, et al. Day-to-day variability of global left ventricular functional and perfusional measurements by quantitative gated SPECT using Tc-99m tetrofosmin in patients with heart failure due to coronary artery disease. J Nucl Cardiol 2004;11:47–52.

[20] Vallejo E, Chaya H, Plancarte G, et al. Variability of serial same-day left ventricular ejection fraction using quantitative gated SPECT. J Nucl Cardiol 2002;9: 377–84.

[21] Williams KA, Lang RM, Reba RC, et al. Comparison of technetium-99m sestamibi-gated tomographic perfusion imaging with echocardiography and electrocardiography for determination of left ventricular mass. Am J Cardiol 1996;77:750–5.

[22] Damrongpipatkij Y, Bella JN, Gorski R, et al. Assessment of left ventricular mass and geometry by cardiac single photon emission computed tomography. Med Sci Monit 2003;9:107–11.

[23] Maruyama K, Hasegawa S, Nakatani D, et al. Left ventricular mass index measured by quantitative gated myocardial SPECT with 99mTc-tetrofosmin: a comparison with echocardiography. Ann Nucl Med 2003; 17:31–9.

[24] Rehr RB, Malloy CR, Filipchuk NG, et al. Left ventricular volumes measured by MR imaging. Radiology 1985;156:717–9.

[25] Longmore DB, Klipstein RH, Underwood SR, et al. Dimensional accuracy of magnetic resonance in studies of the heart. Lancet 1985;1:1360–2.

[26] Katz J, Milliken MC, Stray-Gundersen J, et al. Estimation of human myocardial mass with MR imaging. Radiology 1988;169:495–8.

[27] Grothues F, Smith GC, Moon JC, et al. Comparison of interstudy reproducibility of cardiovascular magnetic resonance with two-dimensional echocardiography in normal subjects and in patients with heart failure or left ventricular hypertrophy. Am J Cardiol 2002;90:29–34.

[28] Bellenger NG, Davies LC, Francis JM, et al. Reduction in sample size for studies of remodeling in heart failure by the use of cardiovascular magnetic resonance. J Cardiovasc Magn Reson 2000;2:271–8.

[29] Plein S, Bloomer TN, Ridgway JP, et al. Steady-state free precession magnetic resonance imaging of the heart: comparison with segmented k-space gradient-echo imaging. J Magn Reson Imaging 2001; 14:230–6.

[30] Lee VS, Resnick D, Bundy JM, et al. Cardiac function:

MR evaluation in one breath hold with real-time true fast imaging with steady-state precession. Radiology 2002;222:835–42.
[31] Myerson SG, Bellenger NG, Pennell DJ. Assessment of left ventricular mass by cardiovascular magnetic resonance. Hypertension 2002;39:750–5.
[32] Spencer KT, Bednarz J, Rafter PG, et al. Use of harmonic imaging without echocardiographic contrast to improve two-dimensional image quality. Am J Cardiol 1998;82:794–9.
[33] Cohen JL, Cheirif J, Segar DS, et al. Improved left ventricular endocardial border delineation and opacification with OPTISON (FS069), a new echocardiographic contrast agent: results of a phase III multicenter trial. J Am Coll Cardiol 1998;32:746–52.
[34] Kitzman DW, Goldman ME, Gillam LD, et al. Efficacy and safety of the novel ultrasound contrast agent perflutren (definity) in patients with suboptimal baseline left ventricular echocardiographic images. Am J Cardiol 2000;86:669–74.
[35] Thomson HL, Basmadjian AJ, Rainbird AJ, et al. Contrast echocardiography improves the accuracy and reproducibility of left ventricular remodeling measurements: a prospective, randomly assigned, blinded study. J Am Coll Cardiol 2001;38:867–75.
[36] Malm S, Frigstad S, Sagberg E, et al. Accurate and reproducible measurement of left ventricular volume and ejection fraction by contrast echocardiography: a comparison with magnetic resonance imaging. J Am Coll Cardiol 2004;44:1030–5.
[37] Hoffmann R, von Bardeleben S, ten Cate F, et al. Assessment of systolic left ventricular function: a multi-centre comparison of cineventriculography, cardiac magnetic resonance imaging, unenhanced and contrast-enhanced echocardiography. Eur Heart J 2005;26:607–16.
[38] Reilly JP, Tunick PA, Timmermans RJ, et al. Contrast echocardiography clarifies uninterpretable wall motion in intensive care unit patients. J Am Coll Cardiol 2000; 35:485–90.
[39] Spencer KT, Bednarz J, Mor-Avi V, et al. Automated endocardial border detection and evaluation of left ventricular function from contrast-enhanced images using modified acoustic quantification. J Am Soc Echocardiogr 2002;15:777–81.
[40] Gopal AS, Keller AM, Rigling R, et al. Left ventricular volume and endocardial surface area by three-dimensional echocardiography: comparison with two-dimensional echocardiography and nuclear magnetic resonance imaging in normal subjects. J Am Coll Cardiol 1993;22:258–70.
[41] Sapin PM, Schroder KM, Gopal AS, et al. Comparison of two- and three-dimensional echocardiography with cineventriculography for measurement of left ventricular volume in patients. J Am Coll Cardiol 1994;24:1054–63.
[42] Gopal AS, Keller AM, Shen Z, et al. Three-dimensional echocardiography: in vitro and in vivo validation of left ventricular mass and comparison with conventional echocardiographic methods. J Am Coll Cardiol 1994;24:504–13.
[43] Sapin PM, Schroeder KD, Smith MD, et al. Three-dimensional echocardiographic measurement of left ventricular volume in vitro: comparison with two-dimensional echocardiography and cineventriculography. J Am Coll Cardiol 1993;22:1530–7.
[44] Gopal AS, Schnellbaecher MJ, Shen Z, et al. Freehand three-dimensional echocardiography for determination of left ventricular volume and mass in patients with abnormal ventricles: comparison with magnetic resonance imaging. J Am Soc Echocardiogr 1997;10:853–61.
[45] Kupferwasser I, Mohr-Kahaly S, Stahr P, et al. Transthoracic three-dimensional echocardiographic volumetry of distorted left ventricles using rotational scanning. J Am Soc Echocardiogr 1997;10:840–52.
[46] Acar P, Maunoury C, Antonietti T, et al. Left ventricular ejection fraction in children measured by three-dimensional echocardiography using a new transthoracic integrated 3D-probe. A comparison with equilibrium radionuclide angiography. Eur Heart J 1998;19:1583–8.
[47] Nosir YF, Fioretti PM, Vletter WB, et al. Accurate measurement of left ventricular ejection fraction by three-dimensional echocardiography: a comparison with radionuclide angiography. Circulation 1996;94: 460–6.
[48] Kuhl HP, Schreckenberg M, Rulands D, et al. High-resolution transthoracic real-time three-dimensional echocardiography: quantitation of cardiac volumes and function using semi-automatic border detection and comparison with cardiac magnetic resonance imaging. J Am Coll Cardiol 2004;43:2083–90.
[49] Gutierrez-Chico JL, Zamorano JL, Perez D, et al. Comparison of left ventricular volumes and ejection fractions measured by three-dimensional echocardiography versus by two-dimensional echocardiography and cardiac magnetic resonance in patients with various cardiomyopathies. Am J Cardiol 2005;95:809–13.
[50] Jenkins C, Bricknell K, Hanekom L, et al. Reproducibility and accuracy of echocardiographic measurements of left ventricular parameters using real-time three-dimensional echocardiography. J Am Coll Cardiol 2004;44:878–86.
[51] Mor-Avi V, Sugeng L, Weinert L, et al. Fast measurement of left ventricular mass with real-time three-dimensional echocardiography: comparison with magnetic resonance imaging. Circulation 2004;110: 1814–8.
[52] Oe H, Hozumi T, Arai K, et al. Comparison of accurate measurement of left ventricular mass in patients with hypertrophied hearts by real-time three-dimensional echocardiography versus magnetic resonance imaging. Am J Cardiol 2005;95:1263–7.
[53] Jugdutt BI. Ventricular remodeling after infarction and the extracellular collagen matrix: when is enough enough? Circulation 2003;108:1395–403.
[54] Kim RJ, Wu E, Rafael A, et al. The use of contrast-

enhanced magnetic resonance imaging to identify reversible myocardial dysfunction. N Engl J Med 2000; 343:1445–53.

[55] Wu E, Judd RM, Vargas JD, et al. Visualisation of presence, location, and transmural extent of healed Q-wave and non-Q-wave myocardial infarction. Lancet 2001;357:21–8.

[56] Bello D, Shah DJ, Farah GM, et al. Gadolinium cardiovascular magnetic resonance predicts reversible myocardial dysfunction and remodeling in patients with heart failure undergoing beta-blocker therapy. Circulation 2003;108:1945–53.

[57] Iida H, Tamura Y, Kitamura K, et al. Histochemical correlates of (15)O-water-perfusable tissue fraction in experimental canine studies of old myocardial infarction. J Nucl Med 2000;41:1737–45.

[58] Knaapen P, Boellaard R, Gotte MJ, et al. Perfusable tissue index as a potential marker of fibrosis in patients with idiopathic dilated cardiomyopathy. J Nucl Med 2004;45:1299–304.

[59] Herschman HR. Molecular imaging: looking at problems, seeing solutions. Science 2003;302:605–8.

[60] Narula J, Haider N, Virmani R, et al. Apoptosis in myocytes in end-stage heart failure. N Engl J Med 1996 335:1182–9.

[61] Olivetti G, Abbi R, Quaini F, et al. Apoptosis in the failing human heart. N Engl J Med 1997;336:1131–41.

[62] Abbate A, Biondi-Zoccai GG, Bussani R, et al. Increased myocardial apoptosis in patients with unfavorable left ventricular remodeling and early symptomatic post-infarction heart failure. J Am Coll Cardiol 2003; 41:753–60.

[63] Chandrashekhar Y, Sen S, Anway R, et al. Long-term caspase inhibition ameliorates apoptosis, reduces myocardial troponin-I cleavage, protects left ventricular function, and attenuates remodeling in rats with myocardial infarction. J Am Coll Cardiol 2004;43:295–301.

[64] Fadok VA, Voelker DR, Campbell PA, et al. Exposure of phosphatidylserine on the surface of apoptotic lymphocytes triggers specific recognition and removal by macrophages. J Immunol 1992;148:2207–16.

[65] Hofstra L, Liem IH, Dumont EA, et al. Visualisation of cell death in vivo in patients with acute myocardial infarction. Lancet 2000;356:209–12.

[66] Narula J, Acio ER, Narula N, et al. Annexin-V imaging for noninvasive detection of cardiac allograft rejection. Nat Med 2001;7:1347–52.

[67] Sosnovik DE, Schellenberger EA, Nahrendorf M, et al. Magnetic resonance imaging of cardiomyocyte apoptosis with a novel magneto-optical nanoparticle. Magn Reson Med 2005;54:718–24.

[68] Dumont EA, Reutelingsperger CP, Smits JF, et al. Real-time imaging of apoptotic cell-membrane changes at the single-cell level in the beating murine heart. Nat Med 2001;7:1352–5.

[69] Bremer C, Tung CH, Weissleder R. In vivo molecular target assessment of matrix metalloproteinase inhibition. Nat Med 2001;7:743–8.

[70] Chen J, Tung CH, Allport JR, et al. Near-infrared fluorescent imaging of matrix metalloproteinase activity after myocardial infarction. Circulation 2005;111: 1800–5.

[71] Su H, Spinale FG, Dobrucki LW, et al. Noninvasive targeted imaging of matrix metalloproteinase activation in a murine model of postinfarction remodeling. Circulation 2005;112:3157–67.

[72] Beltrami AP, Urbanek K, Kajstura J, et al. Evidence that human cardiac myocytes divide after myocardial infarction. N Engl J Med 2001;344:1750–7.

[73] Anversa P, Kajstura J. Ventricular myocytes are not terminally differentiated in the adult mammalian heart. Circ Res 1998;83:1–14.

[74] Schachinger V, Assmus B, Britten MB, et al. Transplantation of progenitor cells and regeneration enhancement in acute myocardial infarction: final one-year results of the TOPCARE-AMI Trial. J Am Coll Cardiol 2004;44:1690–9.

[75] Wollert KC, Meyer GP, Lotz J, et al. Intracoronary autologous bone-marrow cell transfer after myocardial infarction: the BOOST randomised controlled clinical trial. Lancet 2004;364:141–8.

[76] Kraitchman DL, Heldman AW, Atalar E, et al. In vivo magnetic resonance imaging of mesenchymal stem cells in myocardial infarction. Circulation 2003;107:2290–3.

[77] Hill JM, Dick AJ, Raman VK, et al. Serial cardiac magnetic resonance imaging of injected mesenchymal stem cells. Circulation 2003;108:1009–14.

[78] Aicher A, Brenner W, Zuhayra M, et al. Assessment of the tissue distribution of transplanted human endothelial progenitor cells by radioactive labeling. Circulation 2003;107:2134–9.

[79] Hofmann M, Wollert KC, Meyer GP, et al. Monitoring of bone marrow cell homing into the infarcted human myocardium. Circulation 2005;111:2198–202.

[80] Wu JC, Chen IY, Sundaresan G, et al. Molecular imaging of cardiac cell transplantation in living animals using optical bioluminescence and positron emission tomography. Circulation 2003;108:1302–5.

[81] Bengel FM, Schwaiger M. Assessment of cardiac sympathetic neuronal function using PET imaging. J Nucl Cardiol 2004;11:603–16.

[82] Flotats A, Carrio I. Cardiac neurotransmission SPECT imaging. J Nucl Cardiol 2004;11:587–602.

[83] Dilsizian V, Loredo ML, Jagoda EM, Eckelman WC, Shirani J. Scintigraphic and immunohistochemical evidence for localization of angiotensin converting enzyme to myocytes in human ischemic cardiomyopathy. J Am Coll Cardiol 2003;41:427.

ELSEVIER
SAUNDERS

Heart Failure Clin 2 (2006) 129 – 143

HEART
FAILURE
CLINICS

Nuclear Probes for Assessing Myocardial Viability in Heart Failure

James A. Arrighi, MD[a,*], Vasken Dilsizian, MD[b]

[a]*Brown Medical School/Rhode Island Hospital, Providence, RI, USA*
[b]*University of Maryland Medical Center, Baltimore, MD, USA*

Systolic left ventricular dysfunction is the end stage of most cardiovascular disorders that may manifest themselves clinically as heart failure. Among patients who have symptoms of heart failure, most may have coronary artery disease as the underlying cause of the left ventricular dysfunction. Determining whether left ventricular dysfunction is due to the consequences of coronary artery disease or one of the many other etiologies of heart failure is a critical early step. The left ventricular dysfunction may be secondary to previous myocardial infarction or prolonged and repetitive ischemia [1–4]. Substantial data now exist to indicate that prolonged alterations in regional or global left ventricular function may occur when patients are subjected to supply (decreased blood flow) or demand ischemia, and that such dysfunction may be completely reversible. Thus, noninvasive assessment of myocardial ischemia and viability would identify the subgroup of patients who have heart failure that has a potentially reversible degree of left ventricular dysfunction and may benefit from revascularization. Therapeutic interventions that reverse dysfunctional but viable myocardium may improve heart failure symptoms and impact left ventricular remodeling and patient outcome. Moreover, the identification of myocardial ischemia may have implications in secondary prevention strategies, because acute myocardial infarction is a common mechanism of death in patients who have heart failure.

The objective of assessing myocardial viability in heart failure is to optimize selection of patients whose symptoms and prognosis may improve following revascularization. In a recent clinical trial of stable, community-based patients who had heart failure, approximately 70% of patients had evidence for hibernation or stress-induced ischemia in the absence of angina [5]. Thus, a significant subpopulation of patients who have heart failure may benefit from a noninvasive assessment of myocardial ischemia and viability.

Pathophysiologic background

The pathophysiologic concepts of hibernation [2,3], stunning [4], and ischemic preconditioning [5] represent different mechanisms of acute and chronic adaptation to a temporary or sustained reduction in coronary blood flow. Hibernating myocardium refers to persistent regional left ventricular dysfunction that arises from prolonged hypoperfusion at rest. Stunned myocardium refers to the state of persistent regional dysfunction after a transient period of ischemia. Ischemic preconditioning refers to a form of short-term metabolic memory, which is based on the observation that a brief period of ischemia followed by reperfusion lessens the effects of a subsequent long period of ischemia [6]. In an individual patient who has coronary artery disease, one or all of these phenomena may be active. These phenomena are part of the spectrum of myocardial

* Corresponding author. Brown Medical School/Rhode Island Hospital, 593 Eddy Street, Providence, RI 02903.
E-mail address: james_arrighi@brown.edu
(J.A. Arrighi).

1551-7136/06/$ – see front matter
doi:10.1016/j.hfc.2006.02.002

ischemia and reperfusion that represent different mechanisms of adaptation for programmed cell survival (Fig. 1) [7]. As such, procedures that alleviate myocardial ischemia would have salutary effects to all three phenomena with the resultant improvement in left ventricular function, remodeling, arrhythmias, and long-term survival. Therefore, the goal of myocardial viability assessment is to differentiate, prospectively, patients who have potentially reversible left ventricular dysfunction who may benefit from revascularization.

The nuclear techniques for assessing myocardial viability generally involve evaluation of regional myocardial perfusion, cell membrane integrity, or metabolism (Fig. 2). Single photon emission CT (SPECT) radiotracers, such as thallium-201 (^{201}Tl)- and technetium-99m (^{99m}Tc)-labeled sestamibi or tetrofosmin, and the positron emission tomography (PET) radiotracers rubidium-82 (^{82}Rb) and nitrogen-13 (^{13}N) ammonia assess perfusion and cell membrane integrity. Metabolic tracers, such as ^{18}F-2-fluoro-2-deoxyglucose (FDG) or fatty acid analogs, assess some aspect of glucose and fatty acid metabolism for high-energy ATP production in hypoperfused and hypocontractile myocardial regions (Table 1). Evaluation of contractile reserve with dobutamine is another common method of viability assessment. Although dobutamine is used most commonly with echocardiography, it also may be used with gated SPECT or PET to enhance viability detection. Finally, myocardial scar can be delineated by gadolinium-enhanced cardiac MRI.

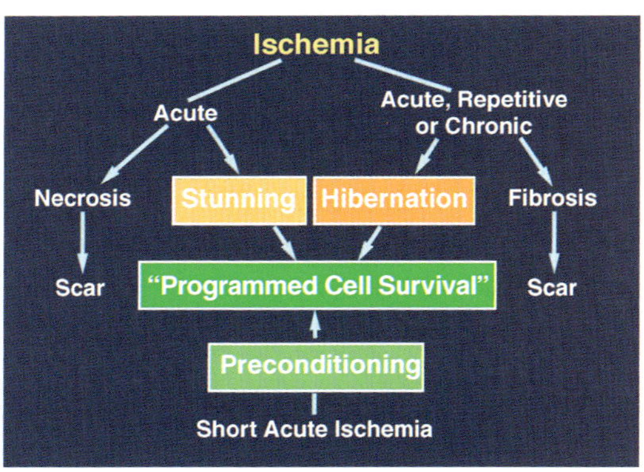

Fig. 1. Myocardial hibernation, stunning, and ischemic preconditioning trigger programmed cell survival, most likely by different mechanisms. Common to all three phenomena is an intact functioning nucleus of the cardiac myocyte. (*Adapted from* Taegtmeyer H. Modulation of responses to myocardial ischemia: metabolic features of myocardial stunning, hibernation, and ischemic preconditioning. In: Dilsizian V, editor. Myocardial viability: a clinical and scientific treatise. Armonk (NY): Futura Publishing Company, Inc.; 2000. p. 32; with permission.)

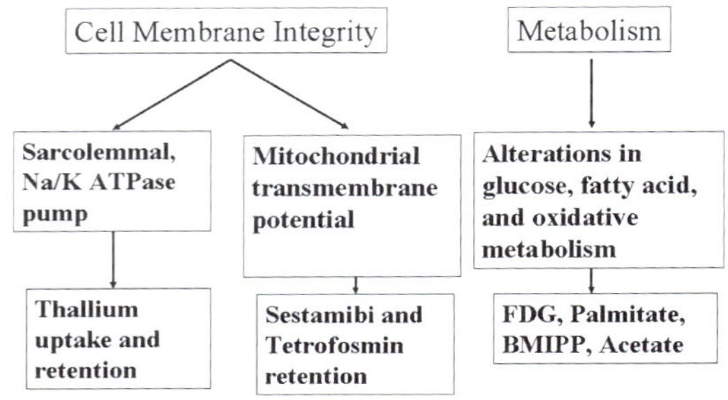

Fig. 2. Schematic physiologic basis for assessing myocardial viability with nuclear radiotracers.

Requirements for cellular viability

The most common definition of myocardial viability in clinical studies is improvement in contractile function of a dysfunctional region after restoration of blood flow. Requirements for cellular viability include adequate myocardial blood flow, intact sarcolemmal and mitochondrial membrane function, and preserved metabolic activity. Myocardial blood flow has to be adequate to deliver oxygen and substrate to the myocyte to be used in the metabolic process, as well as to remove the end products of the metabolic process. Intact sarcolemmal and mitochondrial membrane function to maintain elec-

Table 1
Common nuclear cardiology protocols for the assessment of myocardial viability

Technology	Radiotracer	Common protocols
SPECT	Thallium-201	(1) Stress-3–4-hour redistribution-reinjection
		(2) Stress–reinjection–24-hour redistribution
		(3) Rest-Redistribution
SPECT	^{99m}Tc-sestamibi	(1) Rest-nitrate augmented rest (± stress)
	^{99m}Tc-tetrofosmin	(2) Rest–low-dose dobutamine (with gating)
PET	FDG	(1) Rest FDG PET with glucose-loading; comparison with resting perfusion image with ^{82}Rb or ^{13}N-ammonia PET or SPECT radiotracers

trochemical gradients across the cell membrane is a requirement for myocyte viability. Because cell membrane integrity is highly dependent on preserved intracellular metabolic activity, tracers that reflect sarcolemmal cation flux, such as ^{201}Tl and ^{82}Rb, should parallel the viability information that is provided by markers of metabolic activity, such as FDG. Similarly, tracers that reflect mitochondrial membrane integrity, such as ^{99m}Tc-labeled sestamibi and tetrofosmin, provide information on myocardial viability. Thus, in the setting of reduced regional blood flow and function, techniques that assess intact cellular sarcolemmal or mitochondrial function or metabolic processes provide unique insight into the presence or absence of myocardial viability.

Nuclear probes for myocardial perfusion and cell membrane integrity

Single photon emission CT myocardial perfusion tracers

Thallium-201

Thallium is the first radiotracer that was used widely to assess regional blood flow and sarcolemmal integrity, and hence viability [8]. Although its use declined after the introduction of ^{99m}Tc–based perfusion tracers, it remains a highly effective perfusion and viability tracer. Thallium has the highest first-pass extraction fraction (~85%) of any commonly used perfusion tracer. The usefulness of thallium as a viability tracer is based on its similarities to potassium, in that it is transported across the sarcolemmal membrane by way of an active, energy-dependent transport system that is unaffected by hypoxia, unless irreversible injury is present [9,10]. Thus, the uptake and retention of thallium is dependent on regional blood flow and sarcolemmal membrane integrity.

Early after intravenous injection of thallium (whether during stress or at rest), the distribution of the tracer reflects regional blood. The later distribution of thallium over a 4- to 24-hour period reflects myocardial potassium concentration and is a function of regional blood volume. During the redistribution phase, there is a continuous exchange of thallium between the myocardium and the extracardiac compartments, which is driven by the concentration gradient of the tracer and myocyte viability. Viable myocardium concentrates more thallium over time, whereas scarred myocardium does not. Therefore, preserved viability may be reflected by enhanced regional concentration of thallium from early to delayed images, or by maintenance of a certain degree of uptake in the myocardium. Several thallium protocols have been assessed for the detection of myocardial viability. Among the range of choices, two protocols are optimized for viability detection: stress–4-hour redistribution-reinjection imaging [11] and rest-redistribution imaging [12]. The former assesses myocardial ischemia and viability, whereas the latter assesses only myocardial viability. Other, less commonly used clinical approaches include combined or sequential assessment of thallium uptake and contractile reserve with low-dose dobutamine [13,14] and nitrate-enhanced rest-redistribution thallium SPECT [15].

Technetium-99m–labeled sestamibi and tetrofosmin

The advantages of ^{99m}Tc-labeled perfusion radiotracers over thallium include shorter half-life, less radiation exposure, improved quality of gated images, and more flexibility in imaging times after stress. The extraction fraction of sestamibi is only 60%, and that of tetrofosmin is approximately 54%, both of which are significantly lower than that of thallium. Nonetheless, clinical studies [16,17] showed that the lower extraction fractions of these ^{99m}Tc-labeled perfusion radiotracers do not affect their accuracy for the detection of significant (>70%) coronary artery stenosis. Unlike thallium, neither tracer has significant redistribution, which necessitates two injections of the tracer (exercise and rest) for typical stress-rest protocols.

Experimental studies indicated that sestamibi and tetrofosmin uptake accurately reflects perfusion and viability in a wide range of pathophysiologic states. Studies showed that myocardial uptake and clearance of sestamibi and tetrofosmin are related to mitochondrial transmembrane potential and do not differ from ischemic to nonischemic regions. In addition, experimental studies [18,19] of myocardial infarction, with and without reperfusion, have enhanced the optimism in the clinical use of these tracers for myocardial viability assessment.

Positron emission tomography myocardial perfusion tracers

PET flow agents can be divided into two types: freely diffusible tracers and soluble microspheres. Oxygen-15 (^{15}O)-labeled water is an example of a freely diffusible tracer that allows repeated studies to be carried out in rapid sequence. The rapid physiologic washout clears the tracer from the myocardium and permits a subsequent study to be performed; however, such tracers usually do not give clinically meaningful images. Rather one must perform mathematical modeling at each pixel to arrive at flow values at each pixel. The second type of flow tracer, the so-called "soluble microsphere," usually is easier to scan because the radioactivity is fixed in place for a reasonable length of time. Therefore, optimal counting statistics can be obtained; however, the persistence of binding usually prevents these tracers from being used in sequential studies. In addition, the amount of binding may depend on a biochemical interaction that could change as a function of disease and confound the flow measurement. ^{13}N-ammonia and ^{82}Rb fall more closely into the latter category of flow tracers [20,21]. ^{15}O-water and ^{13}N-ammonia are produced by a cyclotron, which limits their usefulness. ^{82}Rb is produced by a generator, is commercially available, and is used most commonly for rest-stress PET imaging. ^{82}Rb and ^{13}N-ammonia received approval from the U.S. Food and Drug Administration (FDA) and the Centers for Medicare and Medicaid Services.

Certain parameters of perfusion that are measured with PET have been investigated for the assessment of myocardial viability. In one approach, radiotracer uptake and retention may be used as indices of viability. The perfusable tissue index, which is derived from the analysis of dynamic ^{15}O-water studies, measures the proportion of extravascular tissue that is perfusable by water, which is reduced in areas of scar [22,23]. In another approach, measurement of the retention and washout of ^{82}Rb, which has properties similar to thallium, and thus, represents intact cell membrane integrity, has been proposed for the assessment of viability [24,25]. Alternative approaches capitalize on the ability of PET to quantify coronary flow reserve or absolute myocardial blood flow [16,26,27]. Intact coronary flow reserve may indicate preserved viability, and correlates with preserved metabolic activity. It also was demonstrated that absolute myocardial blood flow below a certain level is unlikely to sustain viability, and thus, quantification of flow may be an accurate marker of viable myocardium [26]. These techniques are promising, and add to our understanding of the pathophysiology of hibernating myocardium; however, they require complex image acquisition or processing, and often require cyclotron-produced radiotracers, which limits their widespread applicability at this time.

Nuclear probes for myocardial metabolism

The principle of using a metabolic tracer for assessing myocardial viability is based on the concept that viable tissue in hypoperfused and dysfunctional regions is metabolically active, whereas scarred or fibrotic tissue is metabolically inactive. Under fasting and aerobic conditions, the heart uses free fatty acids as the primary fuel, which accounts for approximately 65% of the oxidative metabolic requirements. Approximately 20% of the total energy supply of the heart comes from glucose. In the fed state, the combined effects of insulin and the increased arterial glucose concentration result in increased myocardial glucose uptake. In the setting of myocardial ischemia, glucose use also increases and free fatty acid use decreases. This shift to increased glucose uptake and use may reflect a shift to pathways of anaerobic glycolysis, which results in the maintenance of myocyte viability at the expense of less efficient substrate use. The observation that ischemic myocardium takes up more glucose and less fatty acids provides opportunities to image viable, ischemic myocardium using metabolic nuclear probes for glucose or fatty acids.

^{18}F-2-fluoro-2-deoxyglucose

FDG is a glucose analog that is phosphorylated by hexokinase into FDG-6-phosphate, a form of deoxyglucose that cannot be metabolized further in the glycolytic pathway. Thus, FDG essentially is trapped in the myocardium, which allows adequate time to image the heart by PET [28]. Its use as a radiotracer for the assessment of myocardial viability has been studied extensively in patients who have chronic ischemic left ventricular dysfunction and heart failure. The myocardial uptake of FDG parallels glucose uptake in fasting and fed states. In the fasting state, FDG uptake is low, and the heart barely can be visualized. During ischemia, FDG uptake may be increased, but its lack of visualization in the fasting state does not distinguish normal from scarred myocardium. The distinction between normal, hibernating, but viable myocardium and scarred myocardium can be accomplished best with FDG in a "fed" or "glucose-loaded" state, which may be achieved with oral glucose loading or intravenous hyperinsulinemic-euglycemic clamp.

Carbon-11 palmitate

Because fatty acids are the primary source of myocardial energy production in the fasting state, early studies focused on imaging fatty acid with carbon-11 (^{11}C)-palmitate, using PET. Once the tracer is in the cell in the form of ^{11}C-acyl-CoA, it enters the endogenous lipid pool or moves by way of the carnitine shuttle to the mitochondria, where rapid degradation by β-oxidation results in the generation of carbon dioxide. Because of its complicated kinetic modeling and confounding effects of the nonesterified arterial fatty acids, hormonal milieu, and backdiffusion of altered tracer in the myocardium, ^{11}C-palmitate has not gained clinical acceptance.

β-Methyl-p-[^{123}I]-iodophenyl-pentadecanoic acid

Fatty acid imaging with radioiodine-labeled fatty acid analogs, such as β-methyl-p-[^{123}I]-iodophenyl-pentadecanoic acid (BMIPP), using SPECT is an investigational area for the assessment of ischemic memory and viability in patients who have chronic coronary artery disease and heart failure. In contrast to ^{11}C-palmitate, BMIPP predominantly is trapped in myocardial cells with limited catabolism. Uptake of BMIPP from the plasma into myocardial cells occurs by way of a CD36 transporter protein that is present on the sarcolemmal membrane. In ischemic conditions, BMIPP uptake can be discrepant and significantly less than that of regional blood flow, as assessed by thallium or ^{99m}Tc perfusion tracer (Fig. 3). Such reduced BMIPP uptake relative to perfusion has been attributed to delayed recovery of myocardial metabolism after ischemic injury, which is termed ischemic memory [29]. Although BMIPP is approved for clinical use in Japan, it has not received FDA approval.

Carbon-11 acetate

^{11}C-acetate is used to assess oxidative metabolism, which requires dynamic image acquisition and analysis of uptake and washout rates. The clinical applicability of ^{11}C-acetate imaging for viability assessment was reported in several studies [30,31]. These techniques are available only at certain research facilities.

Nuclear probes for imaging the tissue angiotensin-converting enzyme receptor system

Angiotensin-converting enzyme (ACE) inhibitors, such as captopril and lisinopril, have been radiolabeled and used in experimental systems to study the tissue ACE receptor system directly [32]. Preliminary observations in explanted hearts from patients who had heart failure showed a relationship between binding of [^{18}F]fluorobenzoyl-linsinopril and collagen replacement; ACE was absent in the collagen-

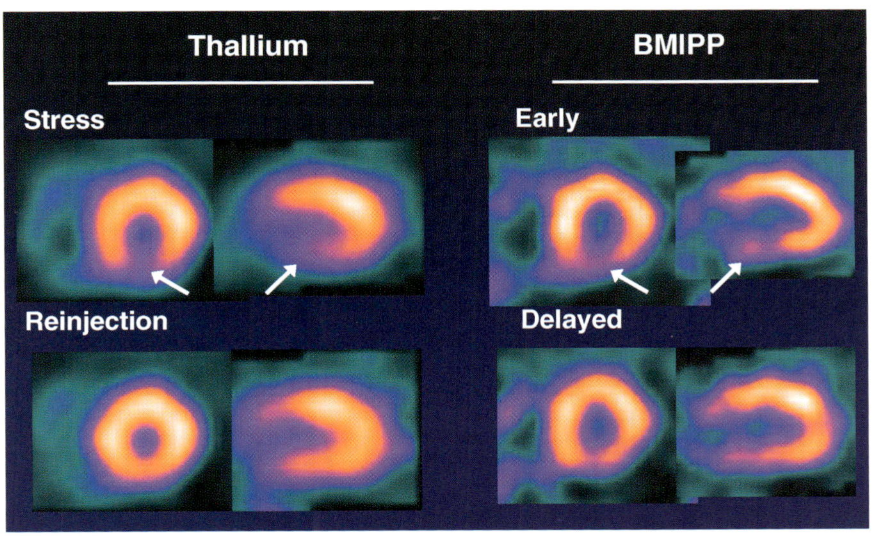

Fig. 3. Metabolic imaging with β-Methyl-*p*-[^{123}I]-Iodophenyl-Pentadecanoic Acid (BMIPP) can successfully demonstrate the metabolic imprint of a stress-induced ischemic episode, also known as *ischemic memory*. Thallium stress and reinjection images following treadmill exercise are displayed in the left panel, in the short-axis and vertical long-axis SPECT tomograms. The thallium images demonstrate a severe reversible inferior defect (*arrows*), consistent with exercise stress-induced ischemia. A similar defect is seen on the early BMIPP images in the same tomographic cuts (*arrows*), with BMIPP injected 22 hours after the stress-induced ischemia. These image data suggest that BMIPP detects prolonged post-ischemic suppression of fatty acid metabolism for up to 22 hours after stress-induced ischemia. (*Adapted from* Dilsizian V, Bateman TM, Bergmann SR, et al. Metabolic imaging with β-methyl-ρ-[^{123}I]-iodophenyl-pentadecanoic acid (BMIPP) identifies ischemic memory following demand ischemia. Circulation 2005;112(14):2169–74; with permission.)

stained areas and was increased in the juxtaposed areas of replacement fibrosis [33–35]. The increased ACE in the juxtaposed areas of replacement fibrosis may be a stimulus for collagen replacement and remodeling. The use of tissue-specific ACE radioligands represents an initial attempt to study ACE in the human heart with chronic ischemic cardiomyopathy and heart failure. If the finding of increased ACE is reversible (eg, with ACE inhibitors), noninvasive imaging with PET would allow monitoring of changes in ACE patterns in vivo, which may reflect progression of disease and the effect of therapies before collagen replacement ensues.

Clinical assessment of myocardial viability in heart failure

Single photon emission CT imaging

A normal stress myocardial perfusion scan in a patient who has heart failure and left ventricular dysfunction is highly predictive for the absence of underlying coronary artery disease as the culprit for the cardiomyopathy. The converse—the presence of any perfusion abnormality—does not necessarily indicate underlying coronary artery disease. Patients who have nonischemic cardiomyopathy may have patchy or larger confluent territories of fibrosis or scarring (confirmed by pathology and cardiac MRI studies) that manifest as fixed defects on myocardial perfusion scans [36]. Although the presence of any perfusion abnormality is not specific for coronary artery disease, the pattern of perfusion abnormality may assist in the differentiation between ischemic and nonischemic cardiomyopathy. The pattern of severe and extensive perfusion defects is more likely to indicate underlying coronary artery disease, whereas smaller and milder defects are more likely to be present in patients who have nonischemic cardiomyopathy [37].

Thallium-201

The extent of defect resolution, from the stress to redistribution images, termed reversible defect, reflects one index of myocardial viability; however, in some patients, stress–3- to 4-hour redistribution imaging may underestimate the amount of ischemic and viable myocardium. Late redistribution imaging—acquired approximately 24 hours after the initial stress thallium injection—allows more time for redistribution to occur, and has good positive predictive value for improvement in function. The negative predictive value is not high, however, because redistribution does not take place in some patients even after a prolonged time, and image quality may be suboptimal [38]. Reinjection of thallium at rest after stress–redistribution imaging improves the identification of ischemic, but viable, myocardium in up to 49% of the apparently irreversible defects on 3- to 4-hour redistribution images [11], and 39% of irreversible defects on 24-hour redistribution images [39]. When regions with reversible thallium defects (demonstration of myocardial ischemia) and success of revascularization (reexamining regional perfusion or vessel patency after revascularization) are taken into consideration, stress-redistribution-reinjection thallium imaging yields excellent positive and negative predictive accuracy (80% to 90% range) for recovery of function after revascularization [11]. Similarly, the concordance of stress-redistribution-reinjection thallium and FDG PET imaging is excellent (up to 88%) when quantitative image analysis is used [40]. In regions that are judged scarred by thallium (severe irreversible defects), metabolic imaging with FDG PET or SPECT may provide incremental information regarding myocardial viability, especially in patients who have severely impaired left ventricular function in whom the effects of thallium attenuation would be particularly prominent [41–43].

Rest-redistribution thallium imaging is an alternative to reinjection imaging after stress in patients who cannot or should not undergo exercise testing. If the clinical question to be addressed is one of the presence and extent of viable myocardium within dysfunctional regions and not inducible ischemia, it is reasonable to perform a rest-redistribution thallium SPECT. A reversible resting defect may identify areas of myocardial hibernation. This finding seems to be an insensitive, although specific, sign of potential improvement in regional function [12]; however, a stress protocol (exercise or pharmacologic) provides important diagnostic and prognostic information regarding inducible ischemia and myocardial viability [44].

Technetium-99m–labeled perfusion tracers

In early clinical studies, sestamibi and tetrofosmin seemed to underestimate defect reversibility and myocardial viability in patients who had chronic coronary artery disease [45,46]. The reason for this underestimation is unclear, but it may involve inadequate tracer delivery because of limited extraction fraction in hypoperfused myocardial regions, blood clearance and lack of significant redistribution, or response to altered metabolic states. More recently, several modifications to the routine rest-stress protocol have emerged that improve the accuracy of

Table 2
Patterns of uptake on positron emission tomography with FDG for the assessment of myocardial viability

Perfusion	FDG uptake	Interpretation
Normal	Present	Normal (regions with normal wall motion) Stunning/viable (regions with abnormal wall motion)
Reduced	Present	Hibernation/viable ("mismatch pattern")
Reduced	Absent	Scar ("matched pattern")

sestamibi and tetrofosmin imaging for the assessment of myocardial viability. These include quantification of the severity of defects [47], nitrate-enhanced rest imaging [48–54], and combined assessment of perfusion and function with gated SPECT [55]. Another approach uses the addition of low-dose dobutamine-gated SPECT, which allows the assessment of contractile reserve combined with sestamibi uptake. This approach may increase specificity to the 85% range, without a significant loss in sensitivity [56]. Finally, attenuation correction may enhance the accuracy of these agents for the assessment of viability [57].

Positron emission tomography imaging

Assessment of myocardial viability with FDG PET usually is performed in conjunction with the assessment of resting perfusion, and in the glucose-loaded state. The perfusion image is used to interpret the FDG image accurately, and several perfusion/metabolism patterns have been recognized as being indicative of scar or viable myocardium (Table 2). If perfusion is normal, regions may be considered viable on this basis alone. Most of these regions also have normal FDG uptake. Some areas may have reduced FDG uptake, which in the setting of acute ischemic myocardial injury with reperfusion, represents scintigraphic pattern of myocardial stunning [58,59]. Among regions with resting hypoperfusion, two patterns of tracer uptake are possible: a concordant reduction in flow and metabolism (termed a flow-metabolism "match"), which is considered to represent myocardial scar; and a discordant increase in FDG uptake compared with flow (termed a flow-metabolism "mismatch"), which is considered to represent hibernating, but viable, myocardium (Fig. 4). The accuracy of such mismatch and match patterns on PET for predicting functional recovery after revascularization is high, with positive and negative predictive values in the 80% to 90% range [60,61]. These findings were confirmed in a multicenter trial that was undertaken in Europe; 178 patients who had coronary artery disease and left ventricular dysfunction underwent FDG PET before revascularization and functional follow-up 4 to 6 months after revascularization [62].

Absolute quantification or regional FDG uptake is possible but it is not clear whether this improves the overall accuracy of FDG PET viability studies. Some studies suggested that FDG uptake alone may be inaccurate in the setting of acute myocardial injury [63]. In the setting of acute myocardial hypoperfusion, increased FDG uptake in the infarcted zones may be secondary to inflammation rather than viability [63]. Conversely, decreased FDG uptake in transiently ischemic zones may be secondary to stunned, but viable, myocardium rather than fibrosis [58,59]. Thus, in general, it is advisable to perform metabolic viability assessment several weeks after an acute myocardial injury. One also should recognize that most publications regarding the salutary results of FDG PET for identifying viable myocardium pertain to patients who have chronic ischemic left ventricular dysfunction and heart failure.

Recently, contrast-enhanced cardiovascular MRI was demonstrated to determine the accurate anatomic localization of scar within the myocardium of patients who had previous infarction. Two studies that involved a small number of patients compared FDG PET with cardiovascular MRI in patients who had chronic coronary artery disease and left ventricular

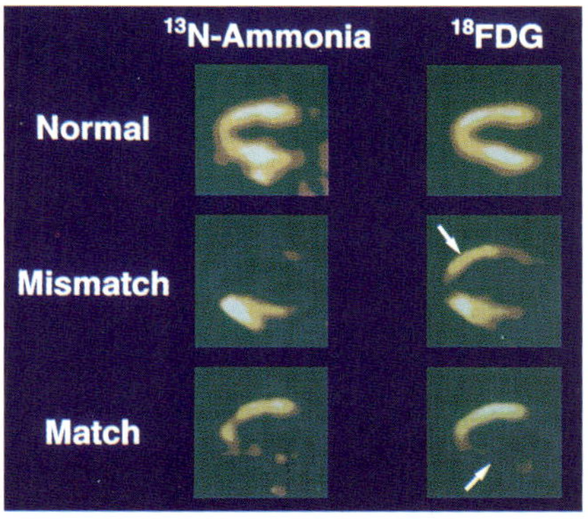

Fig. 4. Cross-sectional vertical long-axis PET images are shown for ^{13}N-ammonia and FDG. Top panel shows examples of normal perfusion and metabolism. Middle panel shows discordance between FDG uptake and ammonia (mismatch defect) in the anterior region that is indicative of hibernating, but viable, myocardium (*arrowhead*). Lower panel shows concordant severely decreased perfusion and metabolism (match defect) in the inferior region that is indicative of scarred myocardium.

dysfunction [64,65]. There was an overall good correlation between grouping of regions as viable and nonviable by the two techniques [64], and an 87% concordance between FDG PET and cardiovascular MRI for predicting functional recovery after revascularization [65]. In the subgroup of segments with discordant findings, most of which were nonviable by PET and viable by cardiovascular MRI, no improvement of function was observed after revascularization. Further prospective studies in larger numbers of patients are needed to evaluate the clinical roles of both techniques. In particular, beyond the dichotomous designation of myocardial regions as viable or scarred, the potential strength of FDG PET rests in its ability to differentiate viable myocardial regions that are hibernating or stunned. Patients who have hibernating, but viable, myocardium may be at higher risk for future cardiac events than are those who have viable myocardium without hibernation [66–70].

Improvement in left ventricular function, symptoms, and prognosis

The clinical usefulness of myocardial viability assessment by any technique rests in its ability to predict improvement of left ventricular function after revascularization, heart failure symptoms, or short- and long-term survival. Ideally, one could then distinguish patients who would benefit from revascularization from those who would not. Definitive, randomized, outcomes-driven data are lacking to prove that an algorithm that includes viability testing is better than clinical and anatomic parameters alone in selecting patients for revascularization. Several studies, however, suggest that viability testing may improve patient selection.

Improvement in left ventricular function

Most initial data on viability studies used left ventricular function as the primary outcome. SPECT and PET techniques perform well in this regard, with positive and negative predictive accuracies for predicting functional recovery in the range of 80%. The restoration of blood flow to viable myocardium, however, may have other important beneficial effects, even in the absence of functional recovery. These effects may include stabilization of the electrical milieu, or the prevention of extensive ventricular remodeling, and improved survival. This potential dissociation between left ventricular function and prognosis was suggested in a study that involved 135 consecutive patients who had ischemic cardiomyopathy and underwent coronary artery bypass surgery based on clinical judgement and not viability testing [71]. Postoperative recovery of global function was observed in approximately two thirds of patients (from 24% ± 5% before to 39% ± 10% after surgery, $P < .005$). Among the one third of patients without improvement in global left ventricular function, the postoperative improvement in angina and heart failure symptoms as well as cardiac death–free survival over the ensuing 32 ± 23 months were comparable to the rates in patients who did exhibit improvement in left ventricular function [71]. These findings support the concept that beyond recovery of left ventricular function, restoration of blood flow to viable myocardium also may have beneficial effects on heart failure symptoms and patient outcome. The interpretation of studies that use left ventricular function as an end point must be made with caution, and with attention to the timing of postrevascularization reassessment of left ventricular function. In patients who have ischemic cardiomyopathy, ischemic episodes may be long-standing, frequent, and severe,

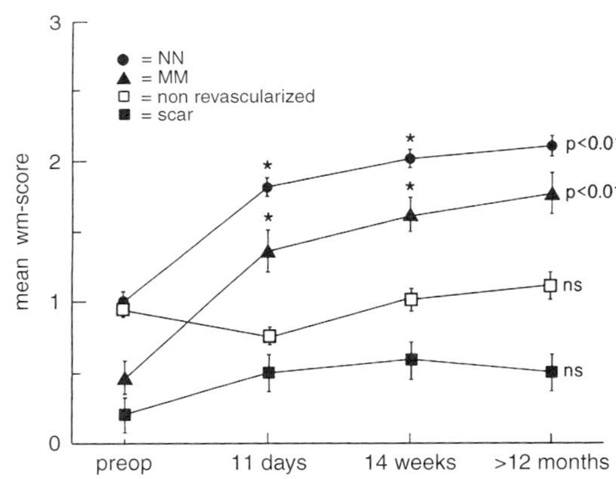

Fig. 5. Time course of functional improvement from 11 days to more than 12 months after revascularization. Categorized by FDG PET imaging, normal segments (black circles), segments with perfusion-metabolism mismatch (black triangles), and segments with scar (black squares) are plotted. Segments that were not revascularized are represented by open squares. MM, flow-metabolism mismatch; NN, normal flow but dysfunctional myocardiom; ns, not significant; wm, wall motion. (*Adapted from* Haas F, Augustin N, Holper K, et al. Time course and extent of improvement of dysfunctioning myocardium in patients with coronary artery disease and severely depressed left ventricular function after revascularization: correlation with positron emission tomographic findings. J Am Coll Cardiol 2000;36(6):1927–34; with permission.)

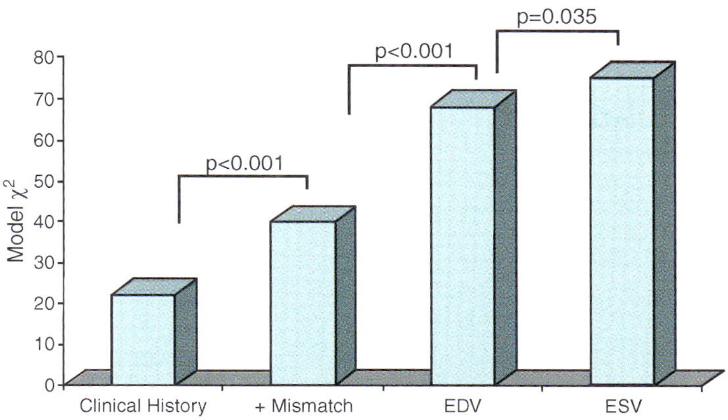

Fig. 6. Incremental value of left ventricular volumes over and above clinical history and PET mismatch data for prediction of recovery of left ventricular function after revascularization. EDV, end-diastolic volume; ESV, end-systolic volume. (*Adapted from* Santana CA, Shaw LJ, Garcia EV, et al. Incremental prognostic value of left ventricular function by myocardial ECG-gated FDG PET imaging in patients with ischemic cardiomyopathy. J Nucl Cardiol 2004;11(5):548; with permission.)

and the recovery of ventricular function after revascularization may be slow or incomplete. In 29 patients who had ischemic cardiomyopathy who underwent preoperative PET viability study, left ventricular function was assessed preoperatively and at 11 days, 14 weeks and more than 12 months after coronary artery bypass surgery [72]. As illustrated in Fig. 5, there is evidence for continued, albeit incomplete, recovery of function in regions that are identified as viable by PET. In contrast, there is no significant functional improvement in regions that are identified as scarred by PET. Thus, the process of functional improvement after revascularization may be prolonged, and at times, incomplete.

Newer generation PET cameras have the capability to perform gated FDG imaging, analogous to gated SPECT. The additional information from gated PET regarding left ventricular function and size may improve the overall accuracy of viability assessment [73]. Among 90 consecutive patients who had ischemic cardiomyopathy and underwent gated FDG PET studies before revascularization, left ventricular functional parameters (eg, ejection fraction, end-diastolic volume, end-systolic volume) had incremental prognostic value over FDG uptake parameters alone (Fig. 6). Thus, beyond the determination of myocardial viability, data on left ventricular size and function may provide additional insight into advanced left ventricular remodeling and measurable improvement of heart failure symptoms after surgery.

Finally, clinical factors other than imaging parameters, such as radiotracer uptake and left ventricular cavity size, may be important to consider in assessing the likelihood of functional recovery. The suitability of target vessels for bypass grafts is one obvious requirement; revascularization should be as complete as possible. Other clinical variables, such as diabetes and time to revascularization, may impact recovery of function, heart failure symptoms, and patient outcome [74,75].

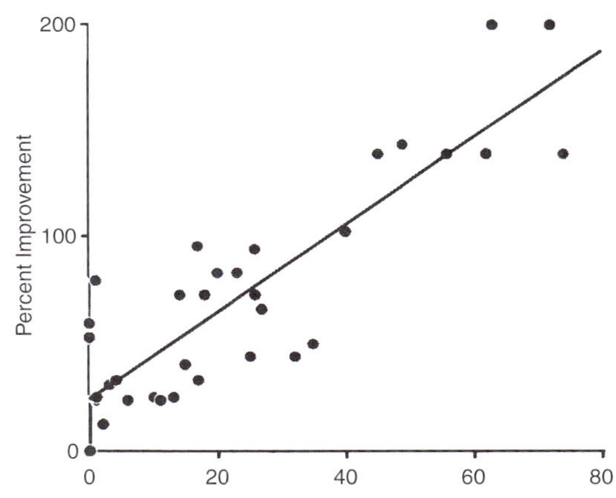

Fig. 7. Scatter plot showing the relation between the anatomic extent of blood flow–metabolism PET mismatch pattern, expressed as percent of the left ventricle, and the change in functional status after coronary artery bypass grafting, expressed as percent improvement in heart failure symptoms from baseline. The greatest improvement in heart failure symptoms occurs in patients with the largest PET mismatch defects. (*Adapted from* Di Carli MF, Asgarzadie F, Schelbert HR, et al. Quantitative relation between myocardial viability and improvement in heart failure symptoms after revascularization in patients with ischemic cardiomyopathy. Circulation. 1995;92(12):3436–44; with permission.)

Improvement in symptoms

Several studies suggested that the amount of viable myocardium that is assessed before revascularization correlates to improvements in functional capacity or symptoms [63–65]. Among patients who underwent PET viability imaging before revascularization, and exercise treadmill testing before and after revascularization, exercise capacity after revascularization improved to a greater extent in patients who had multiple areas of FDG PET viability compared with in patients who had less viable myocardium [76]. In a second study, among patients who had ischemic cardiomyopathy and underwent surgical revascularization, there was a linear relationship between the anatomic extent of perfusion/metabolism PET mismatch pattern and the change in functional status after revascularization [77]. The greatest improvement in heart failure symptoms occurred in patients who had the largest mismatch defects on PET images (Fig. 7). A more recent study showed a significant reduction in hospital admissions for congestive heart failure in patients who had large areas of viable myocardium on PET who underwent revascularization compared with those who were treated with medical therapy alone [78]. These data suggest a strong relationship between the amount of viable myocardium assessed before revascularization and improvement in symptoms and functional capacity after revascularization. None of these studies, however, directly evaluated a viability-driven approach versus a clinically-driven approach for the selection of patients for revascularization.

Prognosis

Several studies suggested that viability assessment may be useful in identifying patients who have ischemic cardiomyopathy who will derive the most prognostic benefit from revascularization, while sparing patients who will not benefit from high-risk procedures. The importance of perfusion-metabolism mismatch on PET imaging was demonstrated in several studies comprising over 400 total patients and an average follow-up of at least 1 year [66–70,78–80]. The findings consistently showed that in the presence of significant myocardial viability, patients who undergo revascularization have a much more favorable prognosis than do those who are treated medically. In contrast, in the absence of significant myocardial viability, the prognosis in patients who are managed medically is comparable to those who undergo revascularization. Similar findings were reported with thallium imaging [64,70,81]. A similar accuracy for predicting outcomes was shown in one study with sestamibi [82]. These studies are limited, however, in that they are nonrandomized, have small numbers of patients, and were not designed to evaluate specifically a viability-driven approach to patient selection for revascularization. One retrospective study among patients who underwent surgical revascularization demonstrated a higher 1-year survival in the group of patients in which PET was part of their preoperative assessment, compared with

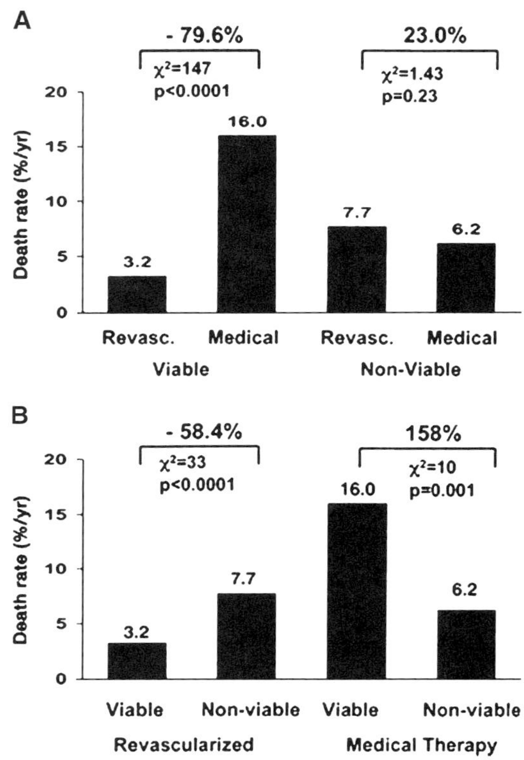

Fig. 8. Prognostic implications of myocardial viability testing derived from meta-analysis of 3088 patients who had coronary artery disease and left ventricular dysfunction and who underwent viability testing. Death rates for patients with and without myocardial viability treated by revascularization or medical therapy are shown in (*A*) and (*B*). In patients with viable myocardium, there is 79.6% reduction in mortality among those who were treated with revascularization ($P < .0001$). In contrast, among patients without evidence of viable myocardium, there was no significant difference in mortality with revascularization versus medical therapy. Revasc., revascularization. (*Adapted from* Allman KC, Shaw LJ, Hachamovitch R, et al. Myocardial viability testing and impact of revascularization on prognosis in patients with coronary artery disease and left ventricular dysfunction: a meta-analysis. J Am Coll Cardiol 2002;39(7): 1151–8; with permission.)

the group that did not have PET (97% versus 79% survival, respectively) [83]. This study could not determine how clinicians used the PET data preoperatively, but it does suggest that the evaluation of myocardial viability before revascularization may be beneficial.

A recent pooled-analysis of 24 studies using thallium or FDG scintigraphy, and dobutamine echocardiography summarized the published data in 3088 patients who had viability testing [84]. Revascularization was associated with an 80% reduction in annual mortality compared with medical therapy in patients who had preserved myocardial viability (3% versus 16% annual mortality, revascularization versus medical therapy, $P<.05$). In contrast, patients who had predominantly nonviable myocardium had similar annual mortality rates whether they were revascularized or were treated medically (7.7% versus 6.2%, respectively, P=NS) (Fig. 8). A randomized, controlled trial, the Surgical Treatment for Ischemic Heart Failure trial, is underway to help determine further the role for viability testing in patients who have ischemic cardiomyopathy.

Viability assessment in candidates for cardiac transplantation

In selected patients who have advanced ischemic cardiomyopathy, the decision to refer for cardiac transplantation may be difficult, based on target vessel anatomy and severity of left ventricular dysfunction. Several studies suggest that assessment of viability with PET may identify a subset of patients—perhaps up to 25%—that has extensive viability and may be referred for higher risk revascularization with acceptable outcome [85,86]. Additional studies are needed to confirm these preliminary findings.

Selection of patients who have heart failure for viability assessment

Over the past several decades, a large number of studies demonstrated that myocardial viability may be assessed accurately using a variety of radionuclide-based techniques. These include SPECT imaging with ^{201}Tl- or ^{99m}Tc-labeled perfusion tracers, as well as glucose use with FDG PET. Using these techniques, it is possible to predict which patients are likely to have improvement in left ventricular function after revascularization, as well as improvement in heart failure symptoms and patient outcome. In patients who have heart failure and active angina, the American College of Cardiology/American Heart Association guidelines suggest referring these patients directly for angiography, because they will benefit from revascularization, in terms of natural history [87]. Conversely, in patients who have known coronary artery disease and left dysfunction without angina, the American College of Cardiology/American Heart Association/American Society of Nuclear Cardiology guidelines consider radionuclide assessment of myocardial viability as a class I indication for consideration of revascularization [37].

References

[1] Heyndrickx GR, Baig H, Nelkins P, et al. Depression of regional blood flow and wall thickening after brief coronary occlusions. Am J Physiol 1978;234:H653–9.

[2] Rahimtoola SH. A perspective on the three large multicenter randomized clinical trials of coronary bypass surgery for chronic stable angina. Circulation 1985;72(Suppl V):V123–35.

[3] Braunwald E, Rutherford JD. Reversible ischemic left ventricular dysfunction: evidence for the "hibernating myocardium." J Am Coll Cardiol 1986;8:1467–70.

[4] Matsuzaki M, Gallagher KP, Kemper WS, et al. Sustained regional dysfunction, produced by prolonged coronary stenosis: gradual recovery after reperfusion. Circulation 1983;68:170–82.

[5] Cleland JG, Pennell DJ, Ray SG, et al. Carvedilol hm: myocardial viability as a determinant of the ejection fraction response to carvedilol in patients with heart failure (CHRISTMAS trial): randomised controlled trial. Lancet 2003;362:14–21.

[6] Murray CE, Jennings RB, Reimer KA. Preconditioning with ischemia: a delay of lethal cell injury in ischemic myocardium. Circulation 1986;74:1124–36.

[7] Taegtmeyer H. Modulation of responses to myocardial ischemia: metabolic features of myocardial stunning, hibernation, and ischemic preconditioning. In: Dilsizian V, editor. Myocardial viability: a clinical and scientific treatise. Armonk (NY): Futura Publishing Company, Inc.; 2000. p. 25–36.

[8] Pohost GM, Zir LM, Moore RH, et al. Differentiation of transiently ischemic from infarcted myocardium by serial imaging after a single dose of thallium-201. Circulation 1977;55:294–302.

[9] Leppo JA, Macneil PB, Moring AF, et al. Separate effects of ischemia, hypoxia, and contractility on thallium-201 kinetics in rabbit myocardium. J Nucl Med 1986;27:66–74.

[10] Leppo JA. Myocardial uptake of thallium and rubidium during alterations in perfusion and oxygenation in isolated rabbit hearts. J Nucl Med 1987;28:878–85.

[11] Dilsizian V, Rocco TP, Freedman NM, et al. Enhanced detection of ischemic but viable myocardium by the reinjection of thallium after stress-redistribution imaging. N Engl J Med 1990;323:141–6.

[12] Ragosta M, Beller GA, Watson DD, et al. Quantitative planar rest-redistribution ^{201}Tl imaging in detection of myocardial viability and prediction of improvement in left ventricular function after coronary artery bypass surgery in patients with severely depressed left ventricular function. Circulation 1993;87:1630–41.

[13] Dellegrottaglie S, Perrone-Filardi P, Pace L, et al. Prediction of long-term effects of revascularization on regional and global left ventricular function by dobutamine echocardiography and rest Tl-201 imaging alone and in combination in patients with chronic coronary artery disease. J Nucl Cardiol 2002;9(2):174–82.

[14] Bax JJ, Maddahi J, Poldermans D, et al. Sequential (201)Tl imaging and dobutamine echocardiography to enhance accuracy of predicting improved left ventricular ejection fraction after revascularization. J Nucl Med 2002;43(6):795–802.

[15] Tadamura E, Mamede M, Kubo S, et al. The effect of nitroglycerin on myocardial blood flow in various segments characterized by rest-redistribution thallium SPECT. J Nucl Med 2003;44(5):745–51.

[16] Kiat H, Maddahi J, Roy LT, et al. Comparison of technetium-99m methoxy isobutyl isonitrile and thallium 201 for evaluation of coronary artery disease by planar and tomographic methods. Am Heart J 1989; 117:1–11.

[17] Kahn JK, McGhie I, Akers MS, et al. Quantitative rotational tomography with T1-201 and Tc-99m 2-methoxy-isobutyl-isonitrile: a direct comparison in normal individuals and patients with coronary artery disease. Circulation 1989;79:1282–93.

[18] Verani MS, Jeroudi MO, Mahmarian JJ, et al. Quantification of myocardial infarction during coronary occlusion and myocardial salvage after reperfusion using cardiac imaging with technetium-99m hexakis 2-methoxybutyl isonitrile. J Am Coll Cardiol 1988;12:1573–81.

[19] Gibbons RJ, Verani MS, Behrenbeck T, et al. Feasibility of tomographic technetium-99m-hexakis-2-methoxy-2-methylpropyl-isonitrile imaging for the assessment of myocardial area at risk and the effect of acute treatment in myocardial infarction. Circulation 1989;80:1277–86.

[20] Lodge MA, Braess H, Mahmood F, et al. Developments in nuclear cardiology: transition from single photon emission computed tomography to positron emission tomography-computed tomography. J Invasive Cardiol 2005;17(9):491–6.

[21] Kitsiou AN, Bacharach SL, Bartlett ML, et al. ^{13}N-ammonia myocardial blood flow and uptake: relation to functional outcome of asynergic regions after revascularization. J Am Coll Cardiol 1999;33:678–86.

[22] Iida H, Kanno I, Takahashi A, et al. Measurement of absolute myocardial blood flow with O-15 water and dynamic positron emission tomography. Circulation 1988;78:104–15.

[23] Yamamoto Y, de Silva R, Rhodes CG, et al. A new strategy for the assessment of viable myocardium and regional myocardial blood flow using 15O-water and dynamic positron emission tomography. Circulation 1992;86:167–78.

[24] Gould KL, Yoshida K, Hess MJ, et al. Myocardial metabolism of fluorodeoxyglucose compared to cell membrane integrity for the potassium analogue rubidium-82 for assessing infarct size in man by PET. J Nucl Med 1991;32:1–9.

[25] vom Dahl J, Muzik O, Wolfe ER, et al. Myocardial rubidium-82 tissue kinetics assessed by dynamic positron emission tomography as a marker of myocardial cell membrane integrity and viability. Circulation 1996;93:238–45.

[26] Gewirtz H, Fischman AJ, Abraham S, et al. Positron emission tomographic measurements of absolute regional myocardial blood flow permits identification of nonviable myocardium in patients with chronic myocardial infarction. J Am Coll Cardiol 1994;23: 851–9.

[27] Bennett SK, Smith MF, Gottlieb SS, et al. Effect of metoprolol on absolute myocardial blood flow in patients with heart failure secondary to ischemic or non-ischemic cardiomyopathy. Am J Cardiol 2002;89:1431–4.

[28] Phelps ME, Schelbert HR, Mazziotta JC. Positron computer tomography for studies of myocardial and cerebral function. Ann Intern Med 1983;98:339–59.

[29] Dilsizian V, Bateman TM, Bergmann SR, et al. Metabolic imaging with β-methyl-ρ-[^{123}I]-iodophenyl-pentadecanoic acid (BMIPP) identifies ischemic memory following demand ischemia. Circulation 2005;112(14): 2169–74.

[30] Gropler RJ, Geltman EM, Sampathkumaran K, et al. Functional recovery after coronary revascularization for chronic coronary artery disease is dependent on maintenance of oxidative metabolism. J Am Coll Cardiol 1992;20:569–77.

[31] Wolpers HG, Burchert W, van den Hoff J, et al. Assessment of myocardial viability by use of 11C-acetate and positron emission tomography. Threshold criteria of reversible dysfunction. Circulation 1997;95: 1417–24.

[32] Lee YHC, Kiesewetter DO, Lang L, et al. Synthesis of 4-[^{18}F]fluorobenzoyllisinopril: a radioligand for angiotensin converting enzyme (ACE) imaging with positron emission tomography. J Labelled Comp Radiopharm 2001;44:S268–70.

[33] Dilsizian V, Shirani J, Lee YHC, et al. Specific binding of [^{18}F] fluorobenzoyl-lisinopril to angiotensin converting enzyme in human heart tissue of ischemic cardiomyopathy. Circulation 2001;104:II-694.

[34] Dilsizian V, Loredo ML, Ferrans VJ, et al. Evidence for increased angiotensin II type I receptor immunoreactivity in peri-infarct myocardium of human explanted hearts. J Am Coll Cardiol 2002;39:365A.

[35] Shirani J, Loredo ML, Eckelman WC, et al. Imaging the renin angiotensin aldosterone system in the heart. Curr Heart Fail Rep 2005;2(2):78–86.

[36] McCrohon JA, Moon JC, Prasad SK, et al. Differentiation of heart failure related to dilated cardiomyopathy and coronary artery disease using gadolinium-enhanced cardiovascular magnetic resonance. Circulation 2003;108:54–9.

[37] Klocke FJ, Baird MG, Bateman TM, et al. ACC/AHA/ASNC guidelines for the clinical use of cardiac radionuclide imaging: a report of the American College of Cardiology/American Heart Association Task Force on Practice Guidelines. Circulation 2003;108(11):1404–18.

[38] Kiat H, Berman DS, Maddahi J, et al. Late reversibility of tomographic myocardial thallium-201 defects: an accurate marker of myocardial viability. J Am Coll Cardiol 1988;12:1456–63.

[39] Kayden DS, Sigal S, Soufer R, et al. Thallium-201 for assessment of myocardial viability: quantitative comparison of 24-hour redistribution imaging with imaging after reinjection at rest. J Am Coll Cardiol 1991;18:1480–6.

[40] Bonow RO, Dilsizian V, Cuocolo A, et al. Identification of viable myocardium in patients with chronic coronary artery disease and left ventricular dysfunction. Comparison of thallium scintigraphy with reinjection and PET imaging with F-18 fluorodeoxyglucose. Circulation 1991;83:26–37.

[41] Srinivasan G, Kitsiou AN, Bacharach SL, et al. ^{18}F-fluorodeoxyglucose single photon emission computed tomography: can it replace PET and thallium SPECT for the assessment of myocardial viability? Circulation 1998;97:843–50.

[42] Dilsizian V, Bacharach SL, Maung KM, et al. Fluorine-18-deoxyglucose SPECT and coincidence imaging for myocardial viability: clinical and technological issues. J Nucl Cardiol 2001;8:75–88.

[43] Shirani J, Lee J, Quigg RJ, et al. Relation of thallium uptake to morphologic features of chronic ischemic heart disease: evidence for myocardial remodeling in non-infarct myocardium. J Am Coll Cardiol 2001;38:84–90.

[44] Kitsiou AN, Srinivasan G, Quyyumi AA, et al. Stress-induced reversible and mild-to-moderate irreversible thallium defects: are they equally accurate for predicting recovery of regional left ventricular function after revascularization? Circulation 1998;98:501–8.

[45] Dilsizian V, Arrighi JA, Diodati JG, et al. Myocardial viability in patients with chronic coronary artery disease: comparison of ^{99m}Tc-sestamibi with thallium reinjection and ^{18}F-fluorodeoxyglucose. Circulation 1994;89:578–87.

[46] Dilsizian V. Technetium-99m labeled myocardial perfusion tracers: blood flow or viability agents? In: Dilsizian V, editor. Myocardial viability: a clinical and scientific treatise. Armonk (NY): Futura Publishing Company, Inc.; 2000. p. 315–48.

[47] Udelson JE, Coleman PS, Metherall JA, et al. Predicting recovery of severe regional ventricular dysfunction: comparison of resting scintigraphy with ^{201}Tl and ^{99m}Tc-sestamibi. Circulation 1994;89:2552–61.

[48] Galli M, Marcassa C, Imparato A, et al. Effects of nitroglycerin by technetium-99m sestamibi tomoscintigraphy on resting regional myocardial hypoperfusion in stable patients with healed myocardial infarction. Am J Cardiol 1994;74:843–8.

[49] Bisi G, Sciagra R, Santoro GM, et al. Sublingual isosorbide dinitrate to improve technetium-99m-teboroxime perfusion defect reversibility. J Nucl Med 1994;35:1274–8.

[50] Senior R, Kaul S, Raval U, et al. Impact of revascularization and myocardial viability determined by nitrate-enhanced Tc-99m sestamibi and Tl-201 imaging on mortality and functional outcome in ischemic cardiomyopathy. J Nucl Cardiol 2002;9(5):454–62.

[51] Sciagra R, Leoncini M, Marcucci G, et al. Technetium-99m sestamibi imaging to predict left ventricular ejection fraction outcome after revascularisation in patients with chronic coronary artery disease and left ventricular dysfunction: comparison between baseline and nitrate-enhanced imaging. Eur J Nucl Med 2001;28(6):680–7.

[52] Giorgetti A, Marzullo P, Sambuceti G, et al. Baseline/post-nitrate Tc-99m tetrofosmin mismatch for the assessment of myocardial viability in patients with severe left ventricular dysfunction: comparison with baseline Tc-99m tetrofosmin scintigraphy/FDG PET imaging. J Nucl Cardiol 2004;11(2):142–51.

[53] Acampa W, Cuocolo A, Petretta M, et al. Tetrofosmin imaging in the detection of myocardial viability in patients with previous myocardial infarction: comparison with sestamibi and Tl-201 scintigraphy. J Nucl Cardiol 2002;9(1):33–40.

[54] Giorgetti A, Pingitore A, Favilli B, et al. Baseline/postnitrate tetrofosmin SPECT for myocardial viability assessment in patients with postischemic severe left ventricular dysfunction: new evidence from MRI. J Nucl Med 2005;46(8):1285–93.

[55] Levine MG, McGill CC, Ahlberg AW, et al. Functional assessment with electrocardiographic gated single-photon emission computed tomography improves the ability of technetium-99m sestamibi myocardial perfusion imaging to predict myocardial viability in patients undergoing revascularization. Am J Cardiol 1999;83:1–5.

[56] Leoncini M, Sciagra R, Bellandi F, et al. Low-dose dobutamine nitrate-enhanced technetium 99m sestamibi gated SPECT versus low-dose dobutamine echocardiography for detecting reversible dysfunction in ischemic cardiomyopathy. J Nucl Cardiol 2002;9(4):402–6.

[57] Slart RH, Bax JJ, Sluiter WJ, et al. Added value of attenuation-corrected Tc-99m tetrofosmin SPECT for the detection of myocardial viability: comparison with FDG SPECT. J Nucl Cardiol 2004;11(6):689–96.

[58] DiCarli MF, Prceevski P, Singh TP, et al. Myocardial blood flow, function, and metabolism in repetitive stunning. J Nucl Med 2000;41:1227–34.

[59] Dilsizian V, Narula J. Nuclear investigation in heart failure and myocardial viability. In: Dilsizian V, Narula

J, editors. Atlas of nuclear cardiology. 2nd edition. Philadelphia: Current Medicine, Inc.; 2006. p. 211–36.

[60] Tillisch JH, Brunken R, Marshall R, et al. Reversibility of cardiac wall-motion abnormalities predicted by positron tomography. N Engl J Med 1986;314:884–8.

[61] Tamaki N, Yonekura Y, Yamashita K, et al. Positron emission tomography using fluorine-18 deoxyglucose in evaluation of coronary artery bypass grafting. Am J Cardiol 1989;64:860–5.

[62] Gerber BL, Ordoubadi FF, Wijns W, et al. Positron emission tomography using(18)F-fluoro-deoxyglucose and euglycaemic hyperinsulinaemic glucose clamp: optimal criteria for the prediction of recovery of post-ischaemic left ventricular dysfunction. Results from the European Community Concerted Action Multicenter study on use of(18)F-fluoro-deoxyglucose Positron Emission Tomography for the Detection of Myocardial Viability. Eur Heart J 2001;22(18): 1691–701.

[63] Schwaiger M, Brunken R, Grover-McKay M, et al. Regional myocardial metabolism in patients with acute myocardial infarction assessed by positron emission tomography. J Am Coll Cardiol 1986;8:800–8.

[64] Kuhl HP, Beek AM, van der Weerdt AP, et al. Myocardial viability in chronic ischemic heart disease: comparison of contrast-enhanced magnetic resonance imaging with (18)F-fluorodeoxyglucose positron emission tomography. J Am Coll Cardiol 2003;41: 1341–8.

[65] Knuesel PR, Nanz D, Wyss C, et al. Characterization of dysfunctional myocardium by positron emission tomography and magnetic resonance: relation to functional outcome after revascularization. Circulation 2003;108:1095–100.

[66] DiCarli MF, Davidson M, Little R, et al. Value of metabolic imaging with positron emission tomography for evaluation prognosis in patients with coronary artery disease and left ventricular dysfunction. Am J Cardiol 1994;73:527–33.

[67] Eitzman D, Al-Aouar Z, Kanter HL, et al. Clinical outcome of patients with advanced coronary artery disease after viability studies with positron emission tomography. J Am Coll Cardiol 1992;20:559–65.

[68] Lee KS, Marwick TH, Cook SA, et al. Prognosis of patients with left ventricular dysfunction, with and without viable myocardium after myocardial infarction: relative efficacy of medical therapy and revascularization. Circulation 1994;90:2687–94.

[69] Gioia G, Powers J, Heo J, et al. Prognostic value of rest-redistribution tomographic thallium-201 imaging in ischemic cardiomyopathy. Am J Cardiol 1995;75: 759–62.

[70] Gioia G, Milan E, Giubbini R, et al. Prognostic value of tomographic rest-redistribution thallium 201 imaging in medically treated patients with coronary artery disease and left ventricular dysfunction. J Nucl Cardiol 1996;3(2):150–6.

[71] Samady H, Elefteriades JA, Abbott BG, et al. Failure to improve left ventricular function after coronary revascularization for ischemic cardiomyopathy is not associated with worse outcome. Circulation 1999; 100(12):1298–304.

[72] Haas F, Augustin N, Holper K, et al. Time course and extent of improvement of dysfunctioning myocardium in patients with coronary artery disease and severely depressed left ventricular function after revascularization: correlation with positron emission tomographic findings. J Am Coll Cardiol 2000;36(6):1927–34.

[73] Santana CA, Shaw LJ, Garcia EV, et al. Incremental prognostic value of left ventricular function by myocardial ECG-gated FDG PET imaging in patients with ischemic cardiomyopathy. J Nucl Cardiol 2004;11(5): 542–50.

[74] Sawada S, Hamoui O, Barclay J, et al. Usefulness of positron emission tomography in predicting long-term outcome in patients with diabetes mellitus and ischemic left ventricular dysfunction. Am J Cardiol 2005; 96(1):2–8.

[75] Beanlands RS, Ruddy TD, deKemp RA, et al. Positron emission tomography and recovery following revascularization (PARR-1): the importance of scar and the development of a prediction rule for the degree of recovery of left ventricular function. J Am Coll Cardiol 2002;40(10):1735–43.

[76] Marwick TH, Nemec JJ, Lafont A, et al. Prediction by postexercise fluoro-18 deoxyglucose positron emission tomography of improvement in exercise capacity after revascularization. Am J Cardiol 1992;69(9):854–9.

[77] Di Carli MF, Asgarzadie F, Schelbert HR, et al. Quantitative relation between myocardial viability and improvement in heart failure symptoms after revascularization in patients with ischemic cardiomyopathy. Circulation 1995;92(12):3436–44.

[78] Rohatgi R, Epstein S, Henriquez J, et al. Utility of positron emission tomography in predicting cardiac events and survival in patients with coronary artery disease and severe left ventricular dysfunction. Am J Cardiol 2001;87(9):1096–9.

[79] Di Carli MF, Maddahi J, Rokhsar S, et al. Long-term survival of patients with chronic coronary artery disease and left ventricular dysfunction: implications for the role of myocardial viability assessment in management decisions. J Thorac Cardiovasc Surg 1998;116: 997–1004.

[80] Desideri A, Cortigiani L, Christen AI, et al. The extent of perfusion-F18-fluorodeoxyglucose positron emission tomography mismatch determines mortality in medically treated patients with chronic ischemic left ventricular dysfunction. J Am Coll Cardiol 2005;46(7): 1264–9.

[81] Pagley PR, Beller GA, Watson DD, et al. Improved outcome after coronary bypass surgery in patients with ischemic cardiomyopathy and residual myocardial viability. Circulation 1997;96(3):793–800.

[82] Siebelink HM, Blanksma PK, Crijns HJ, et al. No difference in cardiac event-free survival between positron emission tomography-guided and single-photon emission computed tomography-guided patient man-

agement: a prospective, randomized comparison of patients with suspicion of jeopardized myocardium. J Am Coll Cardiol 2001;37(1):81–8.

[83] Haas F, Haehnel CJ, Picker W, et al. Preoperative positron emission tomographic viability assessment and perioperative and postoperative risk in patients with advanced ischemic heart disease. J Am Coll Cardiol 1997;30:1693–700.

[84] Allman KC, Shaw LJ, Hachamovitch R, et al. Myocardial viability testing and impact of revascularization on prognosis in patients with coronary artery disease and left ventricular dysfunction: a meta-analysis. J Am Coll Cardiol 2002;39(7):1151–8.

[85] Akinboboye OO, Idris O, Cannon PJ, et al. Usefulness of positron emission tomography in defining myocardial viability in patients referred for cardiac transplantation. Am J Cardiol 1999;83:1271–4.

[86] Auerbach MA, Schoder H, Hoh C, et al. Prevalence of myocardial viability as detected by positron emission tomography in patients with ischemic cardiomyopathy. Circulation 1999;99:2921–6.

[87] Hunt SA, Baker DW, Chin MH. ACC/AHA guidelines for the evaluation and management of chronic heart failure in the adult: executive summary. J Am Coll Cardiol 2001;38:2101–13.

ELSEVIER
SAUNDERS

Heart Failure Clin 2 (2006) 145 – 161

HEART
FAILURE
CLINICS

Cardiovascular Magnetic Resonance Assessment of Ischemic and Nonischemic Cardiomyopathies

Aidan R. Raney, BA, David Bello*,[1]

University of California, Irvine, CA, USA

Cardiomyopathies are defined as diseases of the myocardium associated with cardiac dysfunction. Patients who have cardiomyopathy are classified into ischemic cardiomyopathy (ICM) or nonischemic cardiomyopathy (NICM) categories based on the presence or absence, respectively, of coronary artery disease (CAD). The World Health Organization/International Society and Federation of Cardiology (WHO/ISFC) task force classifies NICM as dilated cardiomyopathy, hypertrophic cardiomyopathy (HCM) (obstructive and nonobstructive), restrictive cardiomyopathy (RCM), and arrhythmogenic right ventricular cardiomyopathy (ARVC) [1]. The "unclassified" cardiomyopathies do not readily fit into any single group, and "specific" cardiomyopathies are associated with specific cardiac or systemic disorders. (eg, hypertensive cardiomyopathy) (Table 1). Patients who have cardiomyopathy and associated heart failure symptoms represent an important epidemiologic problem. Approximately 5 million patients in the United States have heart failure, and over 550,000 patients are diagnosed with heart failure for the first time each year [2]. From 1990 to 1999, the annual number of hospitalizations increased from 810,000 to over 1 million for heart failure as the primary diagnosis and from 2.4 to 3.6 million for heart failure as a primary or secondary diagnosis [3].

There are multiple diagnostic techniques that offer insight into heart failure, and current American College of Cardiology/American Heart Association guidelines for the initial evaluation of heart failure include a patient history, laboratory evaluation, ECG, chest radiography, echocardiography, and coronary angiography. The guidelines state that endomyocardial biopsy is considered reasonable in undiagnosed patients who have certain echocardiographic findings and clinical presentation [4], although this method is invasive and inconclusive in a large number of cases because of the limitations of random sampling of the myocardium. Determining the exact cause is important because the cause is related directly to treatment and patient survival.

Cardiovascular magnetic resonance (CMR) imaging has recently emerged as a noninvasive imaging modality that is capable of providing high-resolution images of the heart. Two important CMR imaging techniques, cine-CMR and delayed contrast enhancement after the administration of gadolinium (DE-CMR), are very valuable in the evaluation of cardiomyopathy. Cine-CMR can be used for the noninvasive evaluation of cardiac function and morphology, and DE-CMR can be used for tissue characterization. These modalities are critical in differentiating ICM from NICM. The presence of gadolinium on T1-weighted images creates higher signal intensity, with areas of high gadolinium concentration appearing brighter; this is also known as "hyperenhancement." This article reviews the potential of CMR to distinguish between ICM and NICM, the

* Corresponding author. Department of Medicine, University of California, Route 81, Building 53, Room 100, Irvine, CA.

E-mail address: dbello@uci.edu (D. Bello).

[1] Present address: Orlando Regional Hospital, Orlando, FL 32806.

1551-7136/06/$ – see front matter
doi:10.1016/j.hfc.2006.01.001

Table 1
World Health Organization/International Society and Federation of Cardiology classification of nonischemic cardiomyopathies

Cardiomyopathy	Characteristics
Dilated	Dilatation and impaired contraction of the left ventricle or both ventricles, nonspecific histology. Arrhythmias, thromboembolism, and sudden death are common.
Hypertrophic	Left and/or right ventricular hypertrophy, which is usually asymmetric and involves the interventricular septum with left ventricular volume, is normal or reduced. Includes myocyte hypertrophy and disarray surrounding areas of increased loose connective tissue. Arrhythmias and premature sudden death are common.
Restrictive	Restrictive filling and reduced diastolic volume of either or both ventricles with normal or near-normal systolic function and wall thickness. Increased interstitial fibrosis may be present. It may be idiopathic or associated with other disease (eg, amyloidosis)
ARVC	Progressive fibrofatty replacement of right ventricular myocardium, initially with typical regional and later global right and some left ventricular involvement, with relative sparing of the septum. Presentation with arrhythmias and sudden death is common, particularly in the young.
Unclassified	Unclassified cardiomyopathies include a few cases that do not fit readily into any group. Some diseases may present with features of more than one type of cardiomyopathy.
Specific	The term specific cardiomyopathies is now used to describe heart muscle diseases that are associated with specific cardiac or systemic disorders (eg, hypertensive cardiomyopathy)

Adapted from Richardson P, McKenna W, Bristow M, et al. Report of the 1995 World Health Organization/International Society and Federation of Cardiology Task Force on the Definition and Classification of cardiomyopathies. Circulation 1996;93(5): 841–2.

differentiation of nonischemic causes, and the clinical implications of these findings.

Cardiac magnetic resonance imaging

CMR imaging is a noninvasive imaging modality capable of providing high-resolution images of the heart without radiation. A typical CMR examination consists of several cardiac sequences that are performed separately during an examination. A sequence refers to certain parameters that can be adjusted during the CMR examination, and each sequence is designed to elicit certain characteristics of cardiac anatomy and function. For example, adjusting certain parameters can create T1- and T2-weighted images. Cine-CMR and DE-CMR have been particularly useful in the evaluation of cardiomyopathy. Cine-CMR provides morphologic and functional characteristics through reconstruction of ECG-gated images. Cine-CMR has been shown to accurately measure ventricular mass and volume, with improved accuracy based on the ability to conduct three-dimensional measurements. Cine-CMR also is accurate in the assessment of cardiac function, including ejection fraction and end-systolic wall stress in abnormal ventricles [5,6]. It also has been shown to have excellent reproducibility in the assessment of global and segmental wall motion [7].

DE-CMR imaging using gadolinium is a key tool for defining the cause of specific cardiomyopathies. DE-CMR can accurately identify microscars that cannot be detected by other imaging techniques, in which the use of inversion recovery sequences increases the signal-to-noise ratio of infarct tissue by up to 500% [8]. The mechanism of myocardial hyperenhancement in the setting of infarction is based on the gadolinium volume of distribution [9]. Gadolinium chelates are extracellular contrast agents that are inert and cannot cross myocyte cell membranes. In normal myocardium, myocytes are densely packed, and thus myocyte intracellular space forms the majority (85%) of the volume. Therefore, the volume of distribution of gadolinium in normal myocardium is small. In the setting of acute infarction, there is myocyte membrane rupture, which allows additional gadolinium to diffuse into what was previously intracellular space. This diffusion in turn results in increased gadolinium concentration and the subsequent hyperenhancement of the damaged myocardium on DE-CMR. In the setting of chronic infarction, myocytes have been replaced with collagenous scar tissue. The interstitial space is expanded in scar tissue, which leads to increased gadolinium concentration and therefore hyperenhancement. DE-CMR can differentiate between ischemic and nonischemic cardiomyopathy based on the presence and pattern of hyperenhancement (Fig. 1). In addition to the ability to differentiate between ischemic and nonischemic cardiomyopathy by detecting the presence, location, and extent of myocardial infarction, DE-CMR has also been found to predict improvement

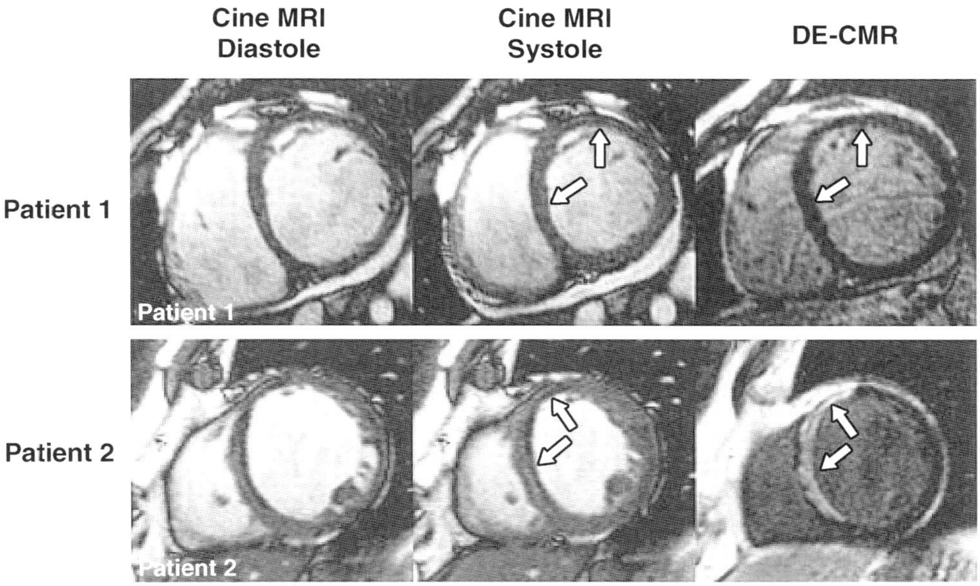

Fig. 1. Cine-MRI and DE-CMR show regional dysfunction (*arrows*) in a patient who has nonischemic cardiomyopathy (Patient 1) and a patient with ischemic cardiomyopathy (Patient 2). Patient 2 shows myocardial hyperenhancement consistent with MI. (*From* Bello D, Shah DJ, Farah GM, et al. Gadolinium cardiovascular magnetic resonance predicts reversible myocardial dysfunction and remodeling in patients with heart failure undergoing beta-blocker therapy. Circulation 2003; 108(16):1950; with permission.)

in contractile function after revascularization and medical therapy in both acute and chronic settings [10,11].

Ischemic cardiomyopathy

Definition of ischemic cardiomyopathy

ICM is determined by the presence of left ventricular systolic dysfunction and one or more of the following criteria: (1) a history of myocardial infarction (MI) diagnosed by ECG (Q waves) or enzyme criteria; (2) a history of revascularization through coronary artery bypass graft surgery, percutaneous transluminal coronary angioplasty (PTCA), or thrombolytic therapy; and (3) angiographic evidence of significant CAD, typically defined as the luminal narrowing greater than 50% of at least one major epicardial artery. Determining whether the cause of left ventricular dysfunction is ischemic or nonischemic has important clinical and therapeutic implications. For example, patients who have ischemic heart disease may benefit from revascularization [10]. Thus, in many centers, coronary angiography is performed routinely. In those patients who do not have significant CAD, NICM usually is diagnosed.

Ischemic cardiomyopathy pattern by cardiac magnetic resonance imaging

Nearly all patients who have ICM exhibit a typical "ischemic" pattern by DE-CMR (see Fig. 1). This pattern can be explained by the pathophysiology of ischemia. After coronary occlusion, a "wave front" of necrosis begins in the subendocardium and grows toward the epicardium over the next few hours. During this period, the region of ischemia remains the same size, but the infarcted region within the ischemic zone increases continuously toward a transmural infarction. Therefore, hyperenhancement that is classified as the "ischemic type" should always involve the subendocardium (ie, subendocardial or transmural) and be located in a region consistent with the perfusion territory of an epicardial coronary artery (Fig. 2) [12].

Detection of MI in patients who have ischemic cardiomyopathy by delayed enhancement cardiac magnetic resonance imaging

In the past decade, several investigators have assessed the usefulness of DE-CMR to differentiate ischemic from nonischemic cardiomyopathy. The studies have found that almost all patients who are

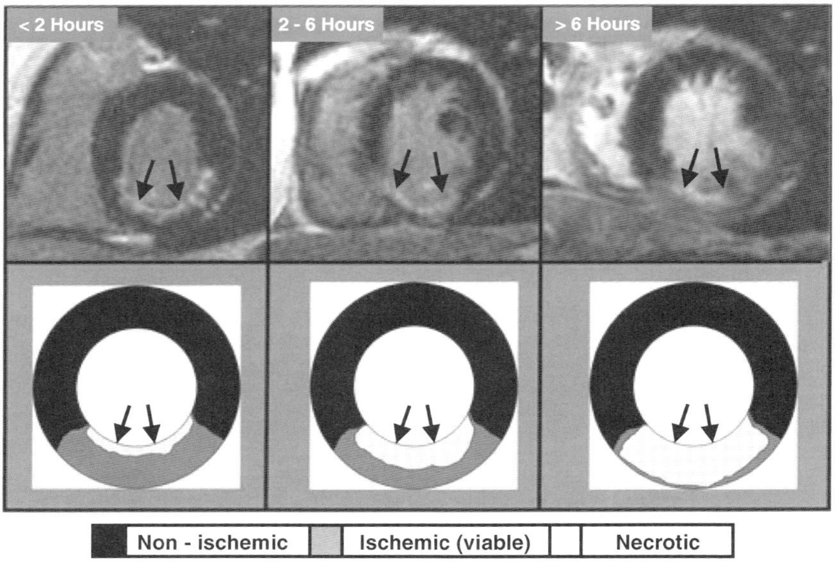

Fig. 2. The typical pattern of ischemic heart disease (*top row*) can be explained by the pathophysiology of ischemia (*bottom row*). Little or no cellular necrosis is found until approximately 15 minutes after occlusion. After 15 minutes, a "wavefront" of necrosis begins subendocardially and grows toward the epicardium over the next few hours. During this period, the infarcted region within the ischemic zone increases continuously toward a transmural infarction. (*From* McCrohon JA, Moon JC, Prasad SK, et al. Differentiation of heart failure related to dilated cardiomyopathy and coronary artery disease using gadolinium-enhanced cardiovascular magnetic resonance. Circulation 2003;108(1):1464; with permission.)

diagnosed with ischemic cardiomyopathy have CMR imaging evidence of myocardial infarction (Table 2) [11,13–16]. In patients diagnosed as having non-ischemic cardiomyopathy (based on negative angiographic findings), up to 13% of patients had an ischemic pattern of hyperenhancement. These findings are consistent with previous pathology studies. Schuster and Bulkley [17] have demonstrated that virtually all patients who have congestive heart failure and significant CAD have gross myocardial scarring at autopsy, even in those without a clinical history of myocardial infarction, angina, or Q waves. The presence of significant CAD in the absence of infarction has also been previously documented [18]

Table 2
Detection of myocardial infarction by cardiovascular magnetic resonance in patients with ischemic and nonischemic cardiomyopathies

		DCM		
First author, year [Ref.]	Ischemic CM	With ischemic pattern	With midwall fibrosis	With no enhancement
Wu, 2001 [15][a]	19/19 = 100%	0/20 = 0%	0/20 = 0%	20/20 = 100%
Bello, 2003 [11][b]	28/28 = 100%	2/17 = 12%	N/A[c]	N/A[c]
Soriano, 2005 [14][d]	21/26 = 81%	4/45 = 9%	4/45 = 9%	37/45 = 82%
McCrohon, 2003 [13]	27/27 = 100%	8/63 = 13%	18/63 = 28%	37/63 = 59%
Bello, 2005 [16]	95/100 = 95%	3/27 = 11%	2/27 = 7%	22/27 = 81%
Total	**190/200 = 95%**	**17/172 = 10%**	**24/155 = 15%**	**116/155 = 75%**

[a] Follow-up at 14 months; 29/32 had hyperenhancement at 3 mo.

[b] A diagnosis of NICM was given to patients with no angiographic evidence of >70% occlusion and assumed to be idiopathic dilated cardiomyopathy. HCM and other cardiomyopathies were not included in this group.

[c] 12% of those without angioraphic evidence had hyperenhancement; the description of midwall or subendocardial was not provided.

[d] Patients were without clinical suspicion of CAD; note that 4/26 (11%) patients who had CAD also had midwall enhancement.

and may be caused by chronic ischemia with appropriate collateralization. In summary, the main finding in patients who have ICM shown by CMR is that nearly all patients have an ischemic (ie, subendocardial or transmural) pattern of hyperenhancement consistent with previous myocardial infarction.

Ischemic cardiomyopathy out of proportion to the extent of coronary artery disease

Another group of patients has cardiomyopathy out of proportion to the extent of CAD. Kaushal and colleagues [16] have shown that 10 of 12 (83%) patients who met criteria for ICM and had left ventricular (LV) dysfunction to a degree that was out of proportion to the extent of CAD showed hyperenhancement characteristic of infarct. None had a history of revascularization or previous myocardial infarction; all had single-vessel coronary artery disease, based on angiography. Myocardial infarction by CMR with scarring in the angiographic territory showing luminal stenosis was seen in all patients. Although these coronary lesions are seen as clinically insignificant and do not undergo revascularization, this finding suggests that the likely mechanism of injury resulting in myocardial infarction in such patients may be from a flow-limiting lesion or lysed thrombus in the area of stenosis. Previous studies have reported recanalization after thrombosis and embolization from minimally stenotic but unstable plaque [19,20]. Thus, for patients who have ischemic cardiomyopathy out of proportion to the extent of CAD, revascularization may be warranted, assuming that there is sufficient viable myocardium.

Nonischemic cardiomyopathy

NICMs are chronic, progressive myocardial diseases with distinct patterns of morphologic, functional, and electrophysiologic changes. The WHO/ISFC task force has classified cardiomyopathies in separate categories that include DCM, HCM (with and without obstruction), RCM, and ARVC [1].

Dilated cardiomyopathy

World Health Organization/International Society and Federation of Cardiology definition

Dilated cardiomyopathy is characterized by dilatation and impaired contraction of the left ventricle or both ventricles. It may be idiopathic, genetic, viral, toxic, or associated with recognized cardiovascular disease in which the degree of myocardial dysfunction is not explained by the abnormal loading conditions or the extent of ischemic damage. Presentation is usually with heart failure, which is often progressive. Arrhythmias, thromboembolism, and sudden death are common and may occur at any stage [1].

Cardiovascular magnetic resonance imaging findings

Cine-MR imaging shows progressive dilation in the right or left ventricle and associated impairment in systolic function. These changes can also occur in ICM, and thus DE-CMR allows for the differentiation of these two main causes of heart failure. DE-CMR findings in patients who are diagnosed with idiopathic dilated cardiomyopathies by clinical criteria are varied and include three main patterns: no hyperenhancement, hyperenhancement with an ischemic pattern (previously described in the section "Ischemic cardiomyopathy"), and midwall hyperenhancement (nonischemic pattern). The majority of patients exhibit no enhancement (see Table 2). Hyperenhancement with an ischemic pattern has been seen in 12% of patients who have a clinical diagnosis of DCM [11]. These findings are consistent with previous autopsy studies, which have shown visible scars in 14% [21] and 12% [18], respectively, of patients who have idiopathic DCM. The mechanisms for myocardial scarring in patients who have nonischemic cardiomyopathy include coronary vasospasm, thrombosis with spontaneous lysis superimposed on minimal atherosclerosis, or coronary emboli. Whether patients who have cardiomyopathy and no angiographic evidence of CAD but with CMR evidence of ischemic pattern should be classified as ICM is subject to debate.

McCrohon and colleagues [13] performed DE-CMR in 27 patients who had idiopathic DCM (n=63) on the basis of coronary angiography and found that 28% had patchy or linear striae of hyperenhancement limited to the mid-myocardium of the ventricular wall (nonischemic pattern) (Fig. 3). These findings are consistent with previous CMR studies that have described similar findings in patients who have dilated cardiomyopathy [14]. Diffuse interstitial fibrosis is common in DCM but does not produce hyperenhancement because the DE-CMR technique works only on focal change [22], and global enhancement is "nulled" by the technique. In light of negative findings for the majority of patients who have DCM, the most significant contribution of DE-CMR may be the absence or presence of infarct

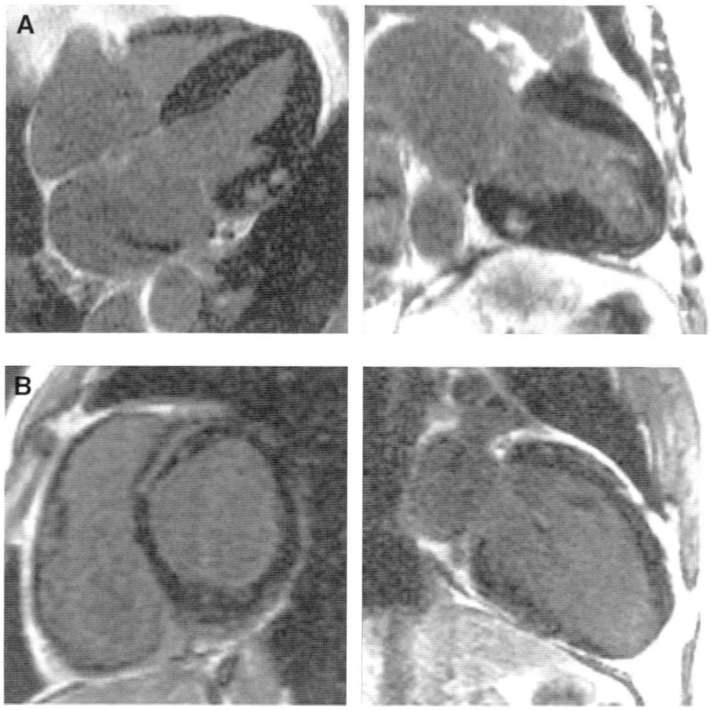

Fig. 3. (*A*) DE-CMR shows patchy foci of midwall enhancement. Patchy gadolinium enhancement involved basal to mid-LV regions. (*B*) DE-CMR shows midwall striae of enhancement. Gadolinium enhancement followed ventricular longitudinal muscle fibers, particularly involving the septum and basal to mid-LV regions. Pattern is clearly different from patients with heart failure related to CAD. (*Adapted from* McCrohon JA, Moon JC, Prasad SK, et al. Differentiation of heart failure related to dilated cardiomyopathy and coronary artery disease using gadolinium-enhanced cardiovascular magnetic resonance. Circulation 2003; 108(1):56–7; with permission.)

and the ensuing influence on treatment and prognosis. These data may have significant clinical implications. For instance, ventricular arrhythmias may be more common in patients who have had a previous myocardial infarction, even in the absence of epicardial coronary artery disease, as the area of MI may serve as an arrhythmogenic substrate.

In summary, the main finding in patients who have idiopathic dilated cardiomyopathy is that the majority of patients have no hyperenhancement, up to 20% have evidence of ischemic pattern of hyperenhancement, and up to 30% have evidence of midwall fibrosis or nonischemic pattern. Whether the presence of hyperenhancement in patients who have NICM has significant prognostic value requires further investigation.

Other nonischemic cardiomyopathy

The studies by Wu and colleagues [15] Bello and colleagues [11,16], Soriano and colleagues [14], and McCrohon and colleagues [13] involved only patients who had ICM or those with idiopathic DCM. Patients who had HCM, myocarditis, or infiltrative disorders were excluded. The following discussion demonstrates that hyperenhancement can occur in these other forms of NICM and describes how the pattern of hyperenhancement and other CMR findings can be used to differentiate between the various causes. A summary of morphologic, functional, and DE-CMR characteristics in patients who have other NICM can be seen in Table 3.

Hypertrophic cardiomyopathy

HCM is characterized by left or right ventricular hypertrophy, which is usually asymmetric and involves the interventricular septum. CMR has been shown to be superior to echocardiography for the quantification of hypertrophied LV mass [23,24], especially in cases of anterior septal thickness of

Table 3
Summary of functional, morphologic, and delayed enhancement characteristics of the cardiomyopathies

Type of CM	Delayed enhancement characteristics	Functional and morphologic characteristics
ARVC	Enhancement in antero-basal region and right ventricular outflow tract; septum typically spared	Fatty deposition shows increased signal on T1-weighted images Thinning and dilation of the right ventricle and outflow tract, aneurysms, and regional wall motion abnormalities
Hypertrophic	Enhancement of septum at RV/LV junction (81%)[a]	LV outflow track obstruction SAM Septal hypertrophy Apical hypertrophy
Myocarditis	Nodular or diffuse epicardial enhancement of lateral free wall or midwall Enhancement may disappear over time	Wall motion abnormalities may be present
Amyloidosis	Global and subendocardial enhancement	Increased interatrial septum and LA or RA wall thickness Pleural and periardial effusions Diastolic dysfunction and depressed contractility
Hemochromatosis	Not typically evaluated on DE	T2 loss of signal in affected regions due to presence of iron[b] Diastolic dysfunction, wall thickening, and ventricular dilatation
AFD	Enhancement in the basal inferolateral wall with sparing of the subendocardium (50%)[c]	Ventricular hypertrophy similar to HCM
Sarcoidosis	Patchy diffuse enhancement Enhancement in basal septum	Increased T2 signal shows inflammation in basal septum Restrictive-type diastolic dysfunction on cine-MRI

The presence of myocardial enhancement in patients with NICM is typically seen in regions not associated with coronary distribution.

[a] 12% of those without angioraphic evidence had hyperenhancement; the description of midwall or subendocardial was not provided.

[b] Patients with ICM or those with idiopathic DCM were excluded (see Table 2).

[c] Patients were without clinical suspicion of CAD; note that 4/26 (11%) patients who had CAD also had midwall enhancement.

greater than 3 mm [25]. MRI is also superior in evaluating apical HCM, which can be difficult to discern by echocardiography [26–28].

HCM can lead to functional impairment of the left ventricular outflow tract (LVOT), and the degree of obstruction in the LVOT can be measured by cine-MRI (Fig. 4). Systolic signal void on cine-MRI [29] and velocity mapping can be used to show increased velocity in the LVOT secondary to obstruction. HCM also causes functional changes in ventricular contraction, with altered regional myocardial function in association with the degree of hypertrophy [30,31]. Diastolic dysfunction secondary to LV asynchrony [32] and increased stiffness of the ventricle may be appreciated. Finally, cine-MRI can discern valvular pathology, including systolic anterior motion (SAM)of the mitral valve, which contributes to LVOT obstruction [29]. Mitral valve regurgitation also may be appreciated.

Typical morphologic changes in HCM include myocyte hypertrophy and disarray surrounding areas of increased loose connective tissue. These areas can be visualized with DE-CMR, where gadolinium concentrates in the increased interstitial space. Hyperenhancement has been found in up to 75% of patients who have HCM [33]. Gadolinium tends to concentrate only in hypertrophied regions [34] and correlates inversely with regional contraction [35]. Enhancement is located primarily in the septal wall [36], with the highest concentration in the region where the right ventricle (RV) is attached to the LV [33,35]. This follows histopathology, which also has the most prominent lesions in this area [37]. HCM typically does not involve the subendocardium. This distribution can also help to discern HCM from amyloidosis, which may present with anatomic findings similar to HCM but usually involves the subendocardium on DE-CMR.

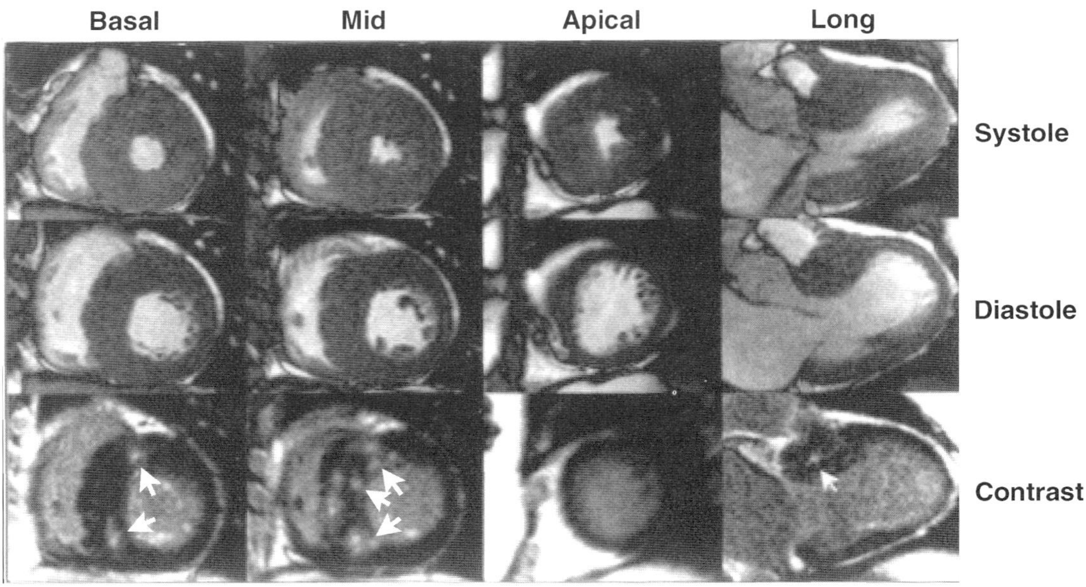

Fig. 4. Patient showing hypertrophy (maximum wall thickness, 27 mm) and scarring. There are multiple foci of scar tissue, which are located predominantly in the mid-myocardial region (*Mid*) and are not present in the lateral free wall. The long-axis (*Long*) cine images demonstrate systolic anterior motion of the mitral valve, systolic flow turbulence in the left ventricular outflow tract, and mitral regurgitation. (*Adapted from* Choudhury L, Mahrholdt H, Wagner A, et al. Myocardial scarring in asymptomatic or mildly symptomatic patients with hypertrophic cardiomyopathy. J Am Coll Cardiol 2002;40(12):2160; with permission.)

The extent of hyperenhancement correlates well with symptoms [34]. In a cohort with a mutation known to cause HCM, Moon and colleagues [38] found 78% of patients who had hypertrophy also had hyperenhancement, whereas those in the same cohort who did not have hyperenhancement did not demonstrate any LV hypertrophy. The presence of hyperenhancement by DE-CMR has important prognostic and therapeutic implications. Premature sudden death is common, especially in the young who have HCM, and the presence of septal scar tissue may provide the substrate for ventricular arrhythmias. Moon and colleagues [39] found that the extent of hyperenhancement was associated with risk factors (ie, extent of LV hypertrophy) for premature death and the occurrence of LV remodeling. CMR can also be useful to guide and monitor the LVOT after alcohol septal ablation [40].

Restrictive and infiltrative cardiomyopathy

Restrictive cardiomyopathy is characterized by restrictive filling and reduced diastolic volume of either or both ventricles with normal or near-normal systolic function and wall thickness, and increased interstitial fibrosis may be present [1]. Restrictive cardiomyopathy may be idiopathic or associated with other disease, including amyloidosis, sarcoidosis, and hemochromatosis. These are also referred to as infiltrative cardiomyopathies, in which the normal myocardium is infiltrated by product from a pathologic process. Cine-MRI shows characteristic findings in restrictive and infiltrative CM, including segmental contraction abnormalities and reduced diastolic filling by the stiffening of tissue. Constrictive pericarditis may present with similar dynamics and should be considered in CMR evaluation.

Amyloidosis

Amyloidosis refers to a group of disorders marked by the deposition of protein secondary to the malformation of B-pleated sheet fibrils. Primary (AL) amyloidosis is the most common form, derived from light-chain immunoglobulin from monoclonal plasma cells. Cardiac involvement is common and is similar to sarcoidosis, the cause of death in most patients [41]. The presence of low-voltage ECG findings and increased cardiac mass on echocardiography are highly suggestive of amyloidosis, although this combination is seen in only 54% of amyloidosis patients [42]. The ability to accurately discern anatomical, functional, and tissue characteristics by CMR allows new insight into the diagnosis of amyloidosis.

Cardiac involvement in amyloidosis may appear similar to hypertrophic cardiomyopathy, with increased thickness of the interatrial septum and ventricles [43,44] as well as increased left or right atrial wall [45]. The thickness of the interatrial septum may help to differentiate between the two, whereas Fattori and colleagues [45] note that interatrial septum or right atrial posterior wall thickness >6.0 mm is unique to amyloidosis. Pleural and pericardial effusions are common in amyloidosis and secondary to amyloid deposition (Fig. 5). They appear as increased intensity on gradient echo sequences and have been detected in 50% and 46%, respectively, of amyloidosis patients [45]. Cardiac function is decreased because amyloid product deposition leads to thickening of the myocardium and results in a stiff and noncompliant ventricle. Diastolic dysfunction is typical, although systolic dysfunction may occur with disease progression. Cine-MRI may show reduced end-diastolic volume, stroke volume, and segmental contraction abnormalities.

The histology of amyloidosis is marked by interstitial expansion with amyloid protein, and heavily involved regions will show hyperenhancement on DE-CMR as gadolinium concentrates in the increased interstitial space. Hyperenhancement has been found in 69% [44] to 76% [46] of amyloidosis patients. The pattern of enhancement is typically subendocardial and global, with the greatest concentration at the midventricular level, and can further assist in differentiation from HCM. A subendocardial pattern is also seen in ischemic heart disease, but the distribution in amyloidosis does not follow any specific coronary artery perfusion territory. The presence of hyperenhancement correlates with increased LV and RV

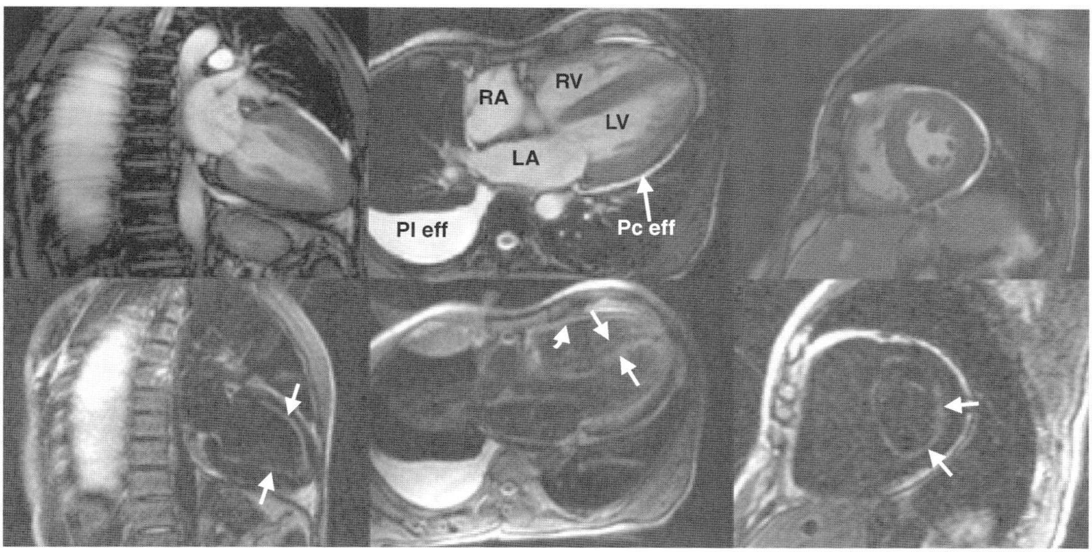

Fig. 5. CMR in a patient with systemic AL amyloidosis. Top row shows diastolic frames from cine images (vertical long axis [*left*], horizontal long axis [*middle*], and short axis [*right*], respectively) showing a thickened LV and pleural effusions (Pl eff) and pericardial effusions (Pc eff) associated with heart failure. Bottom row shows late gadolinium enhancement images in the same planes. The CMR sequence forces myocardium that is remote from the pathology to be nulled (*black*) such that the abnormal region is enhanced. In cardiac amyloidosis, however, the region of greatest abnormality is enhanced because the entire myocardium is affected with amyloid infiltration, and the result is diffuse global subendocardial enhancement (*straight arrows*). The endocardium of the right ventricle (RV) is also heavily loaded with amyloid, and therefore the septum in the horizontal long-axis (*bottom, middle*) view shows biventricular subendocardial enhancement with a dark midwall (zebra-like appearance). The right ventricular free wall is also enhanced (*curved arrow*). Note that the blood pool is dark, which does not occur in other reported conditions, indicating abnormal gadolinium handling in these patients. LA, left atrium; RA, right atrium. (*From* Maceira AM, Joshi J, Prasad SK, et al. Cardiovascular magnetic resonance in cardiac amyloidosis. Circulation 2005;111(2):188; with permission.)

mass index, lower LV ejection fraction, and presence of LV systolic dysfunction [44,46].

Sarcoidosis

The World Health Organization defines sarcoidosis as an unclassified cardiomyopathy. Sarcoidosis is marked by granulomatous infiltration and can affect almost any organ system. Cardiac sarcoidosis usually is clinically silent, but it is apparent at autopsy in 20% to 30% of cases in the United States [47]. Clinical manifestations of cardiac sarcoidosis include heart block, congestive heart failure, ventricular arrhythmias, and sudden death [48].

The early detection of sarcoidosis is critical because cardiac involvement is one of most important factors for prognosis, and initiating corticosteroid therapy before the development of systolic dysfunction results in an improved clinical outcome [49]. CMR can determine small lesions before they are detectable on ECG, echocardiography, or single photon emission-computed tomography [50], and although endomyocardial biopsy has been a mainstay of diagnosis, it is diagnostic in only 20% of cases at autopsy [51]. This is likely because of the fact that the basal septum is not typically sampled in endomyocardial biopsy and represents an area of high involvement in cardiac sarcoidosis. Sarcoidosis has been found to progress through three stages, including edema, granulomatous infiltration, and fibrosis, leading to postinflammatory scarring [47]. CMR provides an excellent tool to observe this progression with different sequences that are useful in detecting each stage, including cine-MRI, T2-weighted images, and delayed enhancement sequences.

CMR is useful in evaluating inflammation, in which associated edema appears brighter on T2-weighted images (Fig. 6). The pattern of T2 enhancement usually is nodular and located in the basal septum. Specific nodules may appear as a central portion with low signal intensity, related to fibrotic tissue, surrounded by high intensity representing edema from inflammation [52]. Late-stage involvement may lead to diffuse myocardial thickening and contraction abnormalities, with areas of focal myocardial thinning, similar to DCM [52]. Cine-MRI typically shows decreased wall motion in areas with increased enhancement, suggesting that these areas reflect the replacement of myocardium by fibrogranulomatous tissue [53]. Cine-MRI also may show features of right-sided heart failure caused by the development of pulmonary fibrosis in patients who have sarcoidosis.

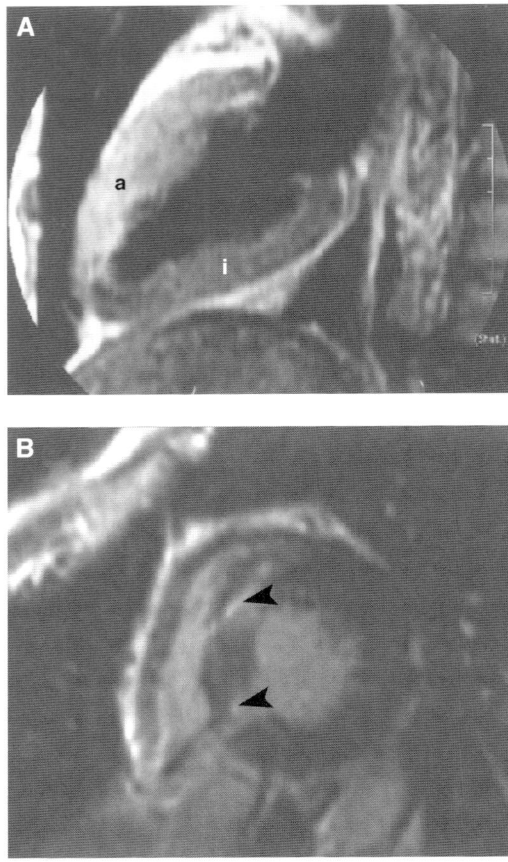

Fig. 6. (*A*) Acute myocardial inflammation caused by multiple organ sarcoidosis in a 37-year-old man with chest pain. Black blood T2-weighted left ventricular long-axis acquisition shows increased signal intensity and myocardial thickening of the anterior wall (a), reflecting myocardial inflammatory edema (compare with normal myocardium in inferior wall [i]). (*B*) Acute myocardial inflammation caused by multiple organ sarcoidosis in a 31-year-old woman with acute chest pain and normal results on coronary angiography. DE-CMR short-axis acquisition shows hyperenhancement of anteroseptal and inferoseptal left ventricular walls (*arrowheads*), suggesting myocardial inflammation with acute necrosis. (*Adapted from* Vignaux O. Cardiac sarcoidosis: spectrum of MRI features. AJR Am J Roentgenol 2005; 184(1):249–50; with permission.)

Two recent studies using DE-CMR have demonstrated a sensitivity of 100% in patients who have biopsy-proven sarcoidosis [50,53]. Enhancement in sarcoidosis is typically patchy and located in the basal septal wall. Vignaux and colleagues [50] postulate that enhancement represents a postinflammatory stage, whereas Tadamura and colleagues [53] have shown evidence of active inflammatory disease.

Further studies will be needed to determine the pathophysiologic process represented by areas of enhancement. Overall, CMR can be used to establish a diagnosis of sarcoidosis and determine prognosis and most recently has been shown to be helpful in monitoring therapy in patients who have sarcoidosis who received corticosteroids [54].

Hemochromatosis

The diagnosis of hemochromatosis is often based on a clinical history of transfusion secondary to thalassemia. Decreased cardiac function is indicative of late-stage cardiac involvement; therefore, early diagnosis is critical because chelation therapy improves clinical outcomes. Other diagnostic techniques, including serum ferritin and endomyocardial biopsy, do not accurately predict myocardial iron overload [55,56], and the biopsy finding may be negative because of subepicardial distribution of iron that is not sampled. The paramagnetic property of iron enables CMR to accurately assess myocardial involvement because local magnetic fields produced by the presence of iron in tissue influence image production and lead to a loss of signal [57]. Gradient echo T2* imaging is the most accurate method for determining the level of myocardial iron deposition and correlates with decreased ejection fraction [56].

Anatomic findings in hemochromatosis include wall thickening and ventricular dilatation. Cine-MRI can assess cardiac dysfunction, in which iron loading and deposition in the myocardium may lead to diastolic dysfunction, characteristic of restrictive cardiomyopathy [58]. Anatomic and functional findings may mimic dilated cardiomyopathy; thus, the main advantage of MRI is the ability to characterize iron-laden tissue through the loss of signal that is created by the presence of iron. CMR is effective in evaluating the reversal of cardiac involvement in patients on chelation therapy [59].

Arrhythmogenic right ventricular cardiomyopathy

Arrhythmogenic right ventricular cardiomyopathy is characterized by the progressive fibro-fatty replacement of right ventricular myocardium, initially with typical regional and later global right and some left ventricular involvement, with relative sparing of the septum. Presentation with arrhythmias and sudden death are common, particularly in the young [1]. ARVC is diagnosed through a combination of criteria, including endomyocardial biopsy, functional and anatomical changes, arrhythmias, and family history [60]. Diagnosis can be difficult, especially at an early stage, and endomyocardial biopsy has a low sensitivity for the detection of ARVC [61,62]. CMR can accurately evaluate functional, anatomical, and tissue characteristics associated with ARVC.

The traditional definition of ARVC includes "fatty" and "fibro-fatty" forms based on histology. The presence of fatty tissue in both forms creates increased signal intensity in the right ventricle on T1-weighted spin-echo sequences, although this mode is not considered diagnostic and may occur in normal or other pathologic conditions. The distinction between forms is important because anatomic and clinical manifestations, including arrhythmias, occur primarily in the fibro-fatty form [63]. The fatty form is characterized by almost complete replacement of the myocardium by fatty tissue, whereas the fibro-fatty form is characterized by fibrosis, fatty infiltration, and myocyte atrophy. Some authors have hypothesized that the fatty and fibro-fatty forms may exist on a continuum, in which the fatty form is transformed into fibro-fatty form through myocarditis or other processes [60].

Cine-MRI can accurately evaluate anatomic and functional changes in the right ventricle, in which the fibro-fatty variant leads to significant thinning and dilation of the right ventricular wall and outflow tract. Involvement of the left ventricle is typically associated with progressive disease [63]. Other common anatomic findings include the presence of aneurysms in the right ventricular wall and outflow tract. Functional changes include early regional contraction abnormalities and global systolic and diastolic dysfunction in later stages. Bomma and colleagues [64] have found that systolic dysfunction involves reduced basal peak filling and emptying rates as well as reduced ejection fraction. Right ventricular volumes increased with the most pronounced change in the midcavity and basal regions. The regional heterogeneity of systolic dysfunction may assist in differentiating ARVC from other sources of right-sided heart failure.

Tandri and colleagues [65] have found a strong correlation between areas of hyperenhancement on DE-CMR and fibro-fatty infiltration on endomyocardial biopsy. The primary location of enhancement was found to be in the anterobasal region of the right ventricle as well as the right ventricle outflow tract. The location of these findings is consistent with previously established histologic distribution of ARVC [66]. Areas of enhancement mirrored regions of right ventricular dysfunction, suggesting a lack of functioning myocardium secondary to fibrosis. The study by Tandri and colleagues shows great potential in the evaluation of ARVC with DE-CMR, although larger studies are needed to validate findings.

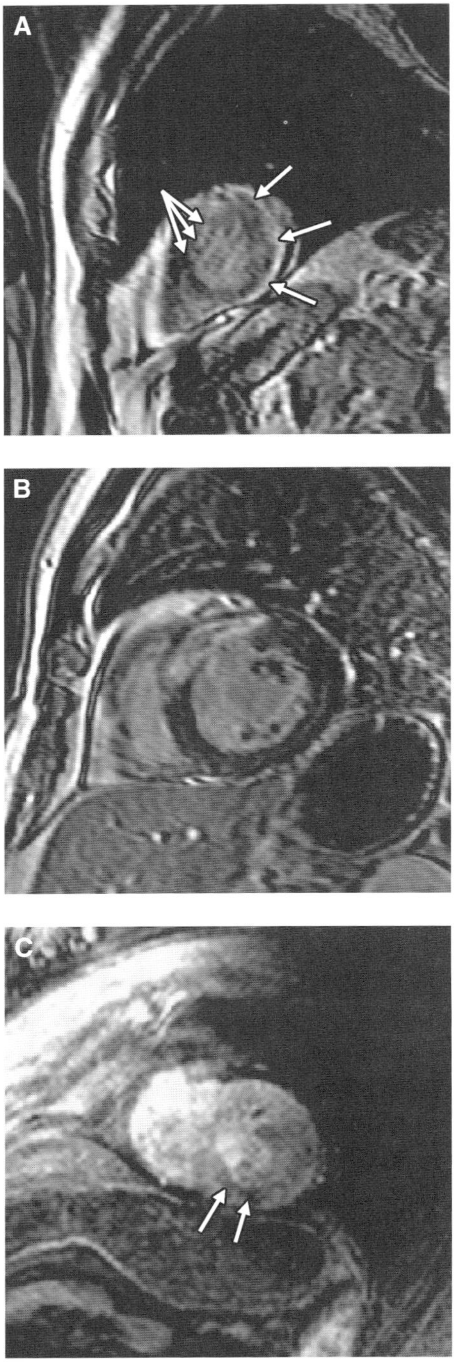

Specific cardiomyopathies

The term "specific cardiomyopathy" is now used to describe heart muscle diseases that are associated with specific cardiac or systemic disorders. The following is brief summary of DE-CMR findings in certain specific cardiomyopathies.

Myocarditis

The presence of myocarditis can be seen in DE-CMR, in which areas of hyperenhancement correlate strongly with areas of histologically proven myocarditis. Hyperenhancement is located primarily in the lateral free wall in the epicardial quartile, which has been shown previously in postmortem evaluations [12]. This finding is important because these regions are not sampled frequently on endomyocardial biopsy. Myocarditis may be considered in the differential for certain presentations of chest pain. Laissy and colleagues found that delayed enhancement in myocarditis was nodular or diffuse and located primarily inferolaterally and subepicardially in nonvascular territories, whereas acute myocardial infarction is associated with early subendocardial perfusion defects and subendocardial or transmural delayed enhancement of a smaller number of segments, all in a vascular distribution (Fig. 7) [67]. DE-CMR imaging of myocarditis may be complicated by the regression or disappearance of hyperenhancement during healing.

Chagas disease

Chagas disease is an inflammatory disease caused by the parasitic protozoan *Trypanosoma cruzi*. Rotchitte and colleagues [68] have demonstrated that DE-CMR is capable of detecting early cardiac involvement in the setting of Chagas disease, in which hyperenhancement was present in a nonischemic-type

Fig. 7. (*A*) Short axis delayed-enhancement T1-weighted multishot gradient-echo IR MR images (3.9/1.4/200, 25° flip angle) of a diffuse form of myocarditis in a 44 year old man. Nodular centromyocardial high enhancement of the anterior wall (*three connected arrows*) associated with band-like or nodular subepicardial high enhancement (*three unconnected arrows*) predominating in the lateral wall of the left ventricle is seen. (*B*) Delayed-enhancement three-dimensional T1-weighted multishot gradient-echo (3.9/1.4/200, 25° flip angle) IR MR images of anterior AMI in 49 year old man. (*C*) The short axis view shows a subendocardial defect (*arrows*) in the inferior wall of the left ventricle. (*From* Laissy JP, Hyafil F, Feldman LJ, et al. Differentiating acute myocardial infarction from myocarditis: diagnostic value of early- and delayed-perfusion cardiac MR imaging. Radiology 2005;237(1):80; with permission.)

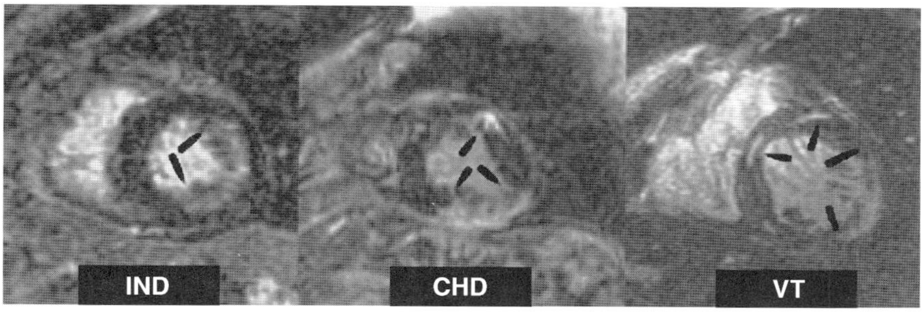

Fig. 8. Myocardial delayed enhancement (*arrowheads*) on left ventricular short-axis slices in different stages of Chagas' disease. IND, indeterminate phase group; CHD, Chagas' heart disease group; VT, Chagas' heart disease with ventricular tachycardia group. (*From* Rochitte CE, Oliveira PF, Andrade JM, et al. Myocardial delayed enhancement by magnetic resonance imaging in patients with Chagas' disease: a marker of disease severity. J Am Coll Cardiol 2005;46(8):1554; with permission.)

pattern. The location typically involved the epicardial or midwall portion of the inferolateral wall (Fig. 8). Other regions may also be affected, and in some patients, the pattern of hyperenhancement may resemble that seen in patients who have coronary artery disease. The extent of enhancement also correlated with decreased cardiac function.

Anderson-Fabry disease

Anderson-Fabry Disease (AFD) is an X-linked recessive storage disorder with variable phenotypes characterized by the accumulation of glycosphingolipid in various tissues. Patients who have cardiac involvement of AFD characteristically show myocardial hypertrophy of the left ventricle. In these patients, the pattern of ventricular hypertrophy caused by AFD may be similar to that seen in HCM. However, the pattern of hyperenhancement seen on DE-CMR appears to be different. Moon and colleagues [69] have recently reported that 50% of patients who have genetically confirmed AFD have myocardial hyperenhancement. In these patients, hyperenhancement was observed most frequently in the basal inferolateral wall, and the subendocardial portion was usually spared.

Unclassified cardiomyopathies

Unclassified cardiomyopathies include a few cases that do not fit readily into any group (eg, fibroelastosis, noncompacted myocardium, systolic dysfunction with minimal dilatation, and mitochondrial involvement). Most recently, CMR has been found to be helpful in identifying noncompacted cardiomyopathy. These unlisted cardiomyopathies as well as some of the specific cardiomyopathies, including valvular, hypertensive, and metabolic cardiomyopathy, are outside of the scope of this chapter.

Clinical applications

Cine-MRI can accurately measure left ventricular mass, myocardial thickness, and left and right ventricular volumes and provides functional assessment of ejection fraction as well as global and segmental wall motion. CMR may be superior in assessing patients who have advanced LV dysfunction caused by technical limitations in other imaging modalities (ie, body habitus). CMR can also evaluate valve function and morphology. Although echocardiography and other imaging techniques have the advantages of quicker scan times, portability, and lower cost, CMR may provide the most optimal assessment of heart function and morphology.

DE-CMR provides tissue characterization, an important tool with which to assess cardiac morphology. For example, a patient who shows normal LV function by multiple gated acquisition imaging may have fat or scar tissue, or both, infiltrating the myocardium. Thus, although the patient's LV function is normal, the patient actually has abnormal heart morphology.

DE-CMR is particularly helpful in the assessment of cardiomyopathy. DE-CMR is capable of differentiating between ischemic and nonischemic forms of CM, and this capability has important clinical and prognostic implications. Revascularization, aggressive lipid therapy, and antiplatelet therapy might be warranted to protect endothelium among all patients who have the ischemic type of hyperenhancement independently of the presence of angiographically proven CAD. DE-CMR tissue characterization can

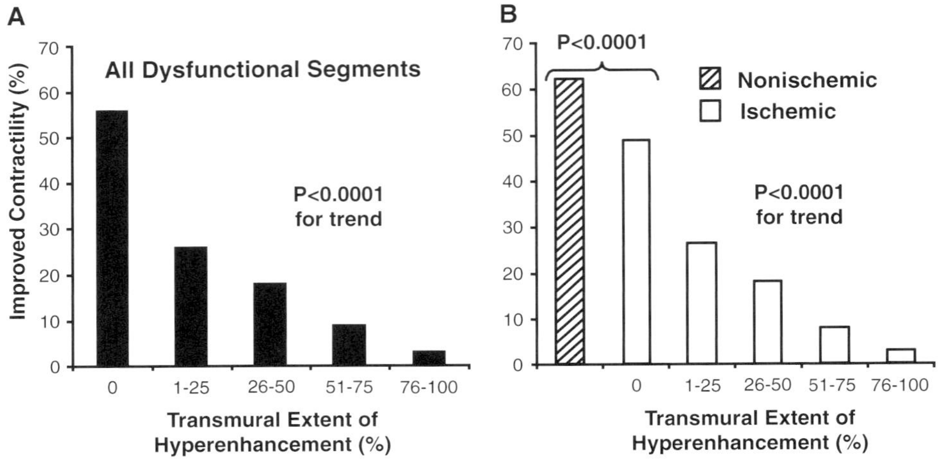

Fig. 9. Relationship between transmural extent of scarring (hyperenhancement) at baseline and the likelihood for improved contractility after β-blocker therapy. Data are shown for all dysfunctional segments (*A*) and when patients with ischemic cardiomyopathy are separated from those with nonischemic cardiomyopathy (*B*). (*From* Bello D, Shah OJ, Farah GM, et al. Gadolinium cardiovascular magnetic resonance predicts reversible myocardial dysfunction and remodeling in patients with heart failure undergoing beta-blocker therapy. Circulation 2003;108(16):1950; with permission.)

assist in the early detection of and initiation of therapy for the nonischemic cardiomyopathies as well. For example, the early diagnosis of cardiac involvement in hemochromatosis and subsequent chelation therapy are likely to improve clinical outcomes. DE-CMR is also effective in monitoring the effects of therapy in diverse cardiomyopathy conditions, including sarcoidosis, myocarditis, hemochromatosis, and ICM.

DE-CMR is capable not only of providing diagnostic information but it can also predict improvement in contractile function after revascularization therapy in both the acute and chronic myocardial infarction [10]. DE-CMR has also been shown to predict the improvement in contractile function after medical therapy (Fig. 9) [11]. DE-CMR provides information on the exact amount of infarct size, and infarct size measured by CMR may have important prognostic implications. Infarct size correlates better than ejection fraction with the induction of ventricular tachyarrhythmia [70]. Furthermore, infarct size has been found to be a better predictor of mortality than ejection fraction [71].

Summary

Cardiac MRI should be considered in all patients who have left ventricular dysfunction. CMR provides superb evaluation of morphologic and functional changes in patients who have cardiomyopathy. In addition, CMR has the ability to characterize tissue through delayed enhancement of gadolinium. CMR provides differentiation of ischemic and nonischemic cardiomyopathies through the evaluation of the presence and characteristic patterns of hyperenhancement. When these patterns are considered in conjunction with morphologic and functional characteristics, they can delineate specific nonischemic cardiomyopathies. In addition to its diagnostic capability, CMR provides important prognostic evaluation and helps to monitor therapy in patients who have cardiomyopathies.

References

[1] Richardson P, McKenna W, Bristow M, et al. Report of the 1995 World Health Organization/International Society and Federation of Cardiology Task Force on the definition and classification of cardiomyopathies. Circulation 1996;93(5):841–2.

[2] American Heart Association. Heart disease and stroke statistics: 2005 update. Dallas (TX): American Heart Association; 2005.

[3] Koelling TM, Chen RS, Lubwama RN, et al. The expanding national burden of heart failure in the United States: the influence of heart failure in women. Am Heart J 2004;147(1):74–8.

[4] Hunt SA, Abraham WT, Chin SH, et al. ACC/AHA 2005 guideline update for the diagnosis and manage-

ment of chronic heart failure in the adult-summary article A report of the American College of Cardiology/ American Heart Association Task Force on Practice Guidelines (Writing Committee to Update the 2001 Guidelines for the Evaluation and Management of Heart Failure). J Am Coll Cardiol 2005;46(6):1116–43.

[5] Doherty III NE, Fujita N, Caputo GR, et al. Measurement of right ventricular mass in normal and dilated cardiomyopathic ventricles using cine magnetic resonance imaging. Am J Cardiol 1992;69(14):1223–8.

[6] Semelka RC, Tomei E, Wagner S, et al. Interstudy reproducibility of dimensional and functional measurements between cine magnetic resonance studies in the morphologically abnormal left ventricle. Am Heart J 1990;119(6):1367–73.

[7] Bellenger NG, Davies LC, Francis JM, et al. Reduction in sample size for studies of remodeling in heart failure by the use of cardiovascular magnetic resonance. J Cardiovasc Magn Reson 2000;2(4):271–8.

[8] Simonetti OP, Kim RJ, Fieno DS, et al. An improved MR imaging technique for the visualization of myocardial infarction. Radiology 2001;218(1):215–23.

[9] Rehwald WG, Fieno DS, Chen EL, et al. Myocardial magnetic resonance imaging contrast agent concentrations after reversible and irreversible ischemic injury. Circulation 2002;105(2):224–9.

[10] Kim RJ, Wu E, Rafael A, et al. The use of contrast-enhanced magnetic resonance imaging to identify reversible myocardial dysfunction. N Engl J Med 2000; 343(20):1445–53.

[11] Bello D, Shah DJ, Farah GM, et al. Gadolinium cardiovascular magnetic resonance predicts reversible myocardial dysfunction and remodeling in patients with heart failure undergoing beta-blocker therapy. Circulation 2003;108(16):1945–53.

[12] Mahrholdt H, Wagner A, Judd RM, et al. Delayed enhancement cardiovascular magnetic resonance assessment of non-ischaemic cardiomyopathies. Eur Heart J 2005;26(15):1461–74.

[13] McCrohon JA, Moon JC, Prasad SK, et al. Differentiation of heart failure related to dilated cardiomyopathy and coronary artery disease using gadolinium-enhanced cardiovascular magnetic resonance. Circulation 2003; 108(1):54–9.

[14] Soriano CJ, Ridocci F, Estornell J, et al. Noninvasive diagnosis of coronary artery disease in patients with heart failure and systolic dysfunction of uncertain etiology, using late gadolinium-enhanced cardiovascular magnetic resonance. J Am Coll Cardiol 2005;45(5): 743–8.

[15] Wu E, Judd RM, Vargas JD, et al. Visualisation of presence, location, and transmural extent of healed Q-wave and non-Q-wave myocardial infarction. Lancet 2001;357(9249):21–8.

[16] Kaushal REA, Fieno D, Radin M, et al. Detection of myocardial infarction in patients with ischemic, non-ischemic and mixed cardiomyopathy by contrast-enhanced MRI. J Cardiovasc Magn Reson 2005;7(1):241.

[17] Schuster EH, Bulkley BH. Ischemic cardiomyopathy: a clinicopathologic study of fourteen patients. Am Heart J 1980;100:506–12.

[18] Uretsky BF, Thygesen K, Armstrong PW, et al. Acute coronary findings at autopsy in heart failure patients with sudden cardiac death: results from the Assessment of Treatment with Lisinopril and Survival (ATLAS) trial. Circulation 2000;102:611–6.

[19] Topol EJ, Yadav JS. Recognition of the importance of embolization in atherosclerotic vascular disease. Circulation 2000;101(5):570–80.

[20] Arroyo LH, Lee RT. Mechanisms of plaque rupture: mechanical and biologic interactions. Cardiovasc Res 1999;41(2):369–75.

[21] Roberts WC, Siefel RJ, McManus BM. Idiopathic dilated cardiomyopathy: analysis of 152 necropsy patients. Am J Cardiol 1987;60:1340–55.

[22] Kim RJ, Judd RM. Gadolinium-enhanced magnetic resonance imaging in hypertrophic cardiomyopathy: in vivo imaging of the pathologic substrate for premature cardiac death? J Am Coll Cardiol 2003;41(9): 1568–72.

[23] Posma JL, Blanksma PK, van der Wall EE, et al. Assessment of quantitative hypertrophy scores in hypertrophic cardiomyopathy: magnetic resonance imaging versus echocardiography. Am Heart J 1996;132(5): 1020–7.

[24] Soler R, Rodriguez E, Rodriguez JA, et al. Magnetic resonance imaging of apical hypertrophic cardiomyopathy. J Thorac Imaging 1997;12(3):221–5.

[25] Devlin AM, Moore NR, Ostman-Smith I. A comparison of MRI and echocardiography in hypertrophic cardiomyopathy. Br J Radiol 1999;72(855):258–64.

[26] Moon JC, Fisher NG, McKenna WJ, et al. Detection of apical hypertrophic cardiomyopathy by cardiovascular magnetic resonance in patients with non-diagnostic echocardiography. Heart 2004;90(6):645–9.

[27] Pons-Llado G, Carreras F, Borras X, et al. Comparison of morphologic assessment of hypertrophic cardiomyopathy by magnetic resonance versus echocardiographic imaging. Am J Cardiol 1997;79(12):1651–6.

[28] Suzuki J, Watanabe F, Takenaka K, et al. New subtype of apical hypertrophic cardiomyopathy identified with nuclear magnetic resonance imaging as an underlying cause of markedly inverted T waves. J Am Coll Cardiol 1993;22(4):1175–81.

[29] Arrive L, Assayag P, Russ G, et al. MRI and cine MRI of asymmetric septal hypertrophic cardiomyopathy. J Comput Assist Tomogr 1994;18(3):376–82.

[30] Sato T, Yamanari H, Ohe T, et al. Regional left ventricular contractile dynamics in hypertrophic cardiomyopathy evaluated by magnetic resonance imaging. Heart Vessels 1996;11(5):248–54.

[31] Kramer CM, Reichek N, Ferrari VA, et al. Regional heterogeneity of function in hypertrophic cardiomyopathy. Circulation 1994;90(1):186–94.

[32] Schwammenthal E, Wichter T, Joachimsen K, et al. Detection of regional left ventricular asynchrony in obstructive hypertrophic cardiomyopathy by magnetic resonance imaging. Am Heart J 1994;127(3):600–6.

[33] Teraoka K, Hirano M, Ookubo H, et al. Delayed contrast enhancement of MRI in hypertrophic cardiomyopathy. Magn Reson Imaging 2004;22(2):155–61.

[34] Bogaert J, Goldstein M, Tannouri F, et al. Original report. Late myocardial enhancement in hypertrophic cardiomyopathy with contrast-enhanced MR imaging. AJR Am J Roentgenol 2003;180(4):981–5.

[35] Choudhury L, Mahrholdt H, Wagner A, et al. Myocardial scarring in asymptomatic or mildly symptomatic patients with hypertrophic cardiomyopathy. J Am Coll Cardiol 2002;40(12):2156–64.

[36] Amano Y, Takayama M, Takahama K, et al. Delayed hyper-enhancement of myocardium in hypertrophic cardiomyopathy with asymmetrical septal hypertrophy: comparison with global and regional cardiac MR imaging appearances. J Magn Reson Imaging 2004;20(4): 595–600.

[37] Kuribayashi T, Roberts WC. Myocardial disarray at junction of ventricular septum and left and right ventricular free walls in hypertrophic cardiomyopathy. Am J Cardiol 1992;70(15):1333–40.

[38] Moon JC, Mogensen J, Elliott PM, et al. Myocardial late gadolinium enhancement cardiovascular magnetic resonance in hypertrophic cardiomyopathy caused by mutations in troponin I. Heart 2005;91(8):1036–40.

[39] Moon JC, McKenna WJ, McCrohon JA, et al. Toward clinical risk assessment in hypertrophic cardiomyopathy with gadolinium cardiovascular magnetic resonance. J Am Coll Cardiol 2003;41(9):1561–7.

[40] Amano Y, Takayama M, Amano M, et al. MRI of cardiac morphology and function after percutaneous transluminal septal myocardial ablation for hypertrophic obstructive cardiomyopathy. AJR Am J Roentgenol 2004;182(2):523–7.

[41] Gertz MA, Rajkumar SV. Primary systemic amyloidosis. Curr Treat Options Oncol 2002;3(3):261–71.

[42] Hamer JP, Janssen S, van Rijswijk MH, et al. Amyloid cardiomyopathy in systemic non-hereditary amyloidosis: clinical, echocardiographic and electrocardiographic findings in 30 patients with AA and 24 patients with AL amyloidosis. Eur Heart J 1992;13(5):623–7.

[43] Celletti F, Fattori R, Napoli G, et al. Assessment of restrictive cardiomyopathy of amyloid or idiopathic etiology by magnetic resonance imaging. Am J Cardiol 1999;83(5):798–801.

[44] Maceira AM, Joshi J, Prasad SK, et al. Cardiovascular magnetic resonance in cardiac amyloidosis. Circulation 2005;111(2):186–93.

[45] Fattori R, Rocchi G, Celletti F, et al. Contribution of magnetic resonance imaging in the differential diagnosis of cardiac amyloidosis and symmetric hypertrophic cardiomyopathy. Am Heart J 1998;136(5): 824–30.

[46] Perugini E, Rapezzi C, Piva T, et al. Noninvasive evaluation of the myocardial substrate of cardiac amyloidosis by gadolinium cardiac magnetic resonance. Heart 2005 [in press].

[47] Silverman KJ, Hutchins GM, Bulkley BH. Cardiac sarcoid: a clinicopathologic study of 84 unselected patients with systemic sarcoidosis. Circulation 1978; 58(6):1204–11.

[48] Yazaki Y, Isobe M, Hiramitsu S, et al. Comparison of clinical features and prognosis of cardiac sarcoidosis and idiopathic dilated cardiomyopathy. Am J Cardiol 1998;82(4):537–40.

[49] Yazaki Y, Isobe M, Hiroe M, et al. Prognostic determinants of long-term survival in Japanese patients with cardiac sarcoidosis treated with prednisone. Am J Cardiol 2001;88(9):1006–10.

[50] Smedema JP, Snoep G, van Kroonenburgh MP, et al. Evaluation of the accuracy of gadolinium-enhanced cardiovascular magnetic resonance in the diagnosis of cardiac sarcoidosis. J Am Coll Cardiol 2005;45(10): 1683–90.

[51] Uemura A, Morimoto S, Hiramitsu S, et al. Histologic diagnostic rate of cardiac sarcoidosis: evaluation of endomyocardial biopsies. Am Heart J 1999;138(2 Pt 1): 299–302.

[52] Vignaux O. Cardiac sarcoidosis: spectrum of MRI features. AJR Am J Roentgenol 2005;184(1):249–54.

[53] Tadamura E, Yamamuro M, Kubo S, et al. Effectiveness of delayed enhanced MRI for identification of cardiac sarcoidosis: comparison with radionuclide imaging. AJR Am J Roentgenol 2005;185(1):110–5.

[54] Vignaux O, Dhote R, Duboc D, et al. Clinical significance of myocardial magnetic resonance abnormalities in patients with sarcoidosis: a 1-year follow-up study. Chest 2002;122(6):1895–901.

[55] Ooi GC, Chen FE, Chan KN, et al. Qualitative and quantitative magnetic resonance imaging in haemoglobin H disease: screening for iron overload. Clin Radiol 1999;54(2):98–102.

[56] Anderson LJ, Holden S, Davis B, et al. Cardiovascular T2-star (T2*) magnetic resonance for the early diagnosis of myocardial iron overload. Eur Heart J 2001; 22(23):2171–9.

[57] Siegelman ES, Mitchell DG, Semelka RC. Abdominal iron deposition: metabolism, MR findings, and clinical importance. Radiology 1996;199(1):13–22.

[58] Kremastinos DT, Tsiapras DP, Tsetsos GA, et al. Left ventricular diastolic Doppler characteristics in beta-thalassemia major. Circulation 1993;88(3):1127–35.

[59] Anderson LJ, Westwood MA, Holden S, et al. Myocardial iron clearance during reversal of siderotic cardiomyopathy with intravenous desferrioxamine: a prospective study using T2* cardiovascular magnetic resonance. Br J Haematol 2004;127(3):348–55.

[60] Fontaine G, Fontaliran F, Frank R. Arrhythmogenic right ventricular cardiomyopathies: clinical forms and main differential diagnoses. Circulation 1998;97(16): 1532–5.

[61] Gemayel C, Pelliccia A, Thompson PD. Arrhythmogenic right ventricular cardiomyopathy. J Am Coll Cardiol 2001;38(7):1773–81.

[62] Kayser HW, van der Wall EE, Sivananthan MU, et al. Diagnosis of arrhythmogenic right ventricular dysplasia: a review. Radiographics 2002;22(3):639–50 [discussion 649–50].

[63] Burke AP, Farb A, Tashko G, et al. Arrhythmogenic right ventricular cardiomyopathy and fatty replacement of the right ventricular myocardium: are they different diseases? Circulation 1998;97(16):1571–80.

[64] Bomma C, Dalal D, Tandri H, et al. Regional differences in systolic and diastolic function in arrhythmogenic right ventricular dysplasia/cardiomyopathy using magnetic resonance imaging. Am J Cardiol 2005; 95(12):1507–11.

[65] Tandri H, Saranathan M, Rodriguez ER, et al. Noninvasive detection of myocardial fibrosis in arrhythmogenic right ventricular cardiomyopathy using delayed-enhancement magnetic resonance imaging. J Am Coll Cardiol 2005;45(1):98–103.

[66] Angelini A, AngBasso C, Nava A, et al. Endomyocardial biopsy in arrhythmogenic right ventricular cardiomyopathy. Am Heart J 1996;132(1 Pt 1):203–6.

[67] Laissy JP, Hyafil F, Feldman LJ, et al. Differentiating acute myocardial infarction from myocarditis: diagnostic value of early- and delayed-perfusion cardiac MR imaging. Radiology 2005;237(1):75–82.

[68] Rochitte CE, Oliveira PF, Andrade JM, et al. Myocardial delayed enhancement by magnetic resonance imaging in patients with Chagas' disease: a marker of disease severity. J Am Coll Cardiol 2005;46(8):1553–8.

[69] Moon JC, Sachdev B, Elkington AG, et al. Gadolinium enhanced cardiovascular magnetic resonance in Anderson-Fabry disease: evidence for a disease specific abnormality of the myocardial interstitium. Eur Heart J 2003;24(23):2151–5.

[70] Bello D. Infarct morphology identifies patients with substrate for sustained ventricular tachycardia. J Am Coll Cardiol 2005;45(7):1104–8.

[71] Bello D, Fieno D, Kim R, et al. Cardiac MRI: infarct size is an independent predictor of mortality in patients with coronary artery disease. J Am Coll Cardiol 2005; 45(3):288A.

ELSEVIER
SAUNDERS

Heart Failure Clin 2 (2006) 163 – 178

HEART
FAILURE
CLINICS

Comprehensive Echocardiographic Assessment of Diastolic Function

Mario J. Garcia, MD*

Cleveland Clinic Lerner College of Medicine, Cleveland, OH, USA

It is now recognized that 30% to 50% of patients who have symptomatic congestive heart failure have preserved left ventricular (LV) ejection fraction [1,2]. Abnormalities in diastolic function not only assume a fundamental role in these but also relate to the severity of symptoms and prognosis in all heart failure patients, regardless of the cause [3,4].

Two-dimensional (2D) and Doppler echocardiography are the most important clinical tools available for the diagnosis of diastolic dysfunction [5]. Echocardiography is widely available, portable, and biologically safe and is also capable of excluding other important causes of heart failure, such as valvular disease. The recent integration of new Doppler modalities in many cases can establish the specific pathophysiologic abnormalities involved and can provide reasonably accurate quantification. In most cases, a comprehensive integration of clinical data, 2D structural information, and Doppler physiologic data is required to provide a complete evaluation.

Diastolic dysfunction may be defined as the inability of the heart to maintain an adequate cardiac output under normal filling pressure [6]. This inability may manifest early as impaired exercise tolerance or as overt left- and right-sided heart failure at rest. There are numerous physiologic parameters that can affect LV diastolic function. These parameters interact to maintain LV filling under relatively low atrial pressure. Of these parameters, the most important intrinsic parameters are the rate of LV relaxation, the stiffness of the LV chamber, and the contractility of the left atrium (LA) (Box 1). Preload and afterload are also critical extrinsic parameters that will contribute to determining the LV filling pressures and cardiac output.

Left ventricular relaxation

LV relaxation is the most important determinant of the initial phase of diastole. LV relaxation is an energy-dependent process that starts with the reuptake of Ca^{2+} by the sarcoplasmic reticulum, which in turn inactivates the troponin–tropomyosin complex [7], allowing the myocardial fiber to stretch. Rapid relaxation of the LV myocytes generates a force that rapidly decreases the LV intracavitary pressure during early diastole and generates a pressure gradient across the mitral valve, drawing blood from the LA. The onset of LV relaxation is asynchronous, starting earlier in the most apical myocardial segments, leading to the development of a negative intracavitary pressure gradient [8]. In ischemic and dilated cardiomyopathies these gradients are markedly reduced [9]. Increased cardiac mass and conduction abnormalities can also reduce the rate of LV relaxation by slowing the transmission of the depolarizing current. Using high-fidelity pressure recordings, LV relaxation can be estimated from the rate of intracavitary pressure decay during isovolumic relaxation, the period between aortic valve closure and mitral opening. The time constant of isovolumic relaxation (τ) is consid-

* Cardiovascular Imaging, Cleveland Clinic Lerner College of Medicine, 9500 Euclid Avenue, F-15, Cleveland, OH 44195.

E-mail address: garciam@ccf.org

doi:10.1016/j.hfc.2006.01.005

Box 1. Evaluation of diastolic function parameters using combined Doppler indices

Impaired relaxation

E<A
E>A + low v_P or E_M

Increased LV stiffness

Short DT

Decreased LA contractility

Low A + AR

Elevated Filling pressures

Short DT (if LV dilated, low EF)
Increased E/v_P
Increased E/E_M

Abbreviations: A, left ventricular filling pulsed Doppler atrial contraction velocity; AR, pulmonary venous atrial contraction reversed flow velocity; DT, left ventricular early filling pulsed Doppler deceleration time; E, left ventricular early filling pulsed Doppler velocity, E_M, early diastolic myocardial tissue Doppler velocity; v_P, color M-mode Doppler early diastolic left ventricular propagation velocity.

ered the gold standard that defines LV relaxation. The fall in intraventricular pressure follows an exponential curve and is used to determine τ, assuming either zero ($p_0 e^{-t/}\tau$) or nonzero ($p_0 e^{-t/}\tau + p_b$) asymptote [10,11]. A small value of τ indicates rapid relaxation and is related directly to the duration of isovolumic relaxation (*IVRT*), whereas it is related inversely to the magnitude of the difference between LV pressure at aortic closure (P_0) and LV pressure at mitral opening (P_{MV}), as shown in Eq. 1:

$$\tau = IVRT/(\ln P_0 - \ln P_{MV}) \quad (1)$$

Because of its high temporal resolution, M-mode echocardiography can provide precise timing of cardiac events, such as the relationship between the onset of LV contraction and relaxation and the opening and closure of the cardiac valves. M-mode studies may demonstrate changes that occur in LV geometry during isovolumic contraction and relaxation. The velocities of circumferential and longitudinal fiber shortening, as determined from digitized M-mode tracings, are reduced in patients who have cardiomyopathy and hypertensive heart disease with slow LV relaxation [12,13].

2D echocardiography can establish the presence of global and regional LV systolic function abnormalities, increased LV mass, and LA size that are often present in patients who have abnormal LV relaxation. In many patients, regional variability in the magnitude and time of onset of early diastolic endocardial motion may be demonstrated using acoustic quantification for automated boundary detection and color-encoded phase analysis of endocardial motion (color-kinesis) [14,15].

Doppler velocities of LV filling are affected by abnormalities of LV relaxation and preload. Doppler velocities relate to pressure gradients as determined by the Bernoulli flow equation. This equation has three basic components, of which the spectral Doppler component permits obtaining only the convective component (Eq. 2):

$$\left[1/2\rho \times \left(\nu_V{}^2 - \nu_A{}^2\right)\right] \quad (2)$$

Thus, spectral Doppler velocities alone cannot provide a quantitative assessment of the pressure gradients across a nonstenotic mitral valve. Nevertheless, there is a direct relationship between the convective and the total pressure gradient that permits obtaining a *qualitative* relationship. This qualitative relationship is fundamental for explaining the clinical observations that relate LV Doppler filling velocities to normal and abnormal diastolic functions. As the ventricular myocardium relaxes during early diastole, the LV cavity pressure (P_v) falls below LA pressure (P_a). The magnitude of the atrioventricular pressure gradient ($P_a - P_v$) during early LV filling is variable. Rapid relaxation (short τ) generates a low LV minimal pressure, increasing the magnitude of this gradient. On the other hand, an elevated p_a in patients who have heart failure and volume overload has a similar effect. The early atrioventricular pressure gradient accelerates the blood across the mitral valve, generating the early filling (Doppler E) wave. In general, the larger the filling volume during early diastole, the smaller will be the contribution of atrial contraction (Doppler A). During early diastole, the mitral valve opens partially, emptying the LA. Simultaneously, the LA volume is replaced by new blood entering from the pulmonary veins (Doppler D). Reduced E velocity, D velocity, and the E/A ratio may indicate either slow LV relaxation or low preload (Fig. 1). For this reason, these indices alone cannot be used reliably to determine LV relaxation. τ may be estimated from the IVRT, systolic blood pressure (p_s), and capillary wedge pressure (p_w) [16] as shown in Eq. 3:

$$\tau = \{IVRT/\ln(p_s) - \ln(p_w)\} \qquad (3)$$

Although this method requires an invasive assessment of LA pressure, it may have a practical value in patients admitted to the intensive care unit who are undergoing hemodynamic monitoring.

As described elsewhere, standard pulsed-wave Doppler echocardiography provides the temporal distribution of blood flow velocities in a single spatial location. In contrast, color M-mode Doppler echocardiography provides the spatiotemporal distribution of these velocities across a scan line. The information displayed in a color M-mode recording of the LV inflow can be compared with that given by multiple simultaneous pulsed Doppler tracings obtained at different levels from the mitral orifice to the LV apex. The onset of flow at the mitral valve level occurs earlier than at the apical regions. The velocity at which the flow propagates within the ventricle (v_p) is given by the slope of the color wavefront. Studies have shown a negative correlation between v_p and τ in various groups of patients who have coronary disease and cardiomyopathy [17], and in experimental models, v_p has been shown to decrease during ischemia and increase during catecholamine administration [18,19]. In comparison to standard Doppler filling indices, v_p is relatively insensitive to alterations in preload [20,21]. Thus, pulsed Doppler indices are more similar in patients who have normal diastolic function (normal LV relaxation and normal preload) than in those with advanced diastolic dysfunction (abnormal relaxation and elevated preload). In contrast, color M-mode Doppler v_p is significantly reduced in the latter and correlates better with τ. Young, healthy subjects have a color M-mode v_p>55 cm/s. Older patients or those who have left ventricular hypertrophy, normal systolic function, and delayed relaxation have lower v_p and low-pulsed Doppler E velocity and an E/A ratio of <1. Patients who have advanced diastolic dysfunction have low v_p but higher pulsed Doppler E and an E/A ratio of >1. Numerical velocity values can be obtained in addition to spatial and temporal information, allowing a *quantitative* estimate of true pressure gradients using the complete Bernoulli's equation,

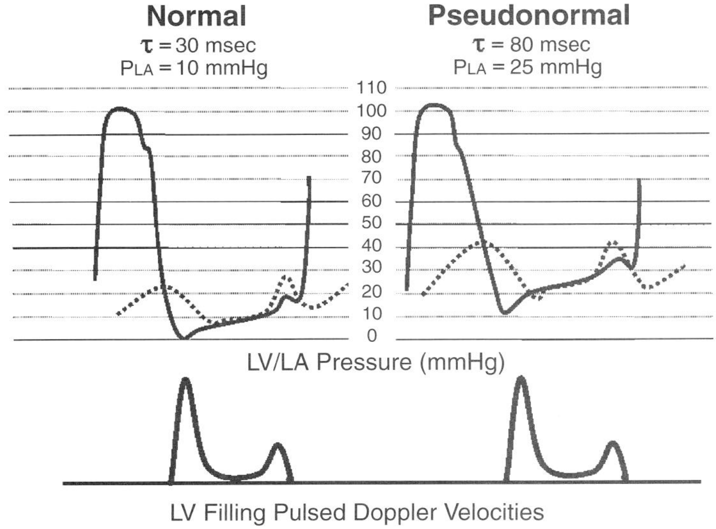

Fig. 1. Influence of preload and relaxation in LV filling pulsed Doppler indices. The normal pattern (*bottom left*) is obtained in the presence of normal relaxation (τ=30 ms) and normal LA pressure (P_{LA}=10 mm Hg). The pseudonormal pattern (*bottom right*) is obtained in the presence of slow LV relaxation (τ=80 ms) and elevated LA pressure (P_{LA}=25 mm Hg). Simultaneous LV pressure (*solid lines*) and LA pressure (*dash lines*) are shown at the top.

including its inertial term [22] (Eq. 4) or the simplified Euler equation [23] (Eq. 5):

$$\rho \int_{A}^{V} \frac{d\vec{v}}{dt} \cdot d\vec{s} \tag{4}$$

$$-\frac{\partial p}{\partial s} = \rho\left[\frac{\partial v}{\partial t} + v\frac{\partial v}{\partial s}\right] \tag{5}$$

This physical relationship explains empirical observations that relate color M-mode indices with LV relaxation, given the association previously described between the generation of intraventricular pressure gradients (IVPG), suction, and relaxation (Fig. 2).

Tissue Doppler echocardiography (TDE) bypasses the high-pass filter and uses low-gain amplification to display the velocities of the myocardium and to eliminate the weaker intensity blood flow signals. TDE velocities may be displayed either in spectral pulsed or color-encoded M-mode or by 2D maps superimposed over structural images [24]. The technical principles and limitations of these modalities are similar to those encountered with standard Doppler flow systems. TDE may provide myocardial velocities at multiple locations of the myocardium using different echocardiographic acoustic windows. Following a positive wave represents ventricular systole (S_M); two waves corresponding to early filling (E_M) and atrial contraction (A_M) appear as a mirror image of the mitral inflow early (E) and atrial (A) filling velocities (Fig. 3). In healthy subjects, the peak of E_M is detected earlier than the peak of LV filling E velocity, suggesting that the rapid relaxation of the myocardium generates a suction force that draws blood into the ventricle. TDE velocities may be affected by translation and rotation of the heart; this is particularly problematic when imaging from the parasternal window. To overcome this limitation, the motion of the LV myocardium can instead be measured in the longitudinal axial plane from the apical acoustic window [25]. Off-line analysis of color M-mode TDE may be used to separate velocity components caused by intrinsic myocardial contraction and relaxation from the translational motion of the heart. One method plots the velocity of each adjacent scan line as the distance from epicardium to endocardium. From a parasternal color M-mode image, the rates of circumferential fiber shortening and lengthening are proportional to the slope of the velocity divided by distance of the regression line. The value of this slope has been referred to as myocardial velocity gradient (MVG). Diastolic MVG have been shown to differentiate myocardial hypertrophy seen in athletes from hypertrophic cardiomyopathy [26]. Another approach obtains the velocity of myocardial segmental systolic thickening and lengthening, or "strain rate," by dividing the difference in velocity ($v_2 - v_1$) between two points by their spatial separation ($s_2 - s_1$). This method can be applied to evaluate the kinetic response of longitudinal or circumferential fibers of the myocardium from the apical or parasternal acoustic imaging views. In healthy subjects, the velocities of the myocardium during diastole are a mirror image of pulsed Doppler

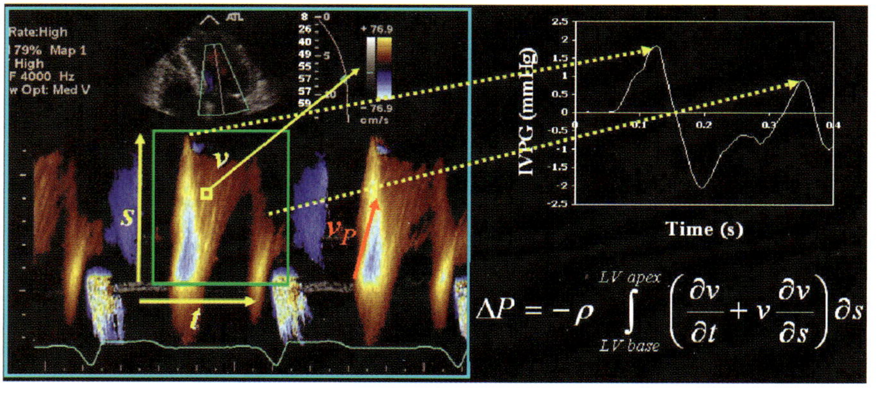

Fig. 2. Color M-mode Doppler assessment of left ventricular filling. v_P represents the slope of the early filling propagation wavefront, measured from the tip of the mitral leaflets to 4 cm distally toward the apex at the first aliasing velocity transition (*red–blue*). The IVPG (*top right*) are determined from computational analysis of velocity (v), space (s) and time (t) using Euler's hydrodynamic equation (*bottom right*). The first positive component corresponds to early diastolic suction. Solid arrows indicate spatial and temporal coordinates. Velocity (v) information is obtained from color table. Dashed arrows point to calculated peak IVPGs during early filling and atrial contraction.

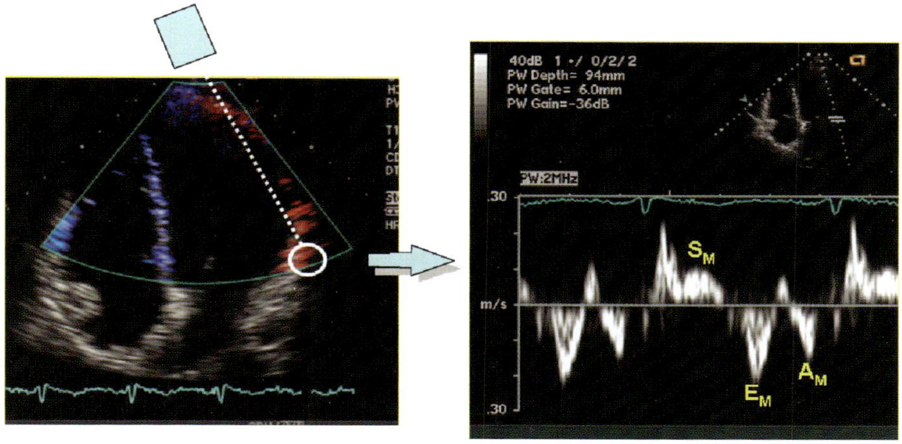

Fig. 3. Tissue Doppler velocities. Color-encoded tissue Doppler velocities obtained in the apical four-chamber view are shown on the left panel. Spectral pulsed Doppler systolic (S_M), early diastolic (E_M), and atrial contraction (A_M) myocardial velocities obtained at the base of the lateral wall are shown on the right image.

transmitral LV filling velocities. Studies have shown an inverse relationship between E_M and LV relaxation (τ) [27,28], both in patients who have normal and those who have elevated preload. Tissue Doppler E_M also appears to be less affected by preload than standard Doppler LV filling indices [27], particularly in the presence of slow ventricular relaxation [29]. Clinical studies suggest that E_M is a better discriminator between patients who have diastolic dysfunction and normal patients, when compared with any other single or combined index of transmitral filling and pulmonary venous Doppler flows [30].

Left ventricular stiffness

When a myocardial fiber is subjected to a given load (stress), it responds by stretching to a given length (strain). The distensibility (strain–stress relationship) of a muscle fiber is typically nonlinear; that is, the force required to stretch a muscle fiber increases geometrically as the fiber is stretched [31]. This property determines a curvilinear relationship between volume and pressure in the ventricle. As the volume of the LV increases during diastole, the intracavitary pressure also increases. The magnitude of pressure change (dP) over a given change in volume (dV) defines the operating stiffness of the LV (S_{LV}). Therefore, with increasing LV filling volume (preload) there is a proportionately larger increase in LV pressure and S_{LV}. Paradoxically, a slow LV relaxation rate decreases the apparent S_{LV} during early filling, because myocardium continues to relax during this period [32], which tends to decrease LV cavity pressure. LV relaxation usually does not affect S_{LV} during late diastole, when it is determined mostly by passive properties. The curvilinear slope of the ventricular pressure volume curve can vary according to myocardial fiber distensibility, elasticity of the connective tissue, LV cavity diameter and wall thickness, the duration of active relaxation, and the effect of pericardial constraint. This slope may be represented as the relative dP/dV ratio for a given LV pressure (P), defining the LV diastolic stiffness constant (K_{LV}) (Fig. 4). A higher proportion of collagen to elastic fibers, as seen with aging, hypertensive heart disease, cardiomyopathies, and after myocardial infarction, results in an increased K_{LV} [33–35]. The external constraining effect of the pericardium increases K_{LV}, a phenomenon that becomes clinically relevant in constrictive pericarditis.

Standard pulsed Doppler velocities of LV filling and pulmonary venous flow may be used to estimate LV stiffness parameters. As the volume of blood enters the LV cavity, LV pressure (P_v) increases and LA pressure (P_a) decreases until the gradient disappears or reverses, causing a deceleration of E. The deceleration time of E (DT) has been shown to be related to the operating stiffness of the LV in clinical studies [36]. In vitro studies have shown that the rate of early transmitral flow deceleration through a restrictive orifice is proportional to net atrioventricular stiffness (S_{NET}) [37,38]. Experiments in an animal model of dilated cardiomyopathy have also

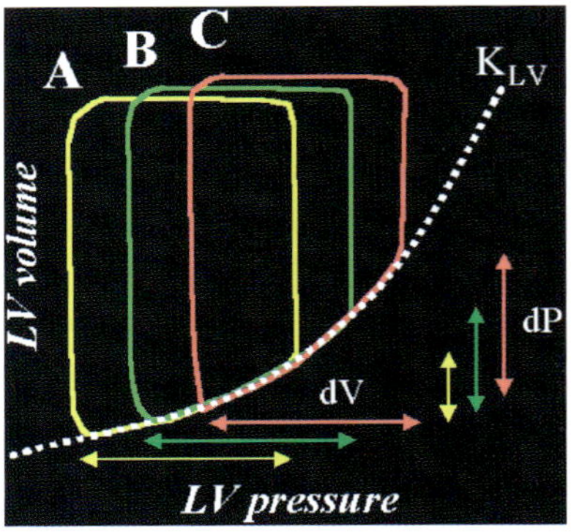

Fig. 4. Calculation of LV stiffness parameters. The LV operating stiffness (S_{LV}) is determined by LV pressure-volume relationship (d) over a cardiac cycle ($S_{LV} = \Delta P/\Delta V$). The $\Delta P/\Delta V$ relationship is load-dependent; at higher LV end-diastolic pressure (from A to B and C) (*horizontal and vertical arrows*), ΔP increases for an equivalent ΔV. The relationship between S_{LV} and end-diastolic volume is determined by the value of the exponential LV stiffness constant (K_{LV}), which may be significantly elevated in patients who have hypertrophic and restrictive cardiomyopathies.

validated an analytical expression applicable to nonrestrictive orifices relating S_{LV} to 1/DT [39,40]. In humans with cardiac disease, Garcia and colleagues [41] demonstrated recently that DT could be applied clinically to provide a quantitative estimate of LV operating stiffness ($S_{LV} = 70/DT^2$). Following LA systole, some amount of blood is propelled backward into the valveless pulmonary veins. The relative duration of the LV filling A wave and pulmonary venous atrial reversal (AR) wave is inversely related to LV end-diastolic stiffness [42].

Left atrium contractility

The left atrium has three important functions. It acts as a reservoir of blood, a passive conduit during early LV filling, and an active pump at end diastole [43]. In young, healthy subjects, its role as a pump is insignificant, contributing to <20% of the total filling volume. In the presence of impaired LV relaxation, the atrial contribution to LV filling increases significantly, at times to over 50%. This is an adaptive mechanism governed by the Frank–Starling law, which states that as the volume and pressure in the LA before its contraction increases, LA contractility also increases. In these patients, LV end-diastolic pressure is elevated, but the mean atrial pressure remains relatively normal at rest. Symptoms are usually absent or minimal unless atrial fibrillation occurs. With worsening LV diastolic function and elevation of LV filling pressure, the LA size increases, losing eventually its mechanical efficiency in advanced stages. Left atrial mechanical function also may be decreased after cardioversion of atrial fibrillation [44].

Following a period of diastasis, the LA contracts, increasing P_a and $P_a - P_v$, accelerating flow across the mitral valve (A wave). The magnitude of the A wave is proportional to the stroke volume and contractility of the LA. The magnitude of the AR flow is also related directly to LA systolic stroke volume, and combining both A and AR, a quantitative estimate of LA

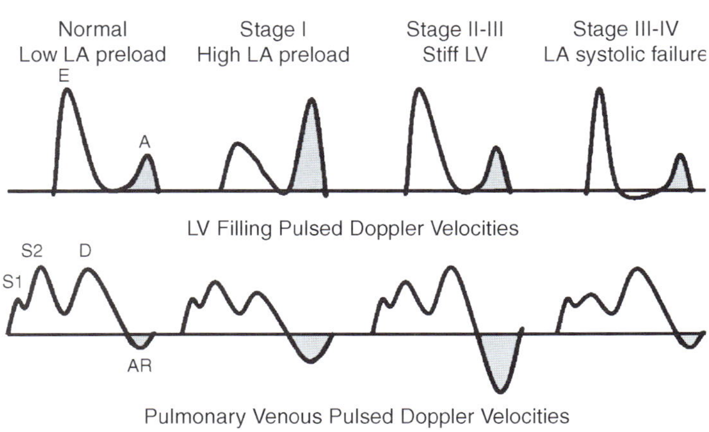

Fig. 5. Evaluation of atrial contractility from LV filling and pulmonary venous pulsed Doppler velocities. The sum of the LV filling atrial (A) area and the pulmonary venous LA reversed flow (AR) area are related directly to the LA contraction stroke volume. A, atrial contraction; D, diastolic; E, early diastolic; S1, first systolic component; S2, second systolic component.

contractility can be obtained (LA dP/dt = 0.1 A_{AC} + 1.8 AR − 4.1 mm Hg) (Fig. 5) [45].

Left ventricular filling pressure

Several investigators have studied the value of Doppler echocardiography for the assessment of LV filling pressures [46–49]. Most of these studies have demonstrated a relationship among mean LA pressure and the pulmonary venous S/D and mitral E/A ratios and IVRT and DT. A difference in the pulmonary venous inflow AR and mitral inflow A wave duration exceeding 30 ms has been shown to be useful in predicting an LV end-diastolic pressure >15 mm Hg [42]. All these previously proposed methods are accurate when applied to groups of patients who have homogeneously impaired LV relaxation, because the methods assume that the reduction in IVRT, atrial filling fraction, pulmonary venous S/D ratio, and DT will occur solely as a consequence of elevated LA pressure. However, when these methods are applied to younger patients and those who have minimal structural heart disease with a normal EF [50,51], the results overestimate actual LV filling pressure, because the methods cannot separate the effect of LV relaxation and preload as confounding variables. Color M-mode and tissue Doppler velocities used as an index of LV relaxation may be combined with standard Doppler flow indices to separate these confounding effects. As discussed previously, LA pressure and LV relaxation are the main determinants of pulsed Doppler E velocity. A positive linear relation between E and LA pressure and a negative but still linear inverse relationship between E and τ have been shown in animal experiments. Because there is a strong (negative) linear correlation between v_p and τ, pulsed and color M-mode Doppler data can be combined to predict LApressure, LAP = 5.27 × (E/v_p) + 4.6 mm Hg ($r = 0.80$, $P < .001$, Standard Error of the Estimate [SEE] = 3.1 mm Hg). This equation has been developed and validated in relatively heterogeneous groups of patients admitted to coronary, medical, and surgical intensive care units. A normal subject who has rapid relaxation under normal preload conditions will have both increased E and v_p. A subject who has impaired relaxation and normal preload will have both reduced E and v_p. In contrast, a patient who has impaired relaxation but elevated preload will exhibit a prominent E but a reduced v_p. Based on the same principles, the combination of standard pulsed Doppler and diastolic myocardial velocities measured by TDE has also been shown to provide an accurate estimation of LV filling pressure [52].

Diastolic function patterns

The general clinical and echocardiographic evaluation of diastolic function recognizes four distinct stages, evolving from normal to advanced disease. These patterns are not unique to a specific disease but represent a spectrum of conditions, which is determined by changing hemodynamic variables.

The normal filling pattern is seen in patients who have normal LV relaxation rate, compliance, and filling pressures. The atrial contribution to LV filling is minimal. Thus, standard Doppler indices of LV filling and pulmunoary venous (PV) flow are characterized by high E, a E/A ratio of <1, IVRT<100 ms, and DT< 220 ms. In healthy, young adults, a rapid relaxation rate results in near-complete LV filling during early diastole, causing a relatively short IVRT and a prominent E. The LA behaves primarily as a reservoir and conduit, and D is prominent because it follows transmitral E. Because the LA volume before atrial contraction is minimal, LA contractility is reduced, resulting in low ejection volume, A and AR velocities, reduced LA relaxation force, and consequently low pulmonary venous systolic relaxation (S1) velocity. As the atrial contribution to LV filling increases with age, A and S become more prominent and the S/D ratio becomes >1. Color M-mode v_p is fast, usually >55 cm/s in younger and >45 cm/s in older adults [53]. Tissue Doppler E_m velocities are >10 and >8 cm/s, respectively.

The delayed relaxation (stage I) pattern of diastolic dysfunction is seen in patients who have a reduced LV relaxation rate but relatively normal compliance and filling pressures. Patients are minimally symptomatic (New York Heart Association [NYHA] class I) or may have mild dyspnea during exercise. Atrial size and its contribution to LV filling are increased, frequently >30% of the stroke volume. The delayed relaxation pattern is characterized by an E/A ratio <1, and IVRT (>100 ms). Ongoing relaxation acts by lowering LV cavity pressure during early LV filling, thus reducing early operating stiffness (S_{LV}). This results in a prolongation of DT (>220 ms). Pulmonary venous flows show S>D, and the AR may be normal or increased depending on the LV end diastolic pressure. Color M-mode v_p is reduced (<45 cm/s), as is E_m (<8 cm/s).

The pseudonormal (stage II) pattern is often the most difficult to recognize because, as its name implies, Doppler filling indices resemble those found in normal subjects. LV relaxation rate is reduced but filling pressure is now increased as a compensatory or over-compensatory mechanism to maintain cardiac output. Patients have mild-to-moderate symptoms

(NYHA class II) of pulmonary vascular congestion and various degrees of LA enlargement, depending on the chronicity of disease. Other echocardiographic evidence of structural heart disease, such as increased LA and LV volumes and mass and reduced ejection fraction, is commonly present. The elevated LA pressure results in an earlier opening of the mitral valve and thus shorter IVRT. Increased S_{LV} causes a rapid increase in LV pressure with cessation of LV filling and a low normal DT (range 150–220 ms). The atrial contribution to LV filling is relatively reduced because of the increased end-diastolic LV stiffness, resulting in reduced mitral inflow A wave, and the pulmonary venous S/D ratio may be normal or <1, depending on the mean LAP. An important diagnostic clue is that the pulmonary venous AR is >35 cm/s, unless atrial mechanical failure is present. Because LV relaxation is impaired, color M-mode v_p remains reduced, <45 cm/s, as does E_m (<8 cm/s).

The restrictive (NYHA stage III–IV) filling pattern is seen in the presence of severely increased S_{LV} and markedly increased filling pressure. LV relaxation is reduced. Patients have overt heart failure (NYHA class III-IV) and moderate-to-severe LA enlargement depending on the chronicity of disease. Echocardiographic features of advanced structural heart disease are invariably present, and LV systolic function is almost always impaired. Standard Doppler filling indices are characterized by an increased E/A ratio (>2), a short DT (<150 ms), and IVRT (<60 ms). Pulmonary venous flow usually shows markedly blunted S. The AR is usually prominent, similar to the pseudonormal stage, unless there is atrial mechanical failure [54]. Color M-mode v_p and E_m are very low, except in patients who have constrictive pericarditis in whom LV relaxation is normal. Reversibility with a Valsalva or other preload-reducing maneuvers differentiates the reversible (stage III) from the irreversible (stage IV) restrictive pattern, which carries a worse prognosis.

Diastolic function assessment in specific cardiac diseases

Most patients who have clinical diastolic dysfunction have hypertensive heart disease. Long-standing arterial hypertension augments LV systolic stress, inducing myocardial fiber hypertrophy and increasing LV wall thickness [55,56]. Genetic and hormonal factors, including circulating angiotensin and insulin levels, may also play a role in the development of cardiac hypertrophy. This physiologic adaptation eventually leads to increased LV chamber stiffness. Ventricular relaxation is also prolonged because of the increased proportion of collagen fibers and because of the slow sequence of electrical repolarization that leads to nonuniform relaxation. Pulsed Doppler filling patterns evolve from a pattern of delayed relaxation to pseudonormal and restrictive filling, with the development of heart failure symptoms [57,58]. Hypertensive cardiomyopathy is responsible for approximately one third of patients who have heart failure who require hospitalization [57,58]. Serial echocardiographic studies are useful for monitoring the effect of antihypertensive therapy causing regression of hypertrophy [59,60].

Ischemia affects relaxation by limiting the availability of energy substrates in the form of ATP. The reabsorption of Ca^{2+} ions by the sarcoplasmic reticulum is an energy-dependent process, which is required for the deactivation of the troponin–tropomyosin complex. In the presence of normal systolic function at baseline, ischemia is manifested by a change to a pattern of impaired LV relaxation. Chronically ischemic or scarred myocardium may become stiffer because of the development of interstitial fibrosis [61,62]. Doppler LV filling patterns will vary according to the extent, duration, and severity of ischemia. These patterns have been shown to carry important prognostic information after an acute myocardial infarction [63] and in chronic ischemic heart disease [50].

The restrictive cardiomyopathies are a group of primary and secondary myocardial diseases characterized by small LV cavity size, abnormal LV relaxation, and increased LV stiffness. These hemodynamic abnormalities lead to chronic elevation of LV filling pressures, decreased cardiac output, and left and right heart failure [64]. Commonly, in restrictive cardiomyopathies, the LV wall thickness is normal or increased because of infiltration or fibrosis, and unlike hypertensive heart disease, cardiomyopathies usually present with low QRS voltage or a pseudoinfarction pattern in the electrocardiogram. The systolic function may be normal or abnormal in advanced stages of the disease. Atrial enlargement is present because of chronic pressure overload. Pulsed Doppler LV filling patterns vary according to the severity of the disease. Initially, a pattern of delayed relaxation is seen, progressing to pseudonormal and finally to restrictive filling patterns in advanced disease. Clinical studies have shown that patients who have amyloidosis and presenting with a restrictive filling pattern have a 50% 1-year mortality rate compared with 10% for those presenting with a pattern of delayed relaxation or pseudonormalization [65]. Pulmonary venous flow demonstrates initially

S > D, progressing later to S < D and a prominent AR. Hepatic vein flow demonstrates similar changes according to the stage, corresponding to a prominent x-axis or y-axis descent or both ("M" pattern) on the central venous pressure tracings. In the advanced stages, the reversed flow (AR and VR) will be increased with inspiration. In cardiac amyloidosis, 2D echocardiography may demonstrate a "sparkling granular" appearance of the myocardium, although this finding is neither highly sensitive nor specific and may be overestimated by the use of tissue harmonic imaging. Increased pericardial thickness and brightness and small pericardial effusions are more specific findings. Abnormal thickening of the cardiac valves and the interatrial septum is often found, as well as mild to moderate valvular regurgitation. The degree of increased LV wall thickness (early, 12–15 mm; advanced, ≥15 mm) may provide important prognostic information in these patients [66].

Hypertrophic cardiomyopathy (HCM) is characterized by a prominent increase in global or segmental LV wall thickness and histologically by myocardial fiber disarray [67]. Diastolic function is characterized by increased LV chamber stiffness and decreased relaxation of variable severity resulting from the asynchronous deactivation of the muscle fibers [68,69]. Patients who have HCM can have symptoms even in the absence of LV outflow tract (LVOT) systolic obstruction, although recent studies suggest that relief of the LVOT gradient after alcohol embolization may be accompanied by an improvement in LV relaxation [70,71]. 2D echocardiography can demonstrate the extension and localization of the hypertrophied myocardium, which frequently has an impaired contractility. Atrial enlargement is common. Pulsed Doppler LV filling usually shows impaired relaxation or pseudonormal patterns and, rarely, the restrictive patterns because of the markedly increased wall thickness and impaired relaxation. Color M-mode Doppler may demonstrate intracavitary flow during isovolumic relaxation because of the asynchronous relaxation. Tissue Doppler echocardiography can identify abnormal regional strain, predominantly in areas of localized hypertrophy (Fig. 6) [72]. These abnormalities can often been found in asymptomatic carriers of hypertrophic cardiomyopathy genetic mutations, even in the absence of phenotypic expression [73].

Left ventricular filling patterns correlate well with functional class and have been shown to carry important and independent prognostic implications in patients who have dilated cardiomyopathy [74]. Diastolic dysfunction is invariably present in these

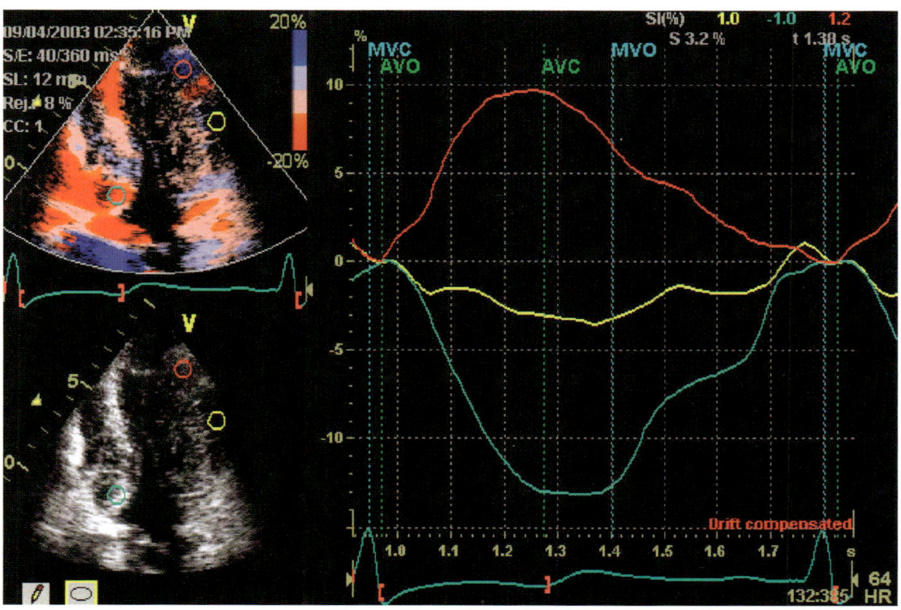

Fig. 6. Regional myocardial systolic strain measured at the anteroapical (*red line*), mid-anterior (*yellow line*) and basal inferior (*blue line*) left ventricular regions obtained from a patient who has apical hypertrophic cardiomyopathy. The basal-inferior systolic strain is within normal range (−13%). The mid-anterior systolic strain is reduced (−3%), whereas the apical-anterior strain is dyskinetic (systolic strain, +10%). Open circles indicate sample volume location.

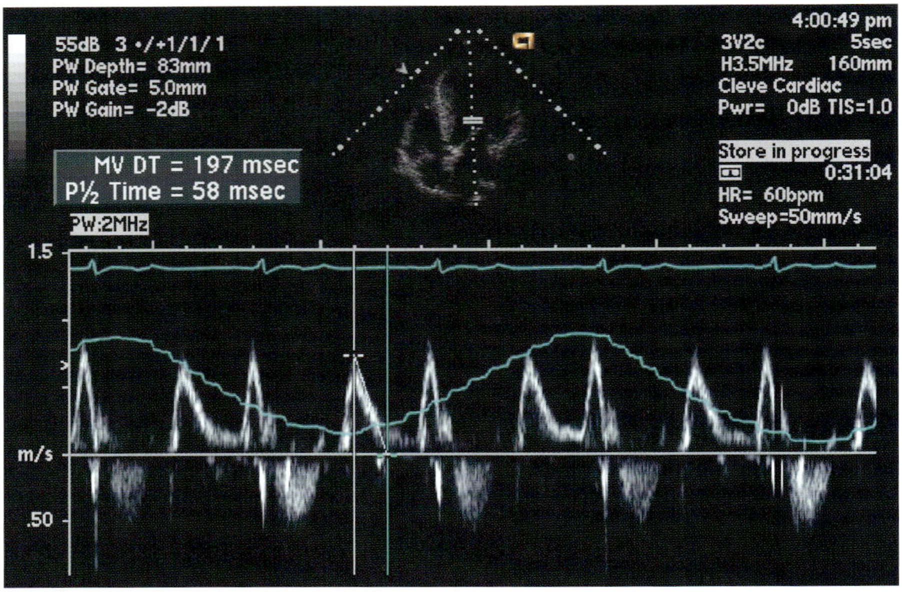

Fig. 7. Measurement of early left ventricular filling pulsed Doppler deceleration time (DT) in a patient who has dilated cardiomyopathy. DT = 197 ms, indicating normal left ventricular operating stiffness.

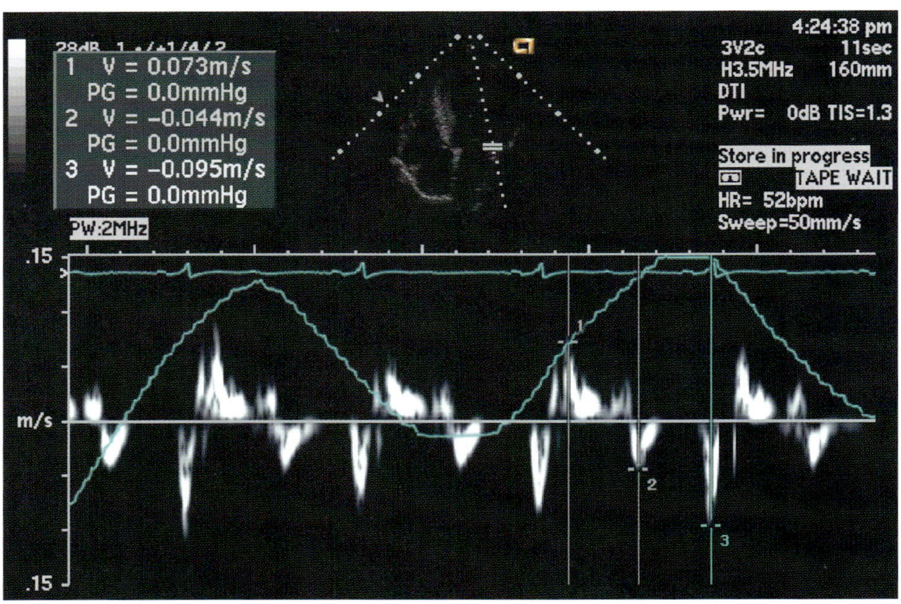

Fig. 8. Measurement of tissue Doppler basal lateral myocardial velocities in a patient who has dilated cardiomyopathy: Early diastolic velocity (E_M) = 4.4 cm/s, indicating abnormal LV relaxation. Combining this index with early left ventricular filling pulsed Doppler velocity (E = 80 cm/s) shown in Fig. 7 yields a E/E_M ratio of 18, equivalent to an estimated mean left atrial pressure of 24 mm Hg.

patients. Because relaxation is invariably impaired, changes in LV filling and pulmonary venous Doppler flow parameters predominantly reflect changes in preload. A high E/A ratio, a low S/D ratio, short IVRT, or short DT indicates elevated LV filling pressures (Figs. 7–9). The role of echocardiography in the follow-up of heart transplant patients has not yet been defined clearly. Echocardiography in acute transplant rejection may demonstrate an increase in LV wall thickness, pericardial effusion, and a decrease in ejection fraction. Alterations in LV filling pattern are seen in up to 80% of the cases of severe rejection, including a reduction in DT and IVRT [75]. It is important to consider that Doppler filling patterns may vary according to the age of the donor heart or the duration of transplantation. Abnormal filling patterns are commonly seen immediately after transplantation. These patterns may lag for up to several weeks and have been associated with the duration of circulatory arrest [76]. Therefore, it is important to analyze serial studies in these patients to interpret anomalies in Doppler filling patterns. Transplant patients who have chronic rejection or coronary artery disease may also exhibit abnormal filling patterns. It has been proposed that serial echocardiographic studies may help in reducing the frequency of surveillance biopsies to detect rejection. Preliminary data suggest that diastolic myocardial velocities measured by TDE are very sensitive for detecting rejection in heart transplant patients [77,78]. Transplant rejection is associated with lymphocytic infiltration and edema, resulting in increased myocardial stiffness and abnormal relaxation. In a recent study, 121 heart transplant recipients underwent pulsed-wave TDE examination at the time of their surveillance endomyocardial biopsies. Peak TDE E_m in 98 nonrejecting allograft recipients was 0.21 ± 0.01 m/s. In 16 patients who had moderate rejection, E_m decreased to 0.14 ± 0.01 m/s and subsequently increased to 0.23 ± 0.01 m/s after successful treatment. No differences, however, were detected in TDE systolic velocities. Using a cutoff value of 0.16 m/s, the authors reported sensitivity, specificity, and negative predictive values of 76%, 88%, and 92%, respectively. One caution that must be taken, however, when interpreting these results, is that factors other than rejection may affect LV relaxation and E_m in these patients, such as the age of the donor heart and the time after transplantation. Thus, lower velocities may not imply rejection if the organ belonged to an older donor or if these velocities are obtained several years after transplantation. One way to circumvent this problem would be to compare the results of serial studies obtained in the same patient.

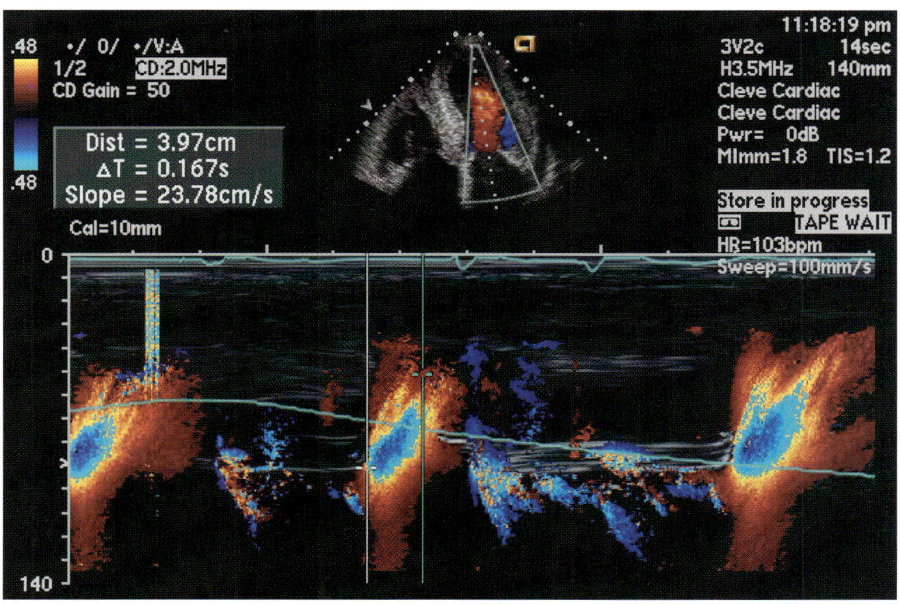

Fig. 9. Measurement of color M-mode early diastolic left ventricular filling propagation velocity (v_P) in a patient with dilated cardiomyopathy. v_P = 24 cm/s, indicating abnormal LV relaxation. Combining this index with early left ventricular filling pulsed Doppler velocity (E = 80 cm/s) shown in Fig. 8 yields a E/v_P ratio of 3.3, equivalent to an estimated mean left atrial pressure of 22 mm Hg.

In most circumstances, however, the diagnosis of rejection requires the integration of clinical data with the detection of several echocardiographic markers such as pericardial effusions, increased wall thickness, and diastolic abnormalities.

Diastolic dysfunction in constrictive pericarditis results from increased pericardial constraint on the LV that is related to the thickness and rigidity of the pericardium. Patients present predominantly with signs and symptoms of right-sided heart failure, including edema, ascites, pleural effusions, and low cardiac output [79]. Echocardiographic studies demonstrate increased pericardial thickness, dilation of hepatic and caval veins, and a prominent interventricular septal bounce. The septal bounce is an abrupt displacement of the interventricular septum toward the LV during inspiration because the onset of RV filling occurs earlier and the expansion the RV free wall is limited by the pericardial constraint. The Doppler LV filling pattern presents a restrictive filling pattern because of the increased S_{LV}, unless the patient is volume-depleted. This pattern corresponds to the "square root sign" in the LV filling pressure tracing and a steep y-axis descent in the central venous pressure. The right ventricular filling pattern shows an increase in E and DT during inspiration because of the decrease in intrathoracic pressure, causing a decrease in pulmonary venous return to the left and augmented venous return to the right heart [80]. During inspiration, intrathoracic pressure decreases. Normally, this change is transmitted to the intrapericardial space and the cardiac chambers, maintaining a relatively constant pressure gradient between the central and pulmonary veins and the atria. In constrictive pericarditis, the rigid pericardium prevents the transmission of this pressure change to the cardiac chambers. The decrease in intrathoracic pressure lowers the pressure in the pulmonary veins, decreasing the pulmonary venous-left atrial pressure gradient and reducing venous return to the left heart, thus lowering the LV inflow E wave velocity. Because of interventricular dependence and limited pericardial space, the right-sided venous return increases with inspiration. During inspiration, Doppler LV filling demonstrates >30% reduction in E and >50% reduction in IVRT [81]. Simultaneously, RV inflow E increases >40%. These changes are observed with the first cardiac cycle after inspiration. The inferior vena cava will be plethoric, the D flow velocities may not increase because of limited filling, and there may be increased reversals during expiration. Superior vena caval (SVC) flow may decrease during inspiration because the SVC is influenced by intrathoracic pressure. This is equivalent to Kussmaul's sign. Pulmonary venous flow decreases during inspiration, predominantly D flow. It is important to consider that the respiratory variability of flows depend on the depth of the inspiratory effort. Under normal conditions, respiratory variability in healthy subjects is <10%. Acute respiratory illnesses can increase intrathoracic pressure swings, also increasing respiratory flow variability, but usually after the first cardiac cycle after inspiration. Excessive preload attenuates the effect of intrathoracic pressure swings and decreases respiratory variability. It may be useful under these conditions to reexamine the patient in a sitting position or after he or she undergoes diuresis. Very low preload can decrease the constraining effect of the pericardium, also masking the characteristic Doppler signs of constriction. The infusion of 1 to 2 L of saline may be useful in these cases [82]. In an important percentage of cases of constriction, respiratory variability may be absent. Tissue Doppler myocardial velocities may be used to differentiate restrictive cardiomyopathy from constrictive pericarditis. These conditions are often difficult to distinguish in the clinical setting using 2D or standard Doppler echocardiography alone. In restrictive cardiomyopathy patients, both relaxation and stiffness are abnormal. On the other hand, relaxation is preserved in purely constrictive pericarditis. Patients who have constrictive pericarditis and normal systolic function have normal or elevated E_M velocities (>8 cm/s), probably reflecting their preserved ventricular relaxation [25,83].

Diastolic dysfunction and exercise intolerance

Several factors are known to determine exercise aerobic capacity, including skeletal muscle fitness, cardiovascular state, pulmonary mechanics, and neuroendocrine factors. In most normal individuals, however, the limiting factors that influence VO_2 max are the skeletal muscle mass and the capacity of the cardiovascular system [84]. During peak exercise, the duration of diastasis is greatly diminished to account for the increase in heart rate. Yet, for the heart to increase the cardiac output, the diastolic mechanics must adjust to the decrease in time to fill [85]. The ability to accommodate high-volume loads has been demonstrated in athletes [86]. This accommodation is carried out at low filling pressures; rather, the early relaxation is increased to provide for a "suction" force and high LV compliance. However, patients who have heart failure may not be able to achieve this necessary increase in diastolic relaxation to accommodate the preload increase [87–89]. Rovner and colleagues [71] recently investigated the relationship between diastolic intraventricular pressure gradients (IVPG) and exercise tolerance in patients who had heart failure using color M-mode Doppler. Echocardiograms were performed before and after metabolic treadmill stress testing in 31 patients who had heart failure and 15 normal subjects. In this study, resting diastolic function indices, including tissue Doppler E_M and color M-mode Doppler v_p, correlated well with metabolic aerobic activity (VO_2 max). A statistically significant increase was observed in v_p and IVPG in both groups after exercise, but the change in IVPG was higher in normal subjects compared with patients who had heart failure (2.6 ± 0.8 versus 1.1 ± 0.8 mm Hg, respectively; $P<.05$). An increase in IVPG correlated with peak VO_2 max ($r=0.8$, $P<.001$) and was the strongest predictor of exercise capacity. This study also demonstrated that in patients who have heart failure, the decreased ability to augment the diastolic relaxation is responsible for the inability to accommodate the increase in estimated preload during exercise, resulting in higher filling pressures.

Summary

The analysis of diastolic function is not only relevant to the evaluation of symptoms in patients who have heart failure and normal ejection fraction it also carries prognostic and therapeutic implications in patients who have systolic heart failure. Echocardiographic indices can establish the diagnosis, severity, and specific mechanism of diastolic heart failure in most patients. Accordingly, it is important for both the clinician and the echocardiographer to acquire in-depth knowledge of conventional and newer echocardiographic indices of diastolic function and to apply these indices in clinical practice.

References

[1] Topol EJ, Traill TA, Fortuin NJ. Hypertensive hypertrophic cardiomyopathy in the elderly. N Engl J Med 1985;312:277–83.

[2] Vasan RS, Larson MG, Benjamin EJ, et al. Congestive heart failure in subjects with normal versus reduced left ventricular ejection fraction: prevalence and mortality in a population-based cohort. J Am Coll Cardiol 1999;33(7):1948–55.

[3] Cohn JN, Johnson G. Heart failure with normal ejection fraction. Circulation 1990;81:III-48–53.

[4] Bonow RO, Udelson JE. Left ventricular diastolic dysfunction as a cause of congestive heart failure. Ann Intern Med 1992;117:502–10.

[5] Cohen GI, Pietrolungo JF, Thomas JD, et al. A practical guide to assessment of ventricular diastolic function using Doppler echocardiography. J Am Coll Cardiol 1996;27:1753–60.

[6] Goldsmith SR, Dick C. Differentiating systolic from diastolic heart failure: pathophysiologic and therapeutic considerations. Am J Med 1993;95:645–55.

[7] Morgan JP. Mechanisms of disease: abnormal intracellular modulation of calcium as a major cause of cardiac contractile dysfunction. N Engl J Med 1991;325:625–32.

[8] Courtois M, Ludbrook PA. Intraventricular pressure transients during relaxation and filling. In: Gaasch WH, LeWinter MM, editors. Left ventricular diastolic dysfunction and heart failure. Philadelphia: Lea & Feibiger; 1994. p. 150–66.

[9] Ling D, Rankin JS, Edwards CH, et al. Regional diastolic mechanics of the left ventricle in the conscious dog. Am J Physiol 1979;236(5):H323–30.

[10] Weiss JL, Frederiksen JW, Weisfeldt ML. Hemodynamic determinants of the time-course of fall in canine left ventricular pressure. J Clin Invest 1976;58:751–60.

[11] Yellin EL, Hori M, Yoran C, et al. Left ventricular relaxation in the filling and non-filling intact canine heart. Am J Physiol 1986;250:H620–9.

[12] Fifer MA, Borow KM, Colan SD, et al. Early diastolic left ventricular function in children and adults with aortic stenosis. J Am Coll Cardiol 1985;5:1147–54.

[13] Van der Mer F, Geboers J, Kestelcot H, et al. The mechanism of disappearance of the physiologic third heart sound with age. Circulation 1986;73:877.

[14] Marangelli V, Pellegrini C, Piccinni G, et al. On-line assessment of left ventricular function by automatic border detection echocardiography during rest and stress conditions. Cardiologia 1993;38:701–12.

[15] Chenzbraun A, Pinto FJ, Popylisen S, et al. Filling patterns in left ventricular hypertrophy: a combined acoustic quantification and Doppler study. J Am Coll Cardiol 1994;23(5):1179–85.

[16] Scalia GM, Greenberg NL, McCarthy PM, et al. Noninvasive assessment of the ventricular relaxation time constant (tau) in humans by Doppler echocardiography. Circulation 1997;95(1):151–5.

[17] Brun P, Tribouilloy C, Duval AM, et al. Left ventricular flow propagation during early filling is related to wall relaxation: a color M-mode Doppler analysis. J Am Coll Cardiol 1992;20:420–32.

[18] Stugaard M, Risoe C, Ihlen H, et al. Intracavitary filling pattern in the failing left ventricle assessed by color M-mode Doppler echocardiography. J Am Coll Cardiol 1994;24:663–70.

[19] Stugaard M, Smiseth OA, Risoe C, et al. Intraventricular early diastolic filling during acute myocardial ischemia: assessment by multigated color M-mode Doppler echocardiography. Circulation 1993;88:2705–13.

[20] Garcia MJ, Palac RT, Malenka DJ, et al. Color M-mode Doppler flow propagation velocity is a relatively preload-independent index of left ventricular filling. J Am Soc Echocardiogr 1999;12:129–37.

[21] Garcia MJ, Smedira NG, Greenberg NL, et al. Color M-mode Doppler flow propagation is a preload insensitive index of left ventricular relaxation: animal and human validation. J Am Coll Cardiol 2000;35: 201–8.

[22] Greenberg NL, Vandervoort PM, Thomas JD. Instantaneous diastolic transmitral pressure differences from color Doppler M mode echocardiography. Am J Physiol 1996;271:H1267–76.

[23] Greenberg NL, Vandervoort PM, Thomas JD. Estimation of diastolic intraventricular pressure gradients from color Doppler M-mode spatiotemporal velocities: analytical Euler equation solution. In: Computers in cardiology. Los Alamitos (CA): IEEE Computer Society Press; 1995. p. 465–8.

[24] Miyatake K, Yamagishi M, Tanaka N, et al. New method for evaluating left ventricular wall motion by color-coded tissue Doppler imaging: in vitro and in vivo studies. J Am Coll Cardiol 1995;25:717–24.

[25] Garcia MJ, Rodriguez L, Ares MA, et al. Differentiation of constrictive pericarditis from restrictive cardiomyopathy: assessment of left ventricular diastolic velocities in the longitudinal axis by tissue Doppler imaging. J Am Coll Cardiol 1996;27:108–14.

[26] Palka P, Lange A, Fleming AD, et al. Differences in myocardial velocity gradient measured throughout the cardiac cycle in patient with hypertrophic cardiomyopathy, athletes and patients with left ventricular hypertrophy due to hypertension. J Am Coll Cardiol 1997;30:760–8.

[27] Sohn DW, Chai IH, Lee DJ, et al. Assessment of mitral annulus velocity by tissue Doppler imaging in the evaluation of left ventricular diastolic function. J Am Coll Cardiol 1997;30(2):474–80.

[28] Oki T, Tabata T, Yamada H, et al. Clinical application of pulsed tissue Doppler imaging for assessing abnormal left ventricular relaxation. Am J Cardiol 1997;79(7):921–8.

[29] Firstenberg MS, Greenberg NL, Main ML, et al. Determinants of diastolic myocardial tissue Doppler velocities: influences of relaxation and preload. J Appl Physiol 2001;90(1):299–307.

[30] Farias CA, Rodriguez L, Garcia MJ, et al. Assessment of diastolic function by tissue Doppler echocardiography: comparison with standard transmitral and pulmonary venous flow. J Am Soc Echocardiogr 1999;12: 609–17.

[31] Factor SM, Flomenbaum M, Zhao MJ, et al. The effect of acutely increased ventricular cavity pressure on intrinsic myocardial connective tissue. J Am Coll Cardiol 1988;12:1582–9.

[32] Templeton GH, Donald IT, Mitchell JH, et al. Dynamic stiffness of papillary muscle during contraction and relaxation. Am J Physiol 1973;224:692–8.

[33] Janicki JS, Matsubara BB. Myocardial collagen and left ventricular diastolic function. In: Gaasch WH, LeWinter MM, editors. Left ventricular diastolic dysfunction and heart failure. Philadelphia: Lea & Febiger; 1994. p. 125–40.

[34] Robinson TF, Factor SM, Sonnenblick EH. The heart as a suction pump. Sci Am 1986;254(6):84–91.

[35] Matsubara BB, Hennigar JR, Janicki JS. Structural and functional role of myocardial collagen. Circulation 1991;84:II212.

[36] Appleton C, Hatle L, Popp R. Demonstration of restrictive ventricular physiology by Doppler echocardiography. J Am Coll Cardiol 1988;11:757–68.

[37] Flachskampf FA, Weyman AE, Guererro JL, et al. Calculation of atrioventricular compliance from the mitral flow profile: analytical and in vitro study. J Am Coll Cardiol 1992;19:998–1004.

[38] Flachskampf FA, Weyman AE, Guerrero JL, et al. Influence of orifice geometry and flow rate on effective valve area: an in vitro study. J Am Coll Cardiol 1990;15:1173–80.

[39] Ohno M, Cheng CP, Little WC. Mechanism of altered patterns of left ventricular filling during the development of congestive heart failure. Circulation 1994; 89:2241–50.

[40] Little WC, Ohno M, Kitzman DW, et al. Determination of left ventricular chamber stiffness from the time for deceleration of early left ventricular filling. Circulation 1995;92:1933–9.

[41] Garcia MJ, Firstenberg MS, Smedira N, et al. Estimation of left ventricular operating stiffness from Doppler early filling deceleration time in humans. Am J Physiol Heart Circ Physiol 2001;280(2):H554–61.

[42] Rossvoll O, Hatle LK. Pulmonary venous flow velocities recorded by transthoracic Doppler ultrasound: relation to left ventricular diastolic pressures. J Am Coll Cardiol 1993;21(7):1687–96.

[43] Nishimura RA, Abel MD, Hatle LK, et al. Relation of pulmonary vein to mitral flow velocities by transesophageal Doppler echocardiography: effect of different loading conditions. Circulation 1990;81(5): 1488–97.

[44] Manning WJ, Leeman DE, Gotch PJ, et al. Pulsed Doppler evaluation of atrial mechanical function after electrical cardioversion of atrial fibrillation. J Am Coll Cardiol 1989;13:617–23.

[45] Nakatani S, Garcia MJ, Firstenberg MS, et al. Noninvasive assessment of LA maximum dP/dt by a combination of transmitral and pulmonary venous flow. J Am Coll Cardiol 1999;34:795–801.

[46] Vanoverschelde JL, Raphael DA, Robert AR, et al. Left ventricular filling in dilated cardiomyopathy: relation to functional class and hemodynamics. J Am Coll Cardiol 1990;15:1288–95.

[47] Stork TV, Muller RM, Piske GJ, et al. Noninvasive measurement of left ventricular filling pressures by means of transmitral pulsed Doppler ultrasound. Am J Cardiol 1989;64:655–60.

[48] Mulvagh S, Quinones MA, Kleiman NS, et al. Estimation of left ventricular end-diastolic pressure

from Doppler transmitral flow velocity in cardiac patients independent of systolic performance. J Am Coll Cardiol 1992;20:112–9.

[49] Vanoverschelde JL, Robert AR, Gerbaux A, et al. Noninvasive estimation of pulmonary arterial wedge pressure with Doppler transmitral flow velocity pattern in patients with known heart disease. Am J Cardiol 1995;75:383–9.

[50] Vanoverschelde JJ, Raphael DA, Robert AR, et al. Left ventricular filling in dilated cardiomyopathy: relation to functional class and hemodynamics. J Am Coll Cardiol 1990;15(6):1288–95.

[51] Nagueh SF, Kopelen HA, Zoghbi WA. Feasibility and accuracy of Doppler echocardiographic estimation of pulmonary artery occlusive pressure in the intensive care unit. Am J Cardiol 1995;75:1256–62.

[52] Nagueh SF, Middleton KJ, Kopelen HA, et al. Doppler tissue imaging: a noninvasive technique for evaluation of left ventricular relaxation and estimation of filling pressures. J Am Coll Cardiol 1997;30(6):1527–33.

[53] Garcia MJ, Thomas JD, Klein AL. New Doppler echocardiographic applications for the study of diastolic function. J Am Coll Cardiol 1998;32:865–75.

[54] Klein AL, Hatle LK, Taliercio CP, et al. Prognostic significance of Doppler measures of diastolic function in cardiac amyloidosis: a Doppler echocardiography study. Circulation 1991;83(3):808–16.

[55] Lorell BH. Left ventricular hypertrophy and diastolic dysfunction. Hosp Pract (Off Ed) 1992;27(10): 189–94.

[56] Hoit BD, Walsh RA. Diastolic function in hypertensive heart disease. In: Gaasch WH, LeWinter MM, editors. Left ventricular diastolic dysfunction and heart failure. Philadelphia: Lea & Febiger; 1994. p. 354–72.

[57] Graettinger WF, Weber MA, Gardin JM, et al. Diastolic blood pressure as a determinant of Doppler left ventricular filling indexes in normotensive adolescents. J Am Coll Cardiol 1987;10(6):1280–5.

[58] Rittoo D, Monaghan M, Sadiq T, et al. Echocardiographic and Doppler evaluation of left ventricular hypertrophy and diastolic function in black and white hypertensive patients. J Hum Hypertens 1990; 4(2):113–5.

[59] Lahiri A, Rodrigues EA, Carboni GP, et al. Effects of long-term treatment with calcium antagonists on left ventricular diastolic function in stable angina and heart failure. Circulation 1990;81(2 Suppl):III130–8.

[60] Myreng Y, Myhre E. Effects of verapamil on left ventricular relaxation and filling dynamics in coronary artery disease: a study by pulsed Doppler echocardiography. Am Heart J 1989;117(4):870–5.

[61] Gaasch WH, Blaustein AS, LeWinter MM. Heart failure and clinical disorders of left ventricular diastolic function. In: Gaasch WW, LeWinter MM, editors. Left ventricular diastolic dysfunction and heart failure. Philadelphia: Lea & Febiger; 1994. p. 245–58.

[62] Carroll JD, Carroll EP. Diastolic function in coronary artery disease. Herz 1991;16(1):1.

[63] Oh JK, Ding ZP, Gersh BJ, et al. Restrictive left ventricular diastolic filling identifies patients with heart failure after acute myocardial infarction. J Am Soc Echocardiogr 1992;5(5):497.

[64] Keren A, Popp RL. Assignment of patients into the classification of cardiomyopathies. Circulation 1992; 86:1622.

[65] Klein AL, Hatle LK, Burstow DJ, et al. Doppler characterization of left ventricular diastolic function in cardiac amyloidosis. J Am Coll Cardiol 1989;13(5): 1017–26.

[66] Cueto-Garcia L, Reeder GS, Kyle RA, et al. Echocardiographic findings in systemic amyloidosis: spectrum of cardiac involvement and relation to survival. J Am Coll Cardiol 1985;6:737–43.

[67] Wigle ED. Diastolic dysfunction in hypertrophic cardiomyopathy. In: Gaasch WH, LeWinter MM, editors. Left ventricular diastolic dysfunction and heart failure. Philadelphia: Lea & Febiger; 1994. p. 373–89.

[68] Brutsaert DL, Rademakers FE, Sys SU. Triple control of relaxation: implications in cardiac disease. Circulation 1984;69(1):190–6.

[69] Brutsaert DL, Sys SU, Gillebert TC. Diastolic failure: pathophysiology and therapeutic implications. J Am Coll Cardiol 1993;22(1):318–25 [Erratum in: J Am Coll Cardiol 1993;22(4):1272].

[70] Nagueh SF, Lakkis NM, Middleton KJ, et al. Changes in left ventricular diastolic function 6 months after nonsurgical septal reduction therapy for hypertrophic obstructive cardiomyopathy. Circulation 1999;99: 344–7.

[71] Rovner A, Smith R, Greenberg NL, et al. Improvement in diastolic intraventricular pressure gradients in patients with HOCM after ethanol septal reduction. Am J Physiol Heart Circ Physiol 2003;285(6): H2492–9.

[72] Yang H, Sun JP, Lever HM, et al. Use of strain imaging in detecting segmental dysfunction in patients with hypertrophic cardiomyopathy. J Am Soc Echocardiog 2003;16(3):233–9.

[73] Ho CY, Sweitzer NK, McDonough B, et al. Assessment of diastolic function with Doppler tissue imaging to predict genotype in preclinical hypertrophic cardiomyopathy. Circulation 2002;105(25): 2992–7.

[74] Xie GY, Berk MR, Smith MD, et al. Prognostic value of Doppler transmitral flow patterns in patients with congestive heart failure. J Am Coll Cardiol 1994;24(1): 132–9.

[75] Desruennes M, Corcos T, Cabrol A. Doppler echocardiography for the diagnosis of acute cardiac allograft rejection. J Am Coll Cardiol 1988;12(1):63–70.

[76] Valantine H, Fowler M, Hatle L, et al. Doppler echocardiographic indices of diastolic function as markers of acute cardiac rejection. Transplant Proc 1987;19(1 Pt 3):2556–9.

[77] Mankad S, Murali S, Mandarino WA, et al. Assessment of acute cardiac allograft rejection by quantitative tissue Doppler echocardiography. Circulation 1997; 96:342.

[78] Puleo JA, Aranda JM, Weston MW, et al. Noninvasive detection of allograft rejection in heart transplant recipients by use of Doppler tissue imaging. J Heart Lung Transpl 1998;17(2):176–84.
[79] Oh JK, Hatle LK, Seward JB, et al. Diagnostic role of Doppler echocardiography in constrictive pericarditis. J Am Coll Cardiol 1994;23(1):154–62.
[80] Hatle L. Diastolic dysfunction in restrictive and constrictive heart disease. In: Gaasch WH, LeWinter MM, editors. Left ventricular diastolic dysfunction and heart failure. Philadelphia: Lea & Febiger; 1994. p. 390–407.
[81] Hatle LK, Appleton CP, Popp RL. Differentiation of constrictive pericarditis and restrictive cardiomyopathy by Doppler echocardiography. Circulation 1989; 79(2):357–70.
[82] Abdalla IA, Murray RD, Lee JC, et al. Does rapid volume loading during transesophageal echocardiography differentiate constrictive pericarditis from restrictive cardiomyopathy? Echocardiography 2002; 19(2):125–34.
[83] Rajogopalan N, Garcia MJ, Rodriguez L, et al. Comparison of new Doppler echocardiographic methods to differentiate constrictive pericardial heart disease and restrictive cardiomyopathy. Am J Cardiol 2001;87(1):86–94.
[84] Vanoverschelde JJ, Essamri B, Vanbutsele R, et al. Contribution of left ventricular diastolic function to exercise capacity in normal subjects. J Appl Physiol 1993;74:2225–33.
[85] Thomas JD, Weyman AE. Numerical modeling of ventricular filling. Ann Biomed Eng 1992;20:19–39.
[86] MacFarlane N, Northridge DB, Wright AR, et al. A comparative study of left ventricular structure and function in elite athletes. Br J Sports Med 1991; 25:45–8.
[87] Coats AJ. Exercise and heart failure. Cardiol Clin 2001;19:517–24.
[88] Higginbotham MB, Morris KG, Conn EH, et al. Determinants of variable exercise performance among patients with severe left ventricular dysfunction. Am J Cardiol 1983:51:52–60.
[89] LeJemtel TH, Liang CS, Stewart DK, et al. Reduced peak aerobic capacity in asymptomatic left ventricular systolic dysfunction. A substudy of the studies of left ventricular dysfunction (SOLVD). SOLVD Investigator. Studies of Left Ventricular Dysfunction. Circulation 1994;90(6):2757–60.

ELSEVIER
SAUNDERS

Heart Failure Clin 2 (2006) 179 – 192

HEART
FAILURE
CLINICS

Myocardial Dyssynchrony and Resynchronization

Theodore P. Abraham, MD[a,*], Albert C. Lardo, PhD[a,b,c], David A. Kass, MD[a,c]

[a]*Division of Cardiology, Johns Hopkins University, Baltimore, MD, USA*
[b]*Department of Radiology, Johns Hopkins University, Baltimore, MD, USA*
[c]*Department of Biomedical Engineering, Johns Hopkins University, Baltimore, MD, USA*

Myocardial dyssynchrony in heart failure

Heart failure is a common cardiovascular condition with more than 500,000 new cases each year and requiring close to 1 billion dollars in health care expenses [1]. During the last decade or so, several publications have noted the prevalence and unfavorable effects of conduction abnormalities in heart failure [2–5]. Conduction delay, most often in the lateral wall, results in early activation and contraction of the septum at a time when the lateral wall is quiescent, and thus in early systole stretches. Subsequent late activation and contraction of the lateral wall occur as the septum is initiating deactivation, resulting in septal bulging. This ventricular dyssynchrony and its associated mechanical abnormalities result in inefficient global contraction and reduced stroke volume [6–8]. Stress is highest in late-activated myocardial regions because of exaggerated prestretch in early systole (secondary to septal contraction) and late systolic contraction against increased afterload [9]. These mechanical perturbations appear to be associated with significant regional molecular changes. Spragg and colleagues [10] demonstrate the regional expression disparities of key proteins involved with stress response (mitogen-activated kinase), calcium handling (eg, phospholamban), and electrophysiology (connexin 43). Dyssynchrony alone, even in the absence of heart failure, results in regionally localized abnormalities in transmural gradients of conduction and repolarization, and in gap junction (connexin 43) myocyte distribution in the late contracting lateral wall [11].

Biventricular pacing, wherein both the right and left ventricles are stimulated simultaneously, was developed in an attempt to "resynchronize" the heart and normalize the mechanical activation sequence [12,13]. Acute hemodynamic studies demonstrated improvements in cardiac output, systolic blood pressure, pulmonary capillary wedge pressure, dP/dtmax, and stroke work [14–19]. Subsequently, several landmark studies showed cardiac resynchronization therapy (CRT) via biventricular pacing reduced symptoms, increased exercise capacity, reduced hospitalizations for heart failure, induced ventricular reverse remodeling, and improved survival in symptomatic heart failure patients refractory to optimal medical therapy [20–25]. Based on the entry criteria employed in these clinical trials, indications for CRT in patients with heart failure are as follows:

- Severe heart failure symptoms on optimal medical therapy (New York Heart Association [NYHA] III or worse)
- Ejection fraction of less than 35%
- Electrocardiographic evidence of conduction abnormality ([QRS] width >120 ms)

Response to cardiac resynchronization therapy

Despite strong evidence of clinical and morphologic improvement after CRT, there appear to be a

* Corresponding author. Division of Cardiology, Johns Hopkins University, 600 North Wolfe Street, Baltimore, MD 21287.
E-mail address: tabraha3@jhmi.edu (T.P. Abraham).

1551-7136/06/$ – see front matter
doi:10.1016/j.hfc.2006.02.001

number of eligible patients who do not respond to this invasive and expensive therapy [26]. Indeed, some patients may experience increased morbidity after CRT [27]. In an attempt to develop better strategies for identifying patients who are most likely to respond to CRT, various clinical, electrocardiographic, and imaging techniques have been, and continue to be, explored.

All the major clinical trials of CRT recruited principally patients with severe heart failure (ie, NYHA class III or greater). There are a few reports of CRT use in less symptomatic patients, but its efficacy in this setting remains less well established. Ongoing studies may help clarify the role of CRT in milder heart failure (Multicenter Automatic Defibrillator Implantation Trial with Cardiac Resynchronization Therapy [MADIT-CRT]) and is currently underway. Reduced ventricular function, as denoted by a low ejection fraction, is an important predictor of response to CRT [18]. Similarly, evidence of conduction abnormality is an important identifier of response to CRT, and improvement from CRT is generally best in individuals with the widest QRS [14,17,28,29]. Conversely, patients with significant heart failure symptoms but without any conduction abnormalities do not seem to benefit from CRT [30]. CRT supposedly corrects mechanical dyssynchrony induced by conduction abnormality (as noted by QRS width). However, there can be a substantial disconnect between electrical synchrony (QRS width) and mechanical synchrony (as determined by MRI or echo-Doppler–based methods) [13]. Almost one third of heart failure patients with narrow QRS complexes may have significant mechanical dyssynchrony, whereas about the same proportion of those with wide QRS complexes may have no mechanical dyssynchrony [31]. These findings have driven recent searches for more reliable identifiers of CRT suitability and responsiveness.

Most recently, Yu and colleagues [32] report that changes in left ventricular (LV) end systolic volume after CRT were strong predictors of long-term survival and heart failure events. A reduction in LV end systolic volume of about 10% had both a sensitivity and specificity of 70% for predicting all-cause mortality, and a sensitivity of 87% and specificity of 69% for predicting cardiovascular mortality. Three to six months after CRT initiation, patients with a 10% reduction in LV end systolic volume had significantly lower all-cause mortality, cardiovascular mortality, and heart failure events, compared with those without similar changes in ventricular volume.

Mechanical synchrony and cardiac resynchronization therapy response

The fundamental abnormality in heart failure patients corrected by CRT is delay in mechanical activation for territories within the LV chamber. It is probably important that early and late regions exist as territories (ie, lateral or posterior wall versus septum) rather than as microdispersed regions throughout the ventricle. Mechanical dyssynchrony can be visually evident by examining regional wall motion, but it is not obvious in most cases. Mechanical dyssynchrony was examined quantitatively by Nelson and colleagues [29] using MRI measures and Yu and colleagues [33] employing tissue Doppler echocardiography. In the former study, global acute hemodynamic response best correlated with mechanical dyssynchrony measured at baseline. In the latter, CRT reduced dyssynchrony quickly, but the dyssynchrony also reappeared quickly after CRT was suspended 3 months later. Thus, both studies support the importance of per-beat delivery of CRT to generate mechanical resynchronization. Some other features of CRT, such as chronic reverse chamber remodeling, behaved differently. Yu and colleagues showed gradual declines in end-systolic and diastolic volumes over the 3 months of CRT that did not change acutely when CRT was then stopped. During the ensuing 4 weeks, gradual chamber dilation reappeared. Sogaard and colleagues [34] and Pitzalis and colleagues [35] subsequently revealed chronic correlations between basal estimated chamber dyssynchrony and chronic reverse remodeling with CRT, the latter serving as a surrogate marker for responsiveness. Bax and colleagues [27] recently found similar predictive value using clinical outcome parameters.

Conventional echocardiography

Conventional and novel echocardiographic techniques have been used to assess both inter- and intraventricular dyssynchrony. Interventricular dyssynchrony denotes mechanical delay in activation of the right and left ventricle. Normally, both ventricles are synchronized and activate almost simultaneously. In heart failure, delayed LV lateral wall activation results in a significant delay in LV ejection, compared with the right ventricle. This interventricular mechanical delay is assessed most commonly by measuring the time delay between onset of flow in the right and left ventricular outflow tracts by pulsed wave Doppler (Fig. 1). Data from the Italian InSync registry [36] suggest that a right-left outflow delay

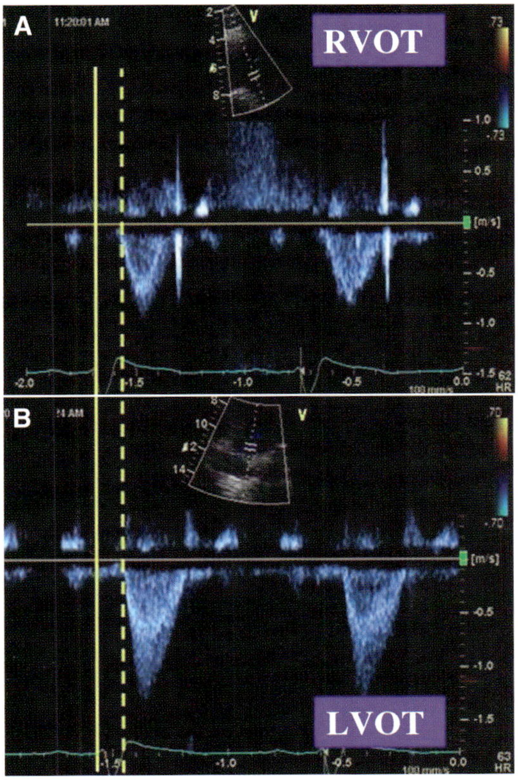

Fig. 1. Measurement of interventricular mechanical delay. A pulsed Doppler flow signal is obtained from outflow tracts of both ventricles. The time from a fiducial point on the EKG (*solid line*) to the onset of flow (*dashed line*) in the right ventricular outflow tract (*A*) and left ventricular outflow tract (*B*) is determined. In this normal example, the onset of flow in both ventricles is simultaneous.

of greater than 45 ms could identify patients with significant dyssynchrony. However, subsequent studies comparing this parameter to measures of intraventricular dyssynchrony found interventricular dyssynchrony to be neither an accurate measure of dyssynchrony nor a reliable predictor of post-CRT improvement [33,35,37].

Conventional echocardiography has also been used to assess intraventricular dyssynchrony. Pitzalis and colleagues [35] used M-mode echocardiography to measure the delay between posterior and septal inward motion (Fig. 2). In this study, septal to posterior wall motion delay (SPWMD) appeared to be a better predictor of reverse remodeling than interventricular mechanical delay by flow Doppler [35]. An improvement in ejection fraction was observed in 79% of patients with SPWMD of greater than 130 ms, compared with 9% in those with SPWMD of less than 130 ms [38]. Although simple, this approach has some disadvantages. Identifying the exact time of peak contraction in a particular wall can be challenging, especially in patients with poor overall wall motion.

Tissue Doppler echocardiography

Tissue Doppler echocardiography (TDE) uses the Doppler principle to track tissue (myocardial motion) rather than blood flow [39–41], employing a pulsed Doppler sample volume or a sample volume within a two-dimensional Doppler sector. Tissue Doppler techniques are used commonly to assess myocardial function in cardiomyopathy and ischemia, and during diastole [42–49]. This method yields the speed at which a particular portion of myocardium moves and its displacement (the absolute distance that the portion of myocardium moves). Using TDE, a tissue

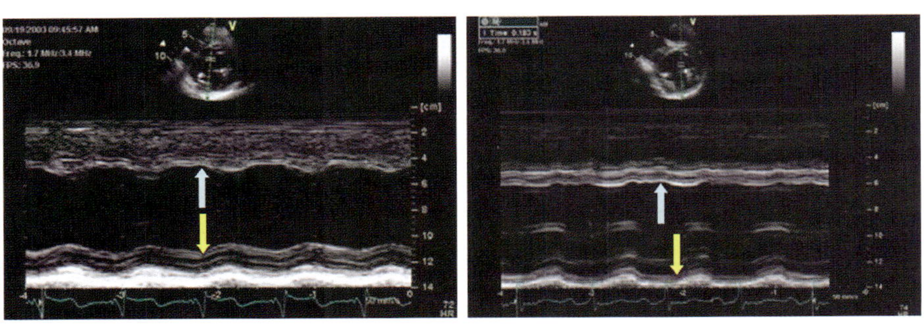

Fig. 2. Septal to posterior wall motion delay by M-mode echocardiography. An M-mode cursor is placed in the midventricular short axis view of the left ventricle. Onset of thickening in the septal and posterior segments is identified. In a normal synchronous heart the onset of thickening is almost simultaneous (*left*); however, in a dyssynchronous heart (*right*) there is a substantial delay in onset of thickening in the posterior wall.

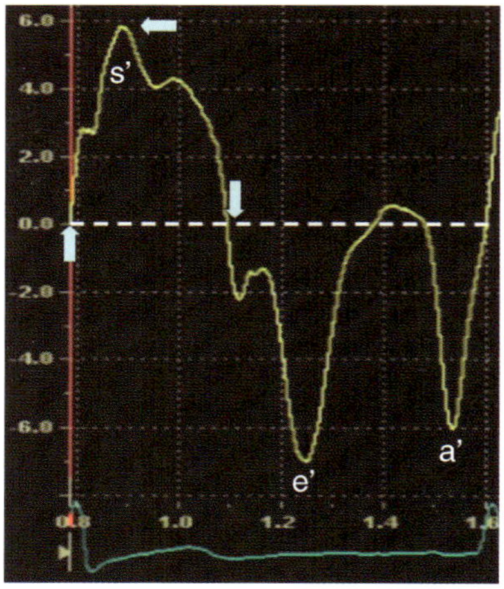

Fig. 3. Tissue velocity tracing obtained from the basal segment of the septum. The initial positive wave denotes systole (*s'*) and the first and second negative waves denote early (*e'*) and late (*a'*) diastolic velocities. The start of contraction occurs when the s' wave leaves the baseline (*up arrow*), peak contraction is the peak amplitude of the s' wave (*left arrow*) and the end of contraction is when the s' wave returns to the baseline (*down arrow*).

velocity tracing is obtained and the integral of tissue velocity yields displacement. In the longitudinal direction (apical views), the apex of the heart is generally immobile while the base moves toward the apex during systole and away from the apex during diastole. A TDE sample placed in the base of the heart would display a positive wave in systole and a negative wave in diastole (Fig. 3). Tissue velocity tracings denote when a segment starts contracting, when the contraction peaks, and when the contraction ends (Fig. 3). Two-dimensional TDE can interrogate mechanical behavior in various portions of the myocardium simultaneously.

TDE data must be synthesized into a dyssynchrony index [50]. The most common approach is to assess the time delay between the tissue velocity systolic peaks at the septal and lateral walls. These curves are usually superimposed in normal hearts, whereas there is substantial delay in heart failure subjects with dyssynchrony (Fig. 4). In addition to the maximal delay between the walls [51], investigators have assessed the variability of delays around the heart, such as the standard deviation of times to peak systolic tissue velocity in 12 basal and midsegments from three standard apical views. This method was suggested by Yu and colleagues as the most predictive of ventricular reverse remodeling [33]. A cutoff value of more than 32 ms predicted improvement after CRT. Another approach is to add delays [52], with a sum of greater than 102 ms predicting an increase in ejection fraction after CRT. More recent studies [27,53] suggest that a maximal intraventricular delay of greater than 65 ms can best identify clinical responders to CRT. According to Bax and colleagues, this cutoff of 65 ms best identified patients who experienced adverse outcomes (mortality and heart failure progression). Most TDE analysis has been performed in the longitudinal direction, although experimental data suggest this may not be the optimal orientation for discerning both dyssynchrony and the impact of CRT [54]. Recent data obtained using angle-corrected TDE in the radial direction suggest radial velocities can also detect dyssynchrony and predict acute response to CRT [55].

The method of measurement of TDE time delays is somewhat time-consuming, especially if multiple

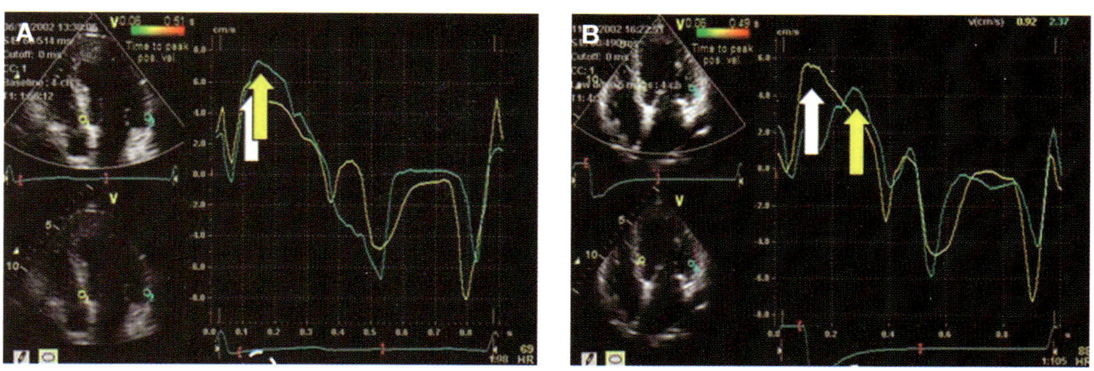

Fig. 4. Representative tissue velocity tracings obtained from the basal septal (*white arrow*) and basal lateral (*yellow arrow*) wall in a 4-chamber apical view of the heart. Systolic tissue velocity peaks almost simultaneously in the normal heart (*A*), whereas there is a delayed lateral systolic peak in the dyssynchronous heart (*B*).

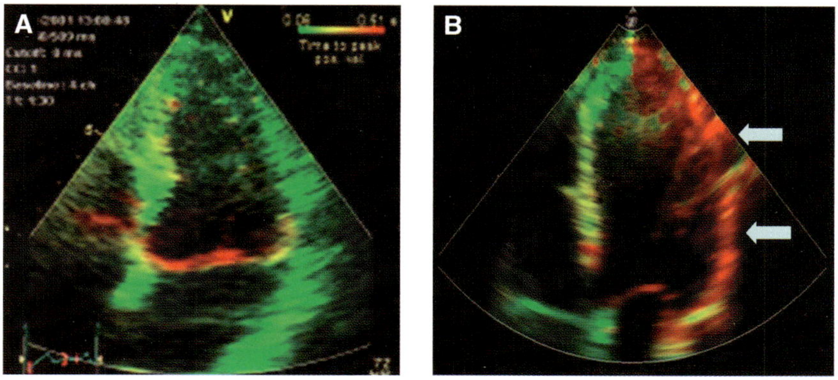

Fig. 5. Color-coded parametric image of time to peak systolic tissue velocity. In this particular program, green indicates normal synchrony (*A*) and red indicates dyssynchrony (*B*). In this example, lateral wall segments colored red (*arrows*) are delayed significantly, compared with the septal wall segments colored green.

segments are interrogated. Therefore, manufacturers have introduced "parametric" imaging techniques that color-code the segments based on the time delay (Fig. 5). These techniques allow physicians to perform a quick initial screen of the color-coded image before making a decision to perform the more laborious manual determination of the absolute time delay [53]. These parametric imaging techniques may allow more routine clinical application of TDE in patient selection for CRT. However, one must remember that the intrinsic signals upon which the imaging is based are the same TDE velocity plots, and the quality of the color-coded image cannot be better than the raw signals upon which it is based.

Strain echocardiography

Tissue velocity measures tissue motion (displacement) at a single point along the ultrasound beam and is therefore susceptible to cardiac translational motion and tethering artifacts. Measurement of strain, on the other hand, depicts regional deformation references typically to diastole, and is less susceptible to such artifacts. Initially, strain was determined noninvasively using MRI [56,57], but now it can be assessed by TDE as well [58–61]. Although one might expect strain analysis to provide information about dyssynchrony that is similar to, if not better than, velocity-based TDE, there are limited data confirming this. Indeed, one study found the opposite to be true [62], although this may be because of the orientation of the Doppler analysis (ie, long axis versus short axis) [54]. Certainly, data from MRI studies in animals and humans have shown that circumferential strain provides a reliable analysis of dyssynchrony. Doppler-derived strain signals are currently noisy. However, advances in technology that improve signal-to-noise ratio and multi-dimensional strain [63] may allow better assessment of the role of SE in dyssynchrony analysis.

Contrast echocardiography

Kawaguchi and colleagues [64] explored the use of echocardiographic contrast to obtain information on regional dyssynchrony. This novel echocardiographic method used contrast variability imaging to quantify dyssynchrony. Thirty to fifty consecutive images of the heart, gated to the cardiac cycle, were obtained before and during contrast injection. At each phase and for each pixel, the temporal average and variance were determined from the total set of cycles. The final pixel intensity was set to the variance/mean ratio and resulted in the contrast variability image. Using this type of imaging, the investigators provided one of the first human demonstrations of a significant decline in spatial and temporal dyssynchrony with LV or biventricular pacing. Decline in dyssynchrony correlated with increase in ejection fraction. This method, however, has not been used widely, given the requirements for injected echocontrast and data processing.

Three-dimensional echocardiography

Real-time three-dimensional echocardiography (3DE) uses a matrix array transducer to obtain a real-time pyramidal volume scan of the heart. Because real-time scan volumes are relatively narrow, acquisition of real-time images of the entire heart is facilitated by widening the sector and acquiring images from every other cardiac cycle. This is called a full volume acquisition. For quantitative analysis of dyssynchrony using 3DE, the system defines a number of 2D slices through the voxel-based 3D data set. In each of the slices, the endocardial border is traced with a semiautomated detection process and a "cast" of the LV cavity is created as a mathematical model, providing time-volume data for the entire cardiac cycle. By dividing this volume into pyramidal subvolumes based around a nonfixed central point, it is possible to gain an estimation of time-volume data corresponding to each of the 16 standard myocardial segments, as defined by the American Society of Echocardiography [65]. A systolic dyssynchrony index (SDI) can be derived from the dispersion of time to minimum regional volume for all 16 LV segments (Fig. 6).

Using real-time 3DE, Zhang and colleagues [66] demonstrated dyssynchrony in heart failure patients with CRT-off compared with CRT-on modes. These 3DE-derived measures of dyssynchrony correlate well with previously validated TDE measures of dyssynchrony (ie, standard deviation of time to peak velocity in 12 segments). Subsequently, Kapetanakis and colleagues [65] studied 89 healthy volunteers and 174 unselected subjects using 3DE. Healthy subjects and cases with normal LV systolic function had a highly synchronized segmental function of 3.5 ± 1.8% with a systolic dyssynchrony index of 4.5 ± 2.4%. However, this index increased with worsening LV systolic function, regardless of QRS duration (mild LV dysfunction, 5.4 ± 0.83%; moderate LV dysfunction, 10.0 ± 2%; severe LV dysfunction, 15.6 ± 1%; *P* for trend <0.001). Using 3DE, the investigators found that 37% of subjects with moderate to severe LV systolic dysfunction had significant dyssynchrony with normal QRS durations (dyssynchrony index of 14.7 ± 1.2%). The 3DE-based index decreased substantially after CRT and responders demonstrated reverse remodeling with a decrease in end-diastolic volume and an increase in LV ejection fraction.

One potential limitation of 3DE is its reduced temporal resolution.

Table 1 summarizes information from clinical studies using all echocardiography techniques.

MRI

MRI allows detailed interrogation of cardiac structure and function with high spatial resolution and is relatively operator independent. Quantitative MRI-based strain techniques have been used to assess myocardial mechanics [56,57]. The potential advantages of MRI-based techniques for dyssynchrony assessment include excellent reproducibility, high spatial resolution, and the ability to obtain three-dimensional information, including mechanics, in the circumferential orientation [67]. Recent data suggest that interrogation of myocardial mechanics in the

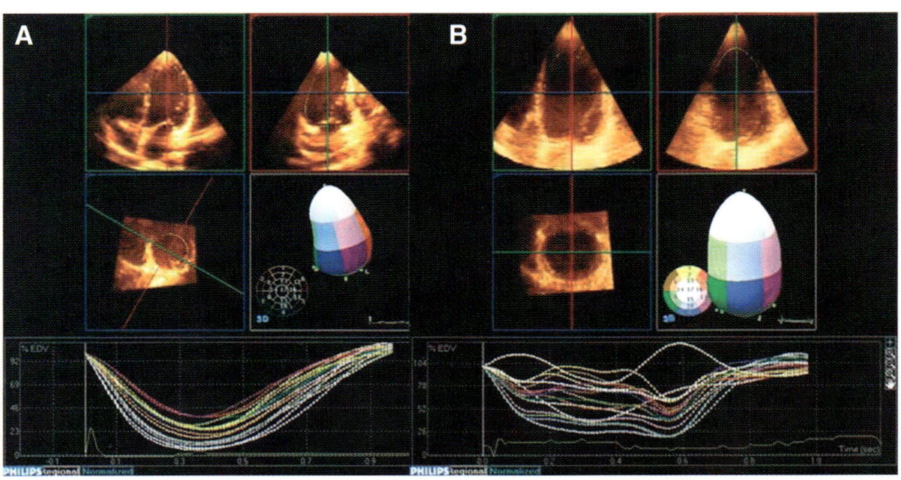

Fig. 6. Three-dimensional echocardiography images illustrating the use of regional volumetry analysis for dyssynchrony assessment. In a normal synchronous ventricle, all segments demonstrate a simultaneous decrease in regional volume (*A*), whereas there is a significant dispersion of time to minimal systolic volume in a dyssynchronous ventricle (*B*).

circumferential direction may be superior to interrogation in the longitudinal direction [54].

Myocardial tagging by MRI allows assessment of regional strain. This technique was described initially more than a decade ago and was the first technique that allowed non-invasive determination of regional mechanics [56,57]. Tagging is the placement of a series of markers (or tags) within the myocardium by using special encoding pulses. The tags appear as dark lines within the image and deform with the myocardium during the cardiac cycle. Analysis of the movement of these tags can help to determine local deformation and strain. Tagging allows determination of strain along three primary orientations – radial, longitudinal, and circumferential (Fig. 7). Current analysis programs for tagged MRI data are time-consuming and may limit its clinical application. However, recent advances in analysis of tagged images have drastically reduced analysis time from several days to a few minutes. Harmonic phase (HARP) analysis of tagged MRI measures motion by filtering certain regions called harmonic peaks in the frequency domain of the images [68,69]. The resulting image is then decomposed into a harmonic magnitude and harmonic phase, which are related to the underlying anatomy of the heart and tag deformation, respectively. The HARP method determines the local strain by measuring the frequency of the tag lines. The number of tags per unit length is called the frequency of the tag pattern. If the tissue contracts, the tag lines become closer to each other and the tag frequency increases in proportion to the contraction, and vice versa (Fig. 8). The HARP technique has been validated and has been used to quantitatively characterize regional function in animals and patients with myocardial infarction [70]. Recently, our laboratory used a two-dimensional HARP analysis to determine the optimal LV pacing site for bi-pacing in a canine model of dyssynchronous heart failure [71]. We have also used it to isolate the effect of infarct extent and location in patients with ischemic dyssynchronous heart failure [72].

Strain-encoded MRI

Strain-encoded (SENC) MRI is a new method of measuring regional strain that requires less complex image processing [73]. As a result, it is faster than HARP analysis, which still requires some postprocessing. SENC imaging is derived from a standard myocardial tagging sequence in which the tissue at end-diastole is tagged with a sinusoidal pattern designed to modulate the longitudinal magnetization orthogonal to the imaging plane. Deformation of tissue during systole will change the local frequency of the pattern in proportion to the through-plane strain component. The distribution of regional contraction (circumferential shortening in long-axis views or longitudinal compression in short-axis views) is then displayed as contrast in the images. Advantages of the SENC technique include

- Instantaneous real-time quantitative strain measurements without the need for user intervention
- Higher spatial resolution over standard tagging as a result of reduced tag spacing
- Acquisition of both circumferential and longitudinal myocardial strain information

Dyssynchrony indices by MRI

Given the more comprehensive strain data generally obtained by MRI methods, a number of approaches have been developed to assess 3-D dyssynchrony. The methods are not specific to this imaging approach, however, and can be employed as well using TDE-derived measurements.

The *regional variance of strain* is determined from the variance of strain magnitude obtained from 28 radially displaced segments for each short-axis section and averaged among slices for each time point. This approach is similar to the commonly used indexes based on TDE [33]. A variation has been to count the total number of regional segments with delayed shortening (expressed as a percentage of total regions examined) [29]. This method has some limitations in that it cannot differentiate between having segments with delayed contraction clustered in one portion of the LV wall (Fig. 9A, *top*), and having them dispersed throughout the heart more homogeneously (Fig. 9A, *bottom*). While the variance of time to peak contraction is identical in both examples, the mechanical consequences on dyssynchrony are very different, with only the former displaying dyssynchrony.

Another approach derives a *regional variance vector of principal strain*, where a unit vector pointing to a given radial position of a segment in a short axis slice is multiplied by a scalar, which can be time at maximal shortening or instantaneous magnitude of shortening (or strain). A vector sum is then determined that will only have significant magnitude if delayed versus early regions are geographically clustered (Fig. 9A, *top*) [54,74].

Lastly, analysis of regional differences in strain at a given moment in time can be used to deter-

Table 1
Summary of representative echocardiographic studies on assessment of dyssynchrony

Investigators	Subjects (n)	Follow-up period (months)	Echo technique	Dyssynchrony parameters	Findings	Sensitivity (%)	Specificity (%)
Pitzalis et al	20	1	M-mode	Septal-to-posterior wall motion delay	Septal-to-posterior delay $\geq$130 ms predicted LV reverse remodeling	100	63
Pitzalis et al	60	14	M-mode	Septal-to-posterior wall motion delay	Septal-to-posterior delay $\geq$130 ms predicted event-free survival	NA	NA
Rose et al	79	6	M-mode	Septal-to-posterior wall motion delay	Septal-to-posterior delay $\geq$130 ms insufficient to predict LV reverse remodeling	24	66
Breithardt et al	34	Acute	2D phase imaging	Difference between the lateral and septal wall motion phase angles	Delayed lateral wall motion predicted acute hemodynamic improvement	NA	NA
Kawaguchi et al	10	9	Contrast echo	Septal and lateral fractional area changes	↑ Septal inward motion, ↓ spatial and temporal LV dyssynchrony by 40%, and correlated with ↑ LVEF	NA	NA
Penicka et al	49	6	Pulsed-wave TDI	Ts(onset) of 3 basal LV and 1 basal RV segments	Summation of inter- and intra(LV)-ventricular delay >102 ms predicted ↑ LVEF	96	71
Ansalone et al	21	1	Pulsed-wave TDI	Systolic dyssynchrony among 5 basal segments	Extensive LV dyssynchrony resulted in ↑ in symptoms, and ↑ LVEF	NA	NA
Garrigue et al	12	12	Pulsed-wave TDI	Ts(onset) between septum and lateral wall	Post-CRT reduction in LV dyssynchrony and improvement in symptoms	NA	NA
Bordachar et al	41	3	Pulsed-wave TDI, M-mode, pulsed-wave Doppler	Maximal difference in 12 LV segments for Ts, Ts(onset), Ts-SD, and DLC	Maximal difference in 12 LV segments for Ts, T(onset), Ts-SD closely correlated with improvement of MR and CO, but not interventricular delay by pulsed-wave Doppler echo	NA	NA
Yu et al	25	3	Color-coded TDI	Ts of 12 LV segments in ejection phase	Improve LV dyssynchrony by delaying Ts in 12 LV segments globally resulting in homogenous Ts	NA	NA
Bax et al	25	Acute	Color-coded TDI	Septal-to-lateral delay of Ts in ejection phase	Septal-to-lateral delay of Ts $\geq$60 ms predicted ↑ LVEF	76	88
Yu et al	30	3	Color-coded TDI	Ts-SD of 12 LV segments in ejection phase	Ts-SD of 12 LV segments >33 ms predicted LV reverse remodeling	NA	NA
Bax et al	85	12	Color-coded TDI	Septal-to-lateral delay of Ts in ejection phase	Septal-to-lateral delay of Ts $\geq$65 ms predicted LV reverse remodeling; and associated with lower event rate	92	92

Notabartolo et al	49	3	Color-coded TDI	Maximal difference in Ts in 6 basal segments (both ejection phase and post-systolic shortening)	Maximal difference in Ts in 6 basal segments >110 ms predicted reverse remodeling	97	55
Yu et al	54	3	Color-coded TDI, SRI	Ts-SD of 12 LV segments in ejection phase (and 17 other parameters)	Ts-SD of 12 LV segments >31 ms predicted LV reverse remodeling	96	78
Sogaard et al	20	12	Color-coded TDI, SRI	DLC	Number of basal segments with DLC predicted ↑ LVEF	NA	NA
Sogaard et al	20	Acute	Color-coded TDI, TT, SRI	TT and DLC	Optimization of V-V timing by TT resulted in ↓ DLC and ↑ LVEF	NA	NA
Breithardt et al	18	Acute	Strain, SRI	Strain and SRI at septal and lateral walls	Baseline: lateral wall strain and strain rate higher than septal; CRT: septal wall strain and strain rate higher than lateral	NA	NA
Sun et al	34	Acute	Displacement, strain, and SRI	Strain, SRI, and displacement at septal and lateral walls	↑ LVEF and ↑ peak strain rate at lateral wall by CRT; ↑ Septal and inferior wall displacement by LV pacing	NA	NA
Popović et al	22	1–12	Displacement and strain	Strain at septal and lateral walls	↑ Global LV peak strain, ↓ coefficient of change in LV strain, no change in septal or lateral wall displacement	NA	NA
Dohi et al	38	Acute	TSI and strain	Peak radial strain septum versus posterior wall	Delay in septal-posterior strain ≥130 ms, predicted ↑ stroke volume	95	88
Gorcsan III et al	29	Acute	TSI	Septal-posterior delay (both ejection phase and post-systolic shortening)	Septal-posterior delay ≥65 ms predicted ↑ stroke volume	87	100
Yu et al	56	3	TSI	Ts-SD of 12 LV segments in ejection phase (inclusion of post-systolic shortening)	Ts-SD of 12 LV segments in ejection phase >34 ms predicted reverse LV remodeling	87	81
Zhang et al	13	3	3D echo	Time to minimal systolic volume (Tmsv) in 6, 12, and 16 LV segments	Improvement of Tmsv parameters during CRT Tmsv of 16 LV segments by 3D echo correlated closely with Ts-SD of 12 LV segments by TDI	NA	NA

Abbreviations: CO, cardiac output; CRT, cardiac resynchronization therapy; DLC, delayed longitudinal contraction; LV, left ventricular; LVEF, left ventricular ejection fraction; MR, mitral regurgitation; NA, not available; RV, right ventricular; SRI, strain rate imaging; TDI, tissue Doppler imaging; TMSV, time to minimal systolic volume; Ts, time to peak myocardial systolic velocity; TSI, tissue synchronization imaging; Ts(onset), time to onset of myocardial systolic velocity; Ts-SD, standard deviation of time to peak myocardial systolic velocity; TT, tissue tracking; V-V, interventricular.

(*Data from* Bax JJ, Abraham T, Barold SS, et al. Cardiac resynchronization therapy: Part 1—issues before device implantation. J Am Coll Cardiol 2005;46:2153–67. Please refer to this publication for details of references quoted in the table.)

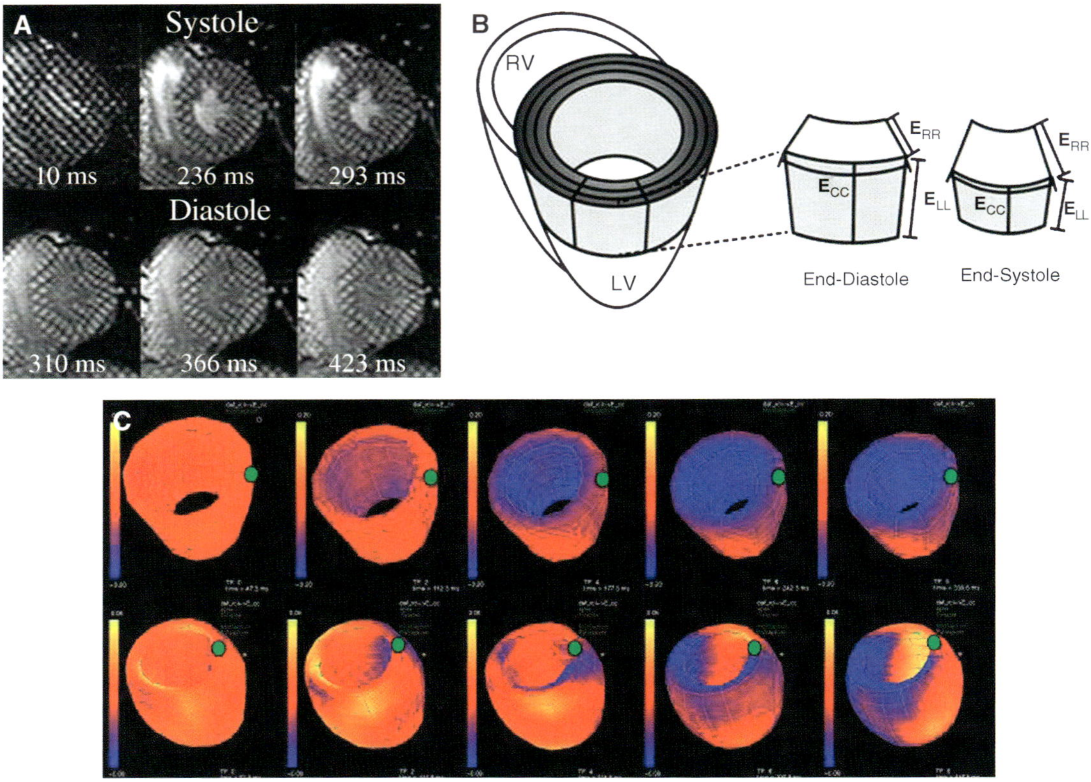

Fig. 7. (*A*) MRI myocardial tagging during systole (*top*) and diastole (*bottom*). (*B*) Direction of myocardial strains. (*C*) Individual phases from the cardiac cycle showing the spatial and temporal evolution of three-dimensional circumferential strain for a normal healthy human heart (*top*) and that of a patient with severe cardiomyopathy and left bundle branch-type conduction delay (*bottom*). Time moves from left (end-diastole) to right (end-systole). During systolic contraction, the spatial and temporal distribution of circumferential strain are visualized by the color changes, where red corresponds to the neutral (end-diastolic) strain, blue is shortening, and yellow is lengthening or stretch. E_{CC}, circumferential strain; E_{LL}, longitudinal strain; E_{RR}, radial strain; LV, left ventricle; RV, right ventricle. (*From* Lardo AC, Abraham TP, Kass DA. Magnetic resonance imaging assessment of ventricular dyssynchrony: current and emerging concepts. J Am Coll Cardiol 2005;46:2224; with permission.)

mine *regional strain uniformity*. Time plots of strain (shortening/stretching) are generated at each of 28 evenly distributed segments around a short-axis slice (Fig. 9B) [13,54]. If segments shorten simultaneously (perfectly synchronous contraction), the plot appears as a straight line. In contrast, regionally clustered dyssynchrony (ie, territory of early versus late activation) generates an undulating plot sort with higher power in the first-order term. The relative ratio of first to zero order magnitudes derived by Fourier analysis generates the index. Two examples corresponding to the hearts in Fig. 9A are shown in Fig. 9C. The heart with clustered regions shows delays in one territory more than the other, so this plot appears more or less sinusoidal. The other example shows more variability around the heart, yielding a higher frequency waveform. If one applies a low-pass filter (ie, relative amplitude of the first harmonic normalized to the mean), then only the former will indicate dyssynchrony; the latter will not. This index is referred to as the circumferential uniformity ratio estimate (CURE). The CURE index compares favorably with vector sum methods [54].

The potential disadvantages of MRI include cost, longer imaging time, lack of availability, complex and long analysis times, and incompatibility with implanted devices. However, advances in technology have significantly reduced cost, imaging time and analysis times. In addition, recent studies suggest that MRI may be safe in patients with implanted devices [75].

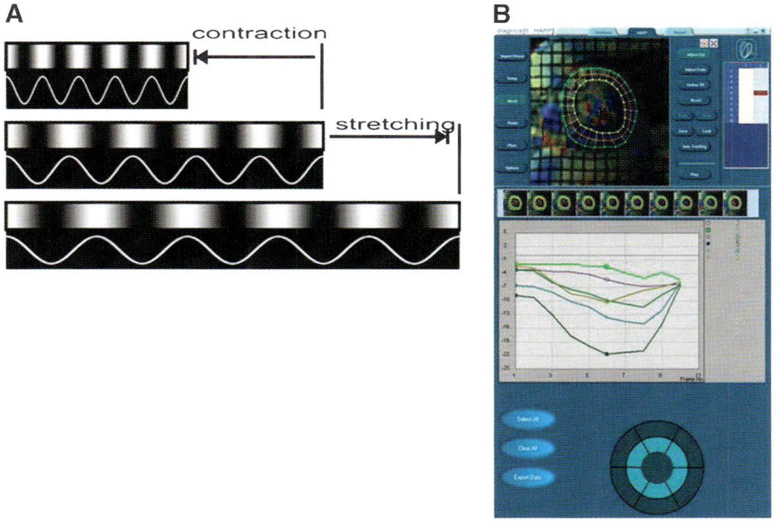

Fig. 8. (*A*) Relationship between local strain and tag frequency for harmonic-phase–based strain measurements. The contraction of a tagged fiber in the middle would increase the tagging frequency (density of tag lines), as shown in the top fiber. Stretching causes a reduction in local frequency. (*B*) Two-dimensional segmentation of the heart and mesh generation (*top*) and regional strain versus time plots over the cardiac cycle (*bottom*). (*From* Lardo AC, Abraham TP, Kass DA. Magnetic resonance imaging assessment of ventricular dyssynchrony: current and emerging concepts. J Am Coll Cardiol 2005;46:2225; with permission.)

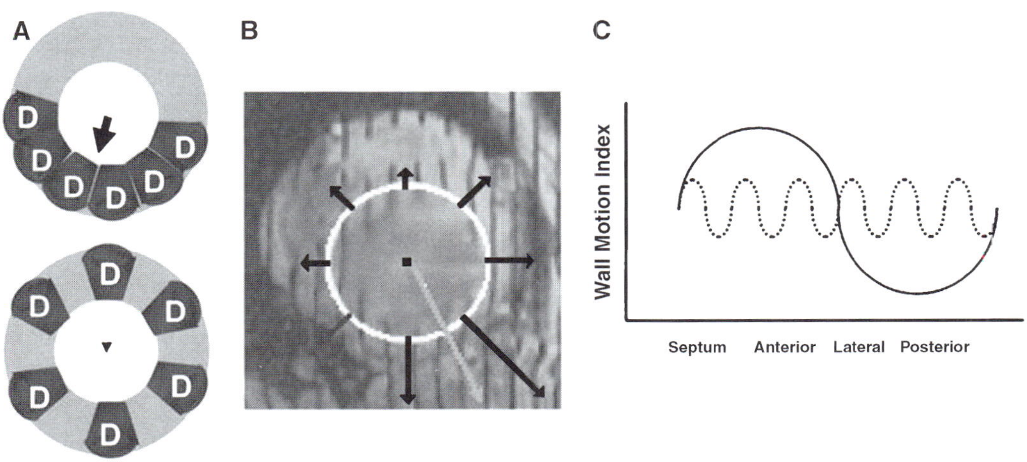

Fig. 9. (*A*) Hearts with delayed segments clustered in one region (*top*) versus distributed evenly about the myocardium (*bottom*). Depending on how one indexes dyssynchrony, the result could be the same for both situations, despite markedly different impacts on dyssynchrony. (*B*) Calculation of a vector-dyssynchrony index. Values of regional shortening (strain) or time of peak shortening are determined at various positions in the cross-section. These are then multiplied by a unit vector pointing in that direction and the vectors are summed to generate the net (gray) vector magnitude. Greater net vector magnitude reflects dyssynchrony. (*C*) Determination of the temporal uniformity of strain or circumferential uniformity ratio estimate index. A measure of wall motion or timing value is plotted against location. Overall dyssynchrony appears as a sine-wave (analogous to the situation shown in top panel of *A*). If delays are dispersed through the wall (*bottom of A*), the plot appears as the dotted line. By determining the low-frequency content of these plots, one derives the dyssynchrony index. (*From* Lardo AC, Abraham TP, Kass DA. Magnetic resonance imaging assessment of ventricular dyssynchrony: current and emerging concepts. J Am Coll Cardiol 2005;46:2227; with permission.)

Summary

Conduction abnormalities are noted in a number of patients with heart failure and are associated with altered ventricular mechanics (mechanical dyssynchrony), resulting in reduced and inefficient systolic function. Correction of mechanical dyssynchrony via biventricular pacing (cardiac resynchronization) is associated with substantial symptomatic benefits, reverse remodeling of the left ventricle, reduced hospitalizations for heart failure, and improved survival. However, approximately 30% of eligible patients undergoing CRT do not experience clinical benefits. Recent published data suggest that assessment of mechanical synchrony with echocardiography, especially newer techniques such as TDE, may be a reliable and accurate means of identifying patients who will best respond to CRT. A septal-to-lateral wall time delay of 65 ms, or a standard deviation of time to peak velocity exceeding 32 ms, appear to be the best predictors of ventricular reverse remodeling. MRI provides three-dimensional information on regional mechanics and may emerge as an important technique for assessment of dyssynchrony. New MRI programs enable faster and less operator-dependent analysis, making MRI more feasible for routine clinical use.

References

[1] American Heart Association. 2000 Heart and Stroke Statistical Update. Dallas, TX. American Heart Association Web site, 2000, 1999. Available at: http://www.americanheart.org. Accessed February 10, 2006.

[2] Askenazi J, Alexander JH, Koenigsberg DI, et al. Alteration of left ventricular performance by left bundle branch block simulated with atrioventricular sequential pacing. Am J Cardiol 1984;53:99–104.

[3] Grines CL, Bashore TM, Boudoulas H, et al. Functional abnormalities in isolated left bundle branch block. The effect of interventricular asynchrony. Circulation 1989;79:845–53.

[4] Xiao HB, Lee CH, Gibson DG. Effect of left bundle branch block on diastolic function in dilated cardiomyopathy. Br Heart J 1991;66:443–7.

[5] Xiao HB, Roy C, Fujimoto S, et al. Natural history of abnormal conduction and its relation to prognosis in patients with dilated cardiomyopathy. Int J Cardiol 1996;53:163–70.

[6] Prinzen FW, Augustijn CH, Arts T, et al. Redistribution of myocardial fiber strain and blood flow by asynchronous activation. Am J Physiol 1990;259:H300–8.

[7] Prinzen FW, Hunter WC, Wyman BT, et al. Mapping of regional myocardial strain and work during ventricular pacing: experimental study using magnetic resonance imaging tagging. J Am Coll Cardiol 1999;33:1735–42.

[8] Wyman BT, Hunter WC, Prinzen FW, et al. Mapping propagation of mechanical activation in the paced heart with MRI tagging. Am J Physiol 1999;276:H881–91.

[9] Curry CW, Nelson GS, Wyman BT, et al. Mechanical dyssynchrony in dilated cardiomyopathy with intraventricular conduction delay as depicted by 3D tagged magnetic resonance imaging. Circulation 2000;101:E2.

[10] Spragg DD, Leclercq C, Loghmani M, et al. Regional alterations in protein expression in the dyssynchronous failing heart. Circulation 2003;108:929–32.

[11] Spragg DD, Akar FG, Helm RH, et al. Abnormal conduction and repolarization in late-activated myocardium of dyssynchronously contracting hearts. Cardiovasc Res 2005;67:77–86.

[12] De Teresa P, Chamoro J. An even more physiological pacing: changing the sequence of ventricular activation. Proceedings, VIIth World Symposium of Cardiac Pacing. Vienna, Austria 1983;95:100.

[13] Leclercq C, Faris O, Tunin R, et al. Systolic improvement and mechanical resynchronization does not require electrical synchrony in the dilated failing heart with left bundle-branch block. Circulation 2002;106:1760–3.

[14] Auricchio A, Stellbrink C, Block M, et al. Effect of pacing chamber and atrioventricular delay on acute systolic function of paced patients with congestive heart failure. The pacing therapies for congestive heart failure study group. The guidant congestive heart failure research group. Circulation 1999;99:2993–3001.

[15] Blanc JJ, Etienne Y, Gilard M, et al. Evaluation of different ventricular pacing sites in patients with severe heart failure: results of an acute hemodynamic study. Circulation 1997;96:3273–7.

[16] Cazeau S, Ritter P, Lazarus A, et al. Multisite pacing for end-stage heart failure: early experience. Pacing Clin Electrophysiol 1996;19:1748–57.

[17] Kass DA, Chen CH, Curry C, et al. Improved left ventricular mechanics from acute VDD pacing in patients with dilated cardiomyopathy and ventricular conduction delay. Circulation 1999;99:1567–73.

[18] Leclercq C, Cazeau S, Le Breton H, et al. Acute hemodynamic effects of biventricular DDD pacing in patients with end-stage heart failure. J Am Coll Cardiol 1998;32:1825–31.

[19] Mansourati J, Etienne Y, Gilard M, et al. Left ventricular-based pacing in patients with chronic heart failure: comparison of acute hemodynamic benefits according to underlying heart disease. Eur J Heart Fail 2000;2:195–9.

[20] Abraham WT, Fisher WG, Smith AL, et al. Cardiac resynchronization in chronic heart failure. N Engl J Med 2002;346:1845–53.

[21] Auricchio A, Stellbrink C, Sack S, et al. Long-term clinical effect of hemodynamically optimized cardiac resynchronization therapy in patients with heart failure and ventricular conduction delay. J Am Coll Cardiol 2002;39:2026–33.

[22] Bakker PF, Meijburg HW, de Vries JW, et al. Biventricular pacing in end-stage heart failure improves functional capacity and left ventricular function. J Interv Card Electrophysiol 2000;4:395–404.

[23] Bristow MR, Feldman AM, Saxon LA. Heart failure management using implantable devices for ventricular resynchronization: Comparison of Medical Therapy, Pacing, and Defibrillation in Chronic Heart Failure (COMPANION) trial. COMPANION Steering Committee and COMPANION Clinical Investigators. J Card Fail 2000;6:276–85.

[24] Cazeau S, Leclercq C, Lavergne T, et al. Effects of multisite biventricular pacing in patients with heart failure and intraventricular conduction delay. N Engl J Med 2001;344:873–80.

[25] Cleland JG, Daubert JC, Erdmann E, et al. The effect of cardiac resynchronization on morbidity and mortality in heart failure. N Engl J Med 2005;352:1539–49.

[26] Abraham WT, Fisher WG, Smith AL, et al. Cardiac resynchronization in chronic heart failure. N Engl J Med 2002;346:1845–53.

[27] Bax JJ, Bleeker GB, Marwick TH, et al. Left ventricular dyssynchrony predicts response and prognosis after cardiac resynchronization therapy. J Am Coll Cardiol 2004;44:1834–40.

[28] Alonso C, Leclercq C, Victor F, et al. Electrocardiographic predictive factors of long-term clinical improvement with multisite biventricular pacing in advanced heart failure. Am J Cardiol 1999;84:1417–21.

[29] Nelson GS, Curry CW, Wyman BT, et al. Predictors of systolic augmentation from left ventricular preexcitation in patients with dilated cardiomyopathy and intraventricular conduction delay. Circulation 2000;101:2703–9.

[30] Gold MR, Feliciano Z, Gottlieb SS, et al. Dual-chamber pacing with a short atrioventricular delay in congestive heart failure: a randomized study. J Am Coll Cardiol 1995;26:967–73.

[31] Yu CM, Lin H, Zhang Q, et al. High prevalence of left ventricular systolic and diastolic asynchrony in patients with congestive heart failure and normal QRS duration. Heart 2003;89:54–60.

[32] Yu CM, Bleeker GB, Fung JW, et al. Left ventricular reverse remodeling but not clinical improvement predicts long-term survival after cardiac resynchronization therapy. Circulation 2005;112:1580–6.

[33] Yu CM, Chau E, Sanderson JE, et al. Tissue Doppler echocardiographic evidence of reverse remodeling and improved synchronicity by simultaneously delaying regional contraction after biventricular pacing therapy in heart failure. Circulation 2002;105:438–45.

[34] Sogaard P, Egeblad H, Kim WY, et al. Tissue Doppler imaging predicts improved systolic performance and reversed left ventricular remodeling during long-term cardiac resynchronization therapy. J Am Coll Cardiol 2002;40:723–30.

[35] Pitzalis MV, Iacoviello M, Romito R, et al. Cardiac resynchronization therapy tailored by echocardiographic evaluation of ventricular asynchrony. J Am Coll Cardiol 2002;40:1615–22.

[36] Zardini M, Tritto M, Bargiggia G. The InSync Italian registry: analysis of clinical outcome and considerations on the selection of candidates to left ventricular resynchronization. Eur Heart J 2000;2:J16–22.

[37] Yu CM, Fung WH, Lin H, et al. Predictors of left ventricular reverse remodeling after cardiac resynchronization therapy for heart failure secondary to idiopathic dilated or ischemic cardiomyopathy. Am J Cardiol 2003;91:684–8.

[38] Pitzalis MV, Iacoviello M, Romito R, et al. Ventricular asynchrony predicts a better outcome in patients with chronic heart failure receiving cardiac resynchronization therapy. J Am Coll Cardiol 2005;45:65–9.

[39] Isaaz K, Ethevenot G, Admant P, et al. A new Doppler method of assessing left ventricular ejection force in chronic congestive heart failure. Am J Cardiol 1989;64:81–7.

[40] Fleming AD, McDicken WN, Sutherland GR, et al. Assessment of colour Doppler tissue imaging using test-phantoms. Ultrasound Med Biol 1994;20:937–51.

[41] Sutherland GR, Stewart MJ, Groundstroem KW, et al. Color Doppler myocardial imaging: a new technique for the assessment of myocardial function. J Am Soc Echocardiogr 1994;7:441–58.

[42] Isaaz K, Thompson A, Ethevenot G, et al. Doppler echocardiographic measurement of low velocity motion of the left ventricular posterior wall. Am J Cardiol 1989;64:66–75.

[43] Nagueh SF, Kopelen HA, Lim DS, et al. Tissue Doppler imaging consistently detects myocardial contraction and relaxation abnormalities, irrespective of cardiac hypertrophy, in a transgenic rabbit model of human hypertrophic cardiomyopathy. Circulation 2000;102:1346–50.

[44] Nagueh SF, Lakkis NM, Middleton KJ, et al. Changes in left ventricular diastolic function 6 months after nonsurgical septal reduction therapy for hypertrophic obstructive cardiomyopathy. Circulation 1999;99:344–7.

[45] Ommen SR, Nishimura RA, Appleton CP, et al. Clinical utility of Doppler echocardiography and tissue Doppler imaging in the estimation of left ventricular filling pressures: A comparative simultaneous Doppler-catheterization study. Circulation 2000;102:1788–94.

[46] Palka P, Lange A, Donnelly JE, et al. Doppler tissue echocardiographic features of cardiac amyloidosis. J Am Soc Echocardiogr 2002;15:1353–60.

[47] Palka P, Lange A, Fleming AD, et al. Age-related transmural peak mean velocities and peak velocity gradients by Doppler myocardial imaging in normal subjects. Eur Heart J 1996;17:940–50.

[48] Tabata T, Oki T, Yamada H, et al. Subendocardial motion in hypertrophic cardiomyopathy: assessment from long- and short-axis views by pulsed tissue Doppler imaging. J Am Soc Echocardiogr 2000;13:108–15.

[49] Tsutsui H, Uematsu M, Shimizu H, et al. Comparative usefulness of myocardial velocity gradient in detecting ischemic myocardium by a dobutamine challenge. J Am Coll Cardiol 1998;31:89–93.
[50] Bax JJ, Abraham T, Barold SS, et al. Cardiac resynchronization therapy: Part 1–issues before device implantation. J Am Coll Cardiol 2005;46:2153–67.
[51] Notabartolo D, Merlino JD, Smith AL, et al. Usefulness of the peak velocity difference by tissue Doppler imaging technique as an effective predictor of response to cardiac resynchronization therapy. Am J Cardiol 2004;94:817–20.
[52] Penicka M, Bartunek J, De Bruyne B, et al. Improvement of left ventricular function after cardiac resynchronization therapy is predicted by tissue Doppler imaging echocardiography. Circulation 2004;109: 978–83.
[53] Gorcsan III J, Kanzaki H, Bazaz R, et al. Usefulness of echocardiographic tissue synchronization imaging to predict acute response to cardiac resynchronization therapy. Am J Cardiol 2004;93:1178–81.
[54] Helm RH, Leclercq C, Faris OP, et al. Cardiac dyssynchrony analysis using circumferential versus longitudinal strain: implications for assessing cardiac resynchronization. Circulation 2005;111:2760–7.
[55] Dohi K, Suffoletto MS, Schwartzman D, et al. Utility of echocardiographic radial strain imaging to quantify left ventricular dyssynchrony and predict acute response to cardiac resynchronization therapy. Am J Cardiol 2005;96:112–6.
[56] Axel L, Dougherty L. MR imaging of motion with spatial modulation of magnetization. Radiology 1989; 171:841–5.
[57] Zerhouni EA, Parish DM, Rogers WJ, et al. Human heart: tagging with MR imaging—a method for noninvasive assessment of myocardial motion. Radiology 1988;169:59–63.
[58] Abraham TP, Laskowski C, Zhan W-Z, et al. Myocardial contractility by strain echocardiography: comparison with physiological measurements in an in vitro model. Am J Physiol Heart Circ Physiol 2003;285: H2599–604.
[59] Greenberg NL, Firstenberg MS, Castro PL, et al. Doppler-derived myocardial systolic strain rate is a strong index of left ventricular contractility. Circulation 2002;105:99–105.
[60] Urheim S, Edvardsen T, Torp H, et al. Myocardial strain by Doppler echocardiography: validation of a new method to quantify regional myocardial function. Circulation 2000;102:1158–64.
[61] Edvardsen T, Gerber BL, Garot J, et al. Quantitative assessment of intrinsic regional myocardial deformation by Doppler strain rate echocardiography in humans: validation against three-dimensional tagged magnetic resonance imaging. Circulation 2002;106: 50–6.
[62] Yu CM, Fung JW, Zhang Q, et al. Tissue Doppler imaging is superior to strain rate imaging and postsystolic shortening on the prediction of reverse remodeling in both ischemic and nonischemic heart failure after cardiac resynchronization therapy. Circulation 2004;110:66–73.
[63] Leitman M, Lysyansky P, Sidenko S, et al. Two-dimensional strain-a novel software for real-time quantitative echocardiographic assessment of myocardial function. J Am Soc Echocardiogr 2004;17:1021–9.
[64] Kawaguchi M, Murabayashi T, Fetics BJ, et al. Quantitation of basal dyssynchrony and acute resynchronization from left or biventricular pacing by novel echo-contrast variability imaging. J Am Coll Cardiol 2002;39:2052–8.
[65] Kapetanakis S, Kearney MT, Siva A, et al. Real-time three-dimensional echocardiography: a novel technique to quantify global left ventricular mechanical dyssynchrony. Circulation 2005;112:992–1000.
[66] Zhang Q, Yu CM, Fung JW, et al. Assessment of the effect of cardiac resynchronization therapy on intraventricular mechanical synchronicity by regional volumetric changes. Am J Cardiol 2005;95:126–9.
[67] Lardo AC, Abraham TP, Kass DA. Magnetic resonance imaging assessment of ventricular dyssynchrony: current and emerging concepts. J Am Coll Cardiol 2005;46:2223–8.
[68] Osman NF, Prince JL. Visualizing myocardial function using HARP MRI. Phys Med Biol 2000;45:1665–82.
[69] Osman NF, McVeigh ER, Prince JL. Imaging heart motion using harmonic phase MRI. IEEE Trans Med Imaging 2000;19:186–202.
[70] Kraitchman DL, Sampath S, Castillo E, et al. Quantitative ischemia detection during cardiac magnetic resonance stress testing by use of FastHARP. Circulation 2003;107:2025–30.
[71] Helm R, Byrne MA, Daya S, et al. Characterization of the optimal left ventricular pacing region in dyssynchronous heart failure implications for biventricular cardiac resynchronization [abstract]. Heart Rhythm 2005;2(Suppl):S8.
[72] Helm R, Wu K, Fernandes V, et al. Quantitative MRI assessment of cardiac dyssynchrony in patients with ischemic cardiomyopathy effect of infarct location. Circulation, in press.
[73] Osman NF, Sampath S, Atalar E, et al. Imaging longitudinal cardiac strain on short-axis images using strain-encoded MRI. Magn Reson Med 2001;46:324–34.
[74] Wyman BT, Hunter WC, Prinzen FW, et al. Effects of single- and biventricular pacing on temporal and spatial dynamics of ventricular contraction. Am J Physiol Heart Circ Physiol 2002;282:H372–9.
[75] Roguin A, Zviman MM, Meininger GR, et al. Modern pacemaker and implantable cardioverter/defibrillator systems can be magnetic resonance imaging safe: in vitro and in vivo assessment of safety and function at 1.5 T. Circulation 2004;110:475–82.

ELSEVIER
SAUNDERS

Heart Failure Clin 2 (2006) 193 – 204

HEART
FAILURE
CLINICS

Noninvasive Imaging of Heart Failure: Neuronal Dysfunction and Risk Stratification

Takahiro Higuchi, MD, PhD, Markus Schwaiger, MD*

Nuklearmedizinische Klinik und Poliklinik, Klinikum rechts der Isar der Technischen Universität München, München, Germany

Congestive heart failure (CHF) is a clinical syndrome of impaired cardiac contractile function resulting from structural damage, and is characterized by a vicious cycle in which reduced cardiac output results in neurohumoral activation. The plasma norepinephrine level, which acts as a major neurotransmitter of the sympathetic nervous system, has been shown to increase in heart failure patients in response to decreased systemic pressure [1]. This hyperadrenergic state in turn causes desensitization and downregulation of cardiac beta-adrenergic receptors and alterations in postsynaptic signal transduction, which causes further impairment of myocardial performance [2]. The close relationship between these alterations of the cardiac autonomic nervous system in heart failure and disease progression, and prognosis, including pump failure and sudden death, has been discussed intensively [3].

Nuclear medicine techniques, such as single photon emission tomography (SPECT) and positron emission tomography (PET), are unique methods of evaluating global and regional myocardial autonomic innervation [4]. These techniques have facilitated and refined substantially the study of the nervous system in both healthy and diseased hearts and have contributed significantly to an improved understanding of heart failure pathophysiology. Radiolabeled catecholamine and catecholamine analogs are available and their tracer physiologic properties are well understood. Additionally, receptor ligands have been introduced that can be combined with presynaptic tracers to gain unique insights into the mechanisms of myocardial biology and pathology (Fig. 1) [5].

Medications, including beta-blockers, angiotensin-II–converting enzyme inhibitors, angiotensin II type-1 receptor blockers, and nonpharmacologic therapy using electrical devices, have been shown to reduce the mortality and morbidity of heart failure patients [6,7]. To maximize the benefit of these available therapies, patients at a high risk of death, such as pump failure death and sudden cardiac death, require accurate risk stratification. Therefore, evaluation of the cardiac autonomic nervous function with noninvasive imaging methods is attractive as a prognostic indicator. This article reviews nuclear cardiology techniques for the imaging of autonomic innervation and discusses the clinical information available regarding their prognostic value in heart failure patients.

Biology of the cardiac autonomic nervous system

The regulation of cardiac function is achieved, in principle, by cardiac muscle fiber length and tension, which depend on ventricular volume and pressure, through the operation of Starling's law of the heart [8]. However, it is well known that the autonomic nervous system is important to cardiac adaptation to the varying demands of daily life [3]. The central nervous system collects data, such as blood pressure, flow, and chemical milieu, via receptors located in the left ventricle, carotid sinus, aortic arch, and brainstem, connected via afferent neurons. Based on the collected information, the autonomic nervous system

* Corresponding author. Klinikum rechts der Isar de Tecnischen Universität München, Ismaninger Str. 22, 81675 München, Germany.

E-mail address: markus.schwaiger@tum.de (M. Schwaiger).

1551-7136/06/$ – see front matter
doi:10.1016/j.hfc.2006.02.003

heartfailure.theclinics.com

Compund	Chemical structures	Type	Main biological target
I-123 metaiodobenzylguanidine (MIBG)	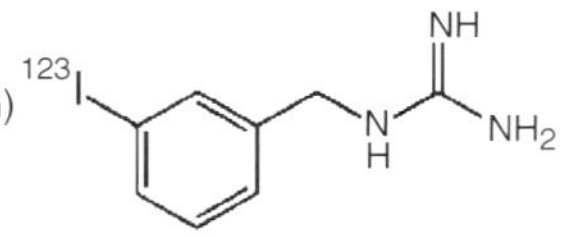	Catecholamine analogue	Presynaptic uptake
C-11 hydorxyepinephrine (HED)	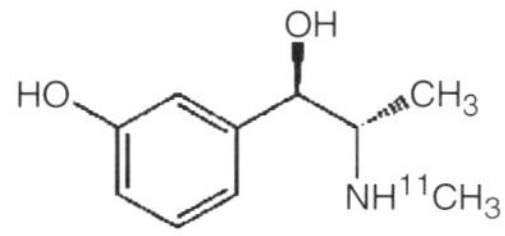	Catecholamine analogue	Presynaptic uptake
C-11 epinephrine (EPI)	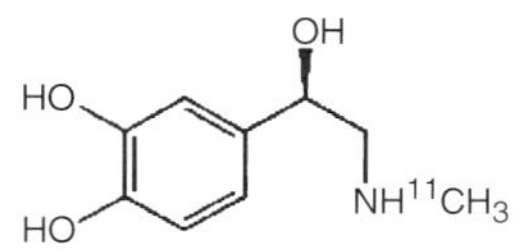	Catecholamine	Presynaptic uptake and strage
C-11 phenylephrine(PHEN)	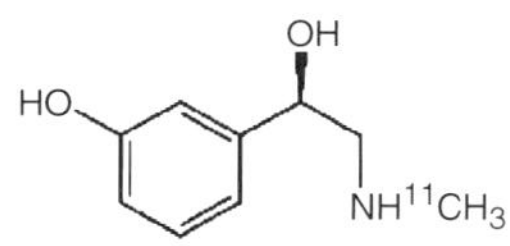	Catecholamine analogue	Presynaptic uptake and metabolism

Fig. 1. Radiotracers for sympathetic nerve imaging of presynaptic level.

controls heart rate, speed, and pattern of ventricular contraction via efferent neurons. The autonomic nervous regulation is also determined by circulating hormonal factors, such as catecholamine, angiotensin II, vasopressin, arterial natriuretic peptide, brain natriuretic peptide, and endotheline-1 [9]. These neuronal activations are usually beneficial in the early stages of heart failure. Adversely, they play an important role in the vicious cycle of advanced heart failure by increasing myocardial energy consumption, afterload, and arrhythmias.

The central component of the cardiac autonomic nervous system is in the medulla, where sensory afferent and efferent neurons form complex network loops. They consist of the sympathetic and parasympathetic nervous systems, with their major neurotransmitters being norepinephrine and acetylcholine, respectively. The sympathetic nervous system exerts positive inotropic effects, whereas the parasympathetic system exerts negative inotropic effects and chronotropic effects.

Sympathetic nervous fibers are distributed throughout the entire myocardium in the human heart. They travel along epicardial vascular structures and penetrate the myocardium with coronary vessels. The sympathetic neurotransmitter norepinephrine is generated from tyrosine in the presynaptic ending of sympathetic nerves, via dihydroxyphenylalanine and dopamine. Norepinephrine is stored in terminal vesicles by energy requiring vesicular amine transporter (VMAT). Voltage-dependent calcium channels, open as a firing impulse, arrive at the synaptic ending, releasing norepinephrine into the synaptic cleft, via exocytosis. Only a small part of the norepinephrine in the cleft binds to adrenoreceptors, including alpha- and beta-adrenoreceptors; $beta_1$-receptors are predominant in cardiac myocytes. Most of the norepinephrine is reabsorbed into the nerve ending via the presynaptic uptake-1 transporter [10]. This uptake-1 mechanism has a high affinity to norepinephrine and is both energy dependent and sodium concentration dependent. The norepinephrine concentration in the synaptic clefts plays an important physiologic and pathophysiologic role in the uptake-1 system in modulations of signal transduction for adrenergic receptors. A portion of the absorbed norepinephrine is restored and released again and the remainder is metabolized by monoamine oxidase (MAO) to 3,4-dihydroxyphenylglycol (DHPG). Most DHPG in systemic circulation is believed to have a neural source because nerve endings do not contain catechol O-methyltransferase (COMT), which would lead to further metabolic processing. There is a second reuptake mechanism into nonneuronal tissue (cardiocyte and vascular endothelial cell) mediated by the so-called "uptake-2 transporter." This uptake-2 mechanism, unlike the uptake-1 mechanism, is not dependent on energy and sodium concentration and is important in ATP depletion conditions such as ischemia. Norepinephrine, which is taken up into the nonneuronal tissue via uptake-2, is metabolized to 3-methoxy-4-hydroxyphenylglycol (MHPG) via normetanephrine (NMN) by COMT and MAO. A small fraction of norepinephrine released into the neural cleft spills over into vascular space and can be measured as norepinephrine level in coronary sinus vein blood. In addition to neuronal stimulation, there are a number of regulatory mechanisms by presynaptic receptors, including the $alpha_2$-adrenergic receptor, that provide negative feedback for exocytosis [11]. Radiolabeled tracers of catecholamine and catecholamine analogs used for SPECT and PET imaging share the same uptake mechanism and endogenous storage characteristics as the true neurotransmitters and can provide information about these nervous system activities [4].

The parasympathetic nervous system acts predominantly against the effects of sympathetic function and is essential for maintaining homeostasis of heart function. Parasympathetic neurons are distributed mainly in the atria and conduction nodules. The density of parasympathetic neurons within the myocardium is low, compared with sympathetic neurons, rendering them a difficult target for nuclear imaging. Acetylcholine is the main neurotransmitter in parasympathetic neurons and is synthesized from chorine at the nerve endings. It is transported via the vesicular acetylcholine transporter (VAChT) into storage vesicles. Upon nerve stimulation, acetylcholine is released from the nerve terminals to the neuronal cleft and binds to muscarinic receptors (M2-subtype) on the myocardium, activating changes in cardiac ion channel function [12].

Imaging of the cardiac autonomic nervous system

There are several radiolabeled tracers for evaluating the sympathetic and parasympathetic nervous systems at pre- and postsynaptic levels. Commonly used SPECT and PET tracers for presynaptic sympathetic innervation are either true catecholamine or catecholamine analogs. Radiolabeled true neurotransmitters follow the entire metabolic pathways, while analogs are resistant to specific steps of metabolisms. The specificity for the presynaptic uptake-1 transporter and vesicular storage inside the nerve terminal varies among currently available tracers.

Tc-99m metaiodobenzylguanidine (MIBG) is a commonly employed SPECT tracer for myocardial sympathetic innervation imaging at the presynaptic level. This agent is an analog of norepinephrine that is modified by the potent neuron blocking agents, guanethidine and bretylium. There are two uptake mechanisms of norepinephrine in the synaptic cleft: uptake-1 (neuronal uptake, a sodium/chloride-dependent transport protein) and uptake-2 (nonneuronal uptake). Administered plasma MIBG that travels to the neural cleft is also believed to undergo heart uptake through these two mechanisms. Although approximately 30% of the heart uptake in rats, mice and dogs is via an unspecific uptake-2 mechanism, most of the heart uptake in humans undergoes specific neuronal uptake [13]. Additionally, MIBG is metabolically resistant to MAO and COMT enzymes, unlike the true neurotransmitter norepinephrine [14]. Thus, the MIBG stored in the vesicle of the nerve ending shows longer retention than norepinephrine, without further metabolism. When a firing impulse arrives at the terminal, stored MIBG is released to the cleft again and is taken up in the neuronal tissue via the uptake-1 transporter or spillover into the blood. MIBG does not show any biologic activity to the noradrenalin receptor. Consequently, possible factors for decreased MIBG uptake and retention are enhancement of norepinephrine release from the nerve ending, deterioration of the uptake-1 transporter (eg, ATP exhaust), decreased density of the sympathetic nerve ending, or competitive inhibition with norepinephrine. Generally, imaging with MIBG includes a planar and SPECT acquisition with a two-step protocol at both 15 to 30 minutes (early phase) and 3 to 4 hours (delayed phase) after MIBG injection. Kinetics can be determined by comparing initial uptake and delayed retention, as well as by the regional distribution of uptake (Table 1) (Fig. 2) [15].

C-11 meta-hydroxyephedrine (HED) is a norepinephrine analog and is the most frequently used PET tracer for sympathetic neuronal imaging in human studies [16]. Plasma HED is transported into cardiac sympathetic nerve terminals mostly via the uptake-1 mechanism. Highly neuronal-specific uptake in the heart has been proved with 92% reduction of myocardial HED uptake by selective neuronal uptake-1 blockage using desipramine. Vesicular storage seems to occur, but binding inside vesicles is low because of a higher lipophilicity of HED, compared with norepinephrine. Similar to MIBG, HED is metabolically

Table 1
Normal values of MIBG scintigraphy from a multicenter study in Japan

Heart to mediastinum ratio	
15 min	2.34 ± 0.35
3–4 h	2.49 ± 0.43
Washout rate	27.74 ± 5.34%

Data from Nishimura T, Sugishita Y, Sasaki Y, et al. Kaku Igaku 1997;34:1139–48.

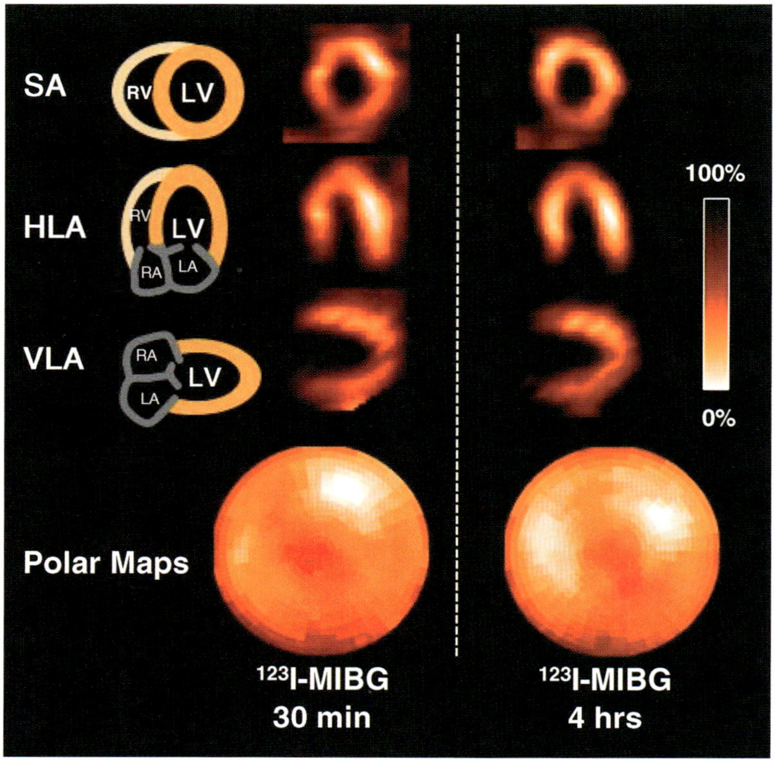

Fig. 2. Regional myocardial distribution of I-123 MIBG in a healthy normal volunteer. SPECT images are acquired 30 minutes and 4 hours after intravenous administration of the tracer. There is homogeneous uptake throughout the left ventricular myocardium in short-axis (SA), horizontal long-axis (HLA), and vertical long-axis (VLA) views; 3-D distribution polar maps show both 30 minute and 4 hour images.

resistant to MAO and COMT enzymes, so the retention in the myocardium mainly reflects a continuing release and reuptake of HED in the sympathetic nerve. HED PET can quantify the retention fraction of HED in myocardial tissue to the arterial input function. PET tracers offer several advantages over single photon approaches such as MIBG in areas such as spatial resolution, sensitivity, and the ability of quantification. In addition, the concentrations of the tracer in blood and in myocardial tissue and their changes over time can be quantified. Therefore, application of tracer kinetics permits modeling-sensitive measurements of the biologic behavior of the tracers.

There are additional PET tracers for sympathetic innervation in the presynaptic level, including C-11 epinephrine (EPI) and C-11 phenylephrine (PHEN) [17]. They are both vulnerable to cytosolic MAO degradation and allow assessment of neuronal uptake and vesicular storage with PET scan. These available C-11–labeled tracers reflect the different mechanisms of the norepinephrine metabolism in sympathetic nerve endings and may be combined to identify more specific pathophysiology on the processes of norepinephrine uptake, vesicular storage, and metabolism in presynaptic adrenergic nerve terminals.

Several postsynaptic receptor ligands have been labeled and proposed as PET tracers for cardiac imaging [5]. However, the clinical use of receptor-targeted tracers has been limited to a few studies and still faces significant challenge. High specific binding, high affinity and hydrophilicity, which avoids binding to internalized inactive receptors, lack of pharmacologic effects, and finally, a simple and reliable tracer synthesis are requirements that have to be met for a widespread application of receptor ligands for cardiac PET. C-11 CGP12177, a hydrophilic nonselective beta-adrenoreceptor antagonist, is still the most widely used tracer for adrenergic receptor imaging [18]. Synthesis of this tracer is not simple and requires C-11 phosgen as a precursor, which has prevented a broader clinical application until now. CGP12177 has high specific affinity and fast plasma clearance, suggesting feasibility for clinical imaging. A graphic method, which adjusts issues related to metabolites, has been established for quantification in humans [19]. This approach requires a dual-injection protocol with doses of high and low specific activity. Beta-adrenergic receptor density (Bmax) measured by C-11 CGP12177 PET correlated well with in vitro measurement of myocardial samples in both healthy volunteers and subjects with congestive cardiomyopathy. C-11 CGP12388 is another recently introduced nonselective beta-adrenergic receptor antagonist. C-11 CGP12388 can be labeled easier than CGP12177 via a 1-pot procedure using 2-C-11-acetone [20]. It is more hydrophilic than C-11 CGP12177 and the biodistribution and retention of CGP12388 is reported to be similar to CGP12177 [21].

F-18 fluoroethoxybenzovesamicol (FEOBV) is a specific tracer that binds to the acetylcholine transporter on parasympathetic neurons [22]. Unfortunately, specific binding in the heart is low and the usefulness of this tracer for clinical cardiac PET imaging is considered limited. PET imaging of cardiac parasympathetic neurons is complicated because of the low density of cholinergic neurons within the ventricular myocardium, and the parasympathetic neurotransmitter mechanism, which is highly specific for acetylcholine, that is very rapidly metabolized in blood. C-11 methylquinuclidinyl benzilate (MQNB) is a tracer for parasympathetic muscarinic receptors [23]. PET studies in healthy volunteers demonstrated rapid plasma clearance and heart uptake mainly in the ventricular septum and in the left ventricular wall, while the atria were not visualized [24].

Autonomic nerve function in heart failure

A huge body of experimental and clinical data has proved that sympathetic tone is heightened in heart failure. High levels of circulating norepinephrine are observed, and increased sympathetic nerve activity has been directly identified by clinical microneurograph. Eisenhofer and colleagues [25] investigated cardiac norepinephrine turnover in subjects with CHF, using titrated norepinephrine. Baseline plasma norepinephrine levels, DHPG levels, and DHPG production rates were higher, but synthesis of norepinephrine itself did not change. Both norepinephrine release and reuptake were increased, but the efficacy of reuptake was reduced. Consequently, in the patient with heart failure, norepinephrine spillover is approximately four times higher and cardiac norepinephrine storage is reduced by approximately 50%, compared with normal subjects. Reduction of functioning local presynaptic catecholamine uptake sites is thus likely to increase the myocardial overexposure to catecholamine.

The mechanisms of sympathetic nerve activation in heart failure patients are not fully understood. Recent clinical trials and experimental studies with new molecular and genetic tools provide additional information regarding the mechanisms of neuronal activation in heart failure [26]. Abnormal inhibitory reflex of sympathetic function, such as arterial baroreflex and cardiopulmonary reflex, had been thought to be responsible for the enhanced sympathetic activation of CHF. However, subsequent animal studies found that sinoaortic baroreceptor denervation and chronic cardiac denervation in CHF showed no differences between the denervated and the nondenervated group [27]. Further evaluation into the impaired inhibitory reflex of the sympathetic function is indicated.

The chemoreflex is an important regulator of sympathetic function [28]. The peripheral chemoreceptors are located in the carotid arteries, and the central chemoreceptors are located in the brainstem. Some animal and human studies have reported increased sensitivity of both peripheral and central chemoreflexes in advanced heart failure. This augmentation of the central chemoreflex is a heightened factor in central sleep apnea, a condition characterized by waxing and waning of ventilation, occurring predominately during non-REM sleep. In addition, in heart failure patients this sleep breathing disorder is a potential contributor to progression of the disease because of the additional enhancement of sympathetic activation as a result of recurrent hypoxemia and hypercapnia [29].

Malliani and colleagues [30] indicated the important role of the emerging excitatory action of cardiovascular sympathetic afferent fibers mediated by the activation of sympathetic activity. The cardiovascular sympathetic afferent fibers originate from all cardiac chambers and the large thoracic vessels. They have positive feedback characteristics and appear to be sensitive to both mechanical and chemical stimulation. In patients who have heart failure, increased wall tension, increased oxygen consumption, and many substances, including bradykinin, potassium, and lactate, stimulate the nerve endings and lead to excitation of the sympathosympathetic reflex. Hypothetically, this process is responsible for sympathetic hyperactivation in the early phase of CHF, characterized by an increase in arterial pressure and heart rate, diastolic dysfunction, and preserved cardiac output, during which no baroreflex deactivation occurs.

Angiotensin II is known to play a role in the acceleration of the sympathetic system and is an important therapeutic target. It has been reported that there are increased angiotensin II concentrations and increased angiotensin II type 1 receptor stimulation in heart failure states [27]. Recently, Wang and colleagues [31] found that in CHF, the increased angiotensin II type 1 receptor in the paraventricular nucleus contributed to the enhanced sympathetic afferent reflex, and blockage of the angiotensin II type 1 receptor resulted in the normalization of this reflex. Nitric oxide, which antagonizes angiotensin II action in many systems, also plays an important role in modulating sympathetic activation in heart failure in several brain areas, including the nucleus tractus solitarius, the paraventricular nucleus, and the rostral ventrolateral medulla. Central nitric oxide synthesis was found to be depressed in the CHF state [27].

Down-regulation of beta-adrenoreceptor is also key to changes in sympathetic function in heart failure [32]. The hyperadrenergic state in CHF causes desensitization and down-regulation of cardiac beta-adrenergic receptors, particularly the beta$_1$-adrenoreceptor located in the postsynaptic junction. It also causes alterations in postsynaptic signal transduction, which impairs myocardial performance. In vitro experimental data have confirmed a reduction of postsynaptic beta-adrenergic receptor density (down-regulation) and an impairment of receptor function (uncoupling), while the inactivating postsynaptic beta-adrenergic receptor kinase-1 was elevated [33]. Additionally, the proportion of beta-adrenergic receptor subtypes seems to change in heart failure, resulting in decreased density of beta$_1$-receptors, but unchanged status of beta$_2$-receptors, located at both sympathetic pre- and postsynaptic junctions, and, therefore, they have a more prominent role in modulating sympathetic signal transduction [34]. Some PET studies with postsynaptic adrenergic receptor ligands have been performed in heart failure. Merlet and colleagues [35] studied subjects with idiopathic cardiomyopathy using GCP-12177, and confirmed that left ventricular beta-adrenergic receptor density was decreased in vivo. More recently, de Jong and colleagues [2], using the alternative adrenergic receptor ligand C-11 CGP12388, also observed lower beta-receptor density in patients with NYHA (New York Heart Association) stage II-III heart failur.

Presynaptic sympathetic nerve imaging in heart failure

Dysfunction of the autonomic nervous system is an inherent feature of heart failure. The pathophysiologic importance of alterations in the autonomic system has been emphasized increasingly. SPECT and PET imaging have contributed significantly to the understanding of the role of autonomic innervation in the failing heart.

A number of clinical studies have reported abnormal MIBG findings, such as impaired early and delayed uptake and enhanced washout from early to delayed uptake, in patients who have heart failure. Imamura and colleagues [36] assessed whether these abnormal findings reflect the severity of heart failure. In their study, MIBG washout correlated with severity of heart failure, based on NYHA classification, independent of the underlying causes, including dilated cardiomyopathy, ischemic cardiomyopathy, and heart failure related to mechanical abnormality. Significant correlation between MIBG washout, heart rate variability, and plasma norepinephrine level has been reported in several studies. Sato and colleagues [37] showed significant correlation between MIBG uptake in the delayed phase and norepinephrine concentrations in the coronary sinus blood at peak exercise in CHF. The mechanism of these abnormal findings of MIBG imaging in heart failure patients is not understood fully. The synaptic endings in the patient with heart failure show enhanced norepinephrine release, decreased efficacy of norepinephrine reuptake, and decreased norepinephrine storage. MIBG shares the same uptake-1 mechanism as norepinephrine, but is resistant to metabolism by MAO and COMT. Therefore, the abnormal findings in the delayed phase and the increased washout may reflect the decrease of MIBG storage, secondary to enhanced MIBG release, and decreased MIBG reuptake via the uptake -1 mechanism.

Vesalainen and colleagues [38] evaluated HED uptake in subjects with stable heart failure due to coronary artery disease or dilated cardiomyopathy, and in healthy control subjects. Global myocardial HED retention in all subjects with stable heart failure was reduced significantly, compared with the subjects with a normal heart. In addition, reduced HED retention was proportional to the head-tilt systolic pressure response and baroreflex control of heart rate, indicating interaction between abnormal myocardial innervation and blood pressure maintenance. In another study, reduced global myocardial HED retention was reported to correlate with clinical markers for heart failure, such as impaired ejection fraction and NYHA classification, as well as elevation of plasma catecholamine levels [39,40]. The abnormality was not only global reduction but also regional deviations of cardiac sympathetic tracer uptake, demonstrated with HED PET. Ungerer and colleagues

[41] investigated transplanted hearts from subjects with heart failure due to cardiomyopathy. They showed marked regional variation in uptake-1 density in the transplanted heart and HED retention before heart transplantation. The density of uptake-1 correlated with HED retention (r = 0.65), but not with affinity of uptake-1, despite the small sample size (n = 9). The uptake reduction was observed primarily in the apex and distal inferolateral area, rather than the proximal wall, reflecting the heterogeneity of the neuronal imaging.

Balance of presynaptic and postsynaptic sympathetic nerves in heart failure

Combined pre- and postsympathetic nerve function using a PET could provide further insights into the pathophysiology of sympathetic nerve function in heart failure. In a pilot study, Link and colleagues [42] measured the balance of pre- and postsynaptic sympathetic function in 9 subjects with ischemic heart failure and 19 normal subjects, using HED and CGP12177 PET. Pre- and postsynaptic function were well matched in the normal group, but were mismatched in the heart failure subjects. In another study, Ungerer and colleagues [43] demonstrated a mismatch in the presynaptic and postsympathetic system in cardiomyopathic heart failure subjects, using PET before heart transplantation. In this study, ex vivo analysis of uptake-1 density and beta-adrenoreceptor kinase of the transplanted heart tissue was performed. The investigators reported that presynaptic sympathetic nervous uptake-1 density did not correlate with beta-adrenoreceptor density, but rather, correlated with the expression of the receptor-inactivating enzyme, beta-adrenoreceptor kinase (Table 2). Regulation of levels and activity of beta-adrenoreceptor kinase were indicated to play an important role in the developing of heart failure. It remains to be determined if the mismatch findings between the presynaptic and postsynaptic nervous function in heart failure patients provide prognostic information.

Risk stratification in heart failure using autonomic nerve imaging

Despite recent improvement in medical treatment, including beta-blockers, angiotensin-II–converting enzyme inhibitors, and angiotensin II receptor blockers, and improved morbidity and mortality rates, the prognosis for advanced heart failure patients is still very poor. Therefore, the importance of risk stratification is still essential to identifying patients who may benefit from aggressive therapy, follow-up, education, and alternative therapies, including heart transplantation [44]. The NYHA classification, malignant arrhythmias, ventricular function, heart rate variability, exercise variables such as peak oxygen consumption, neurohormonal markers such as norepinephrine, atrial natriuretic peptide, and brain natriuretic peptide, and cytokine (eg, IL-6,and so forth) are proposed as important prognostic factors. However, risk stratification of CHF patients is complex because of the pathophysiology of the disease. A combination of several factors is thought to be helpful in increasing the accuracy of the prognostic evaluation.

Assessment of the autonomic nervous system is one of the most sensitive and important factors for prognosis in CHF. Autonomic nervous abnormalities play a central role in initiation and progression of heart failure, which consequently cause pump failure death. The plasma norepinephrine level, which is a sensitive indicator of sympathetic nervous system activity, has been found to be increased significantly in patients with asymptomatic left ventricular dysfunction, and correlates with heart failure progression [45]. Earlier studies have shown that increased plasma norepinephrine level is an indicator of patients' prognoses, independent of deterioration of cardiac function [46]. Plasma brain natriuretic peptide, secreted primarily from the left ventricle in response to myocardial wall tension, was recently proposed as a powerful new prognostic predictor [47]. However, these plasma levels of neurohormonal markers reflect systemic autonomic nervous abnormalities, secondary to cardiac overload, as compen-

Table 2
Relation between pre- and postsynaptic function in heart failure patients

	HED-PET	Uptake-1 density	Beta-receptor density	Beta-ARK-1 level
HED-PET	—	r = 0.65	r = 0.21	r = 0.38
Uptake-1 density	p = .05	—	r = 0.15	r = 0.61
Beta-receptor density	p = 0.4	p = 0.7	—	r = 0.1
Beta-ARK-1 level	p = .07	p = 0.04	p = 0.5	—

Data from Ungerer M, Weig HJ, Kubert S, et al. Eur J Heart Fail 2000;2:23–31.

sation for total circulatory insufficiency. Heart rate variability is another potential prognostic indicator of heart failure as an index of autonomic nerve system, but it mainly reflects abnormal autonomic nervous modulation of sinus node [48]. On the other hand, imaging of the autonomic nervous system with MIBG-SPECT and HED-PET can assess the global and regional presynaptic activity of the myocardium. This seems to have a greater prognostic value.

MIBG imaging is the most widespread sympathetic nerve imaging employed for clinical study and has been reported in some clinical studies to provide adequate information for risk stratification in patients who have heart failure (Table 3) [49–61]. In 1992, Merlet and colleagues [49] reported for the first time the significance of MIBG imaging as a prognostic factor. They assessed MIBG uptake in the delayed phase in 90 subjects with severe heart failure due to cardiomyopathy and ischemic heart disease. Twenty-seven months later, 10 subjects had had a cardiac transplant and 22 had died. The heart to mediastinum uptake ratio of MIBG was less than 1.2, indicating high-risk patients, and was the best predictor of survival (sensitivity 95%, specificity 93%), compared with other indices, such as ejection fraction. This observation was confirmed by the following studies. Nakata and colleagues [50] studied 414 consecutive subjects, including 173 symptomatic heart failure subjects, in a multiple stepwise discriminate analysis, using the Cox proportional hazard model, and proved that the heart to mediastinum uptake ratio in the delayed phase (less than 1.74) was the most powerful predictor for all causes of cardiac death. Compared with other new powerful prognostic indicators, this is an interesting result. Imamura and colleagues [55] found that a background subtracted MIBG washout rate was a better predictor than plasma brain natriuretic peptide level in 171 subjects with CHF due to idiopathic cardiomyopathy (n = 96) and ischemic cardiomyopathy (n = 75). Yamada and colleagues [58] demonstrated in a prospective study that the washout rate in heart failure patients had a higher prognostic value than heart rate variability. The synergistic role of MIBG and other prognostic factors has also been proposed. Kyuma and colleagues [60] assessed the synergistic prognostic value of MIBG imaging and other factors in 158 subjects with heart failure. The hazard ratio for fatal pump failure with brain natriuretic peptide (7.2) or delayed MIBG uptake (10.1) was increased to 34.4 when both indicators were combined. Additionally, PET tracers for sympathetic nerve imaging, such as HED (a PET tracer that shares the same uptake and storage with MIBG) also seem to have a prognostic value, but there are only a few reports in this regard. One paper by Pietila and colleagues [61] retrospectively studied the survival data of 46 CHF subjects who had undergone HED PET. The investigators showed that the degree

Table 3
Summary of the risk for death in heart failure patients evaluated by MIBG sympathetic nerve imaging

Authors	Year	Sex (male/ female)	Mean age (years)	Diagnosis (ischemic/ nonischemic)	Mean LVEF (%)	Follow-up (months)	Survival rate (%) (low risk/ high risk)	*P* value	Criteria for high risk
Merlet et al [49]	1992	76/14	52	24/66	22	27	98/16	<.0001	H/M <1.20
Nakata et al [50]	1998	271/143	61	131/283	49	22	95/85	.0002	H/M <1.74
Cohen-Solal et al [51]	1999	55/38	55	24/69	25	10	70/30	.09	H/M <1.27
Momose et al [52]	1999	52/7	51	0/59	28	24	71/19	<.0001	WR >52
Wakabayashi	2001	62/14	68	76/0	32	54	83/56	.0358	H/M <1.5
et al [53]		43/13	60	0/56	30	55	86/51	.0321	H/M <2.2
Ogita et al [54]	2001	64/15	64	45/34	29	31	100/64	<.001	WR >27
Imamura et al [55]	2001	125/46	63	75/96	27	27	98/15	<.0001	WR >63
Matsui et al [56]	2002	55/19	55	0/74	31	24	83/57	<.05	H/M <1.89
Gerson et al [57]	2003	27/10	48	0/37	27	49	92/28	.0042	H/M <1.54
Yamada et al [58]	2003	51/14	63	41/24	28	34	85/38	<.0012	WR >27
Nakata et al [59]	2003	146/59	61	81/124	34	35	90/72	NA	HM <1.75
Kyuma et al [60]	2004	110/48	64	45/113	41	16	98/70[a]	.006	HM <1.74
Nakata et al [63]	2005	69/19	58	24/64	27	27	75/56	.006	H/M <1.53
Total/mean		1206/459	59	566/1099	31	31	87/47		

Abbreviations: H/M, delayed heart to mediastinal uptake ratio of MIBG; LVEF, left ventricular ejection fraction; NA, not available; WR, washout rate = (early uptake-delayed uptake)/early uptake × 100.

[a] Survival rate for pump failure death.

of HED reduction had prognostic value. Based on these data, further prospective and multicenter studies in larger patient populations are required to establish the clinical usefulness of MIBG or HED imaging for risk stratification in heart failure.

Some studies performed in small patient populations have shown the usefulness of MIBG imaging in the prediction of therapeutic efficacy in patients who have heart failure. Suwa and colleagues [62] performed MIBG imaging in 45 subjects with heart failure due to dilated cardiomyopathy, before initiating beta-blocker therapy, and assessed whether MIBG imaging could predict therapeutic response. They reported that a delayed uptake ratio with a threshold of 1.7 is a good predictor of response to beta-blocker therapy (sensitivity 91%, specificity 92%). Recently, Nakata and colleagues [63] tested whether MIBG imaging could predict an improved prognosis using angiotensin-converting enzyme inhibitors or beta-blockers in 79 subjects with heart failure. They showed that when MIBG uptake was maintained at more than 1.53, the therapies reduced the risk of mortality by twice as much as that of the group with MIBG uptake lower than 1.53. These findings demonstrate an attractive approach to MIBG nerve imaging for the management of heart failure patients, but require further confirmation with larger prospective studies.

Sudden death in heart failure and the sympathetic nervous system

In addition to pump failure, sudden death caused by a cardiac arrhythmia is responsible for morbidity in heart failure patients at a rate of six to nine times higher than in the general population. Indeed, recent large clinical trials have indicated that sudden death by cardiac arrhythmia is a leading cause of death among patients who have heart failure [64].

An abnormal autonomic nervous system appears to be associated with lethal arrhythmias. An earlier study by Meredith and colleagues [65] showed as an index of sympathetic activation a significant increase in cardiac norepinephrine spillover into the plasma in 12 subjects who had recovered from a spontaneous sustained ventricular tachycardia or ventricular fibrillation. Using MIBG or HED imaging in paced heart failure dogs and clinical heart failure subjects, there is evidence that neuronal dysfunction is not spread uniformly across the myocardium [41,66]. Regional heterogeneity of innervation has been shown in patients with previous ventricular arrhythmias, using MIBG imaging [67]. Cao and colleagues [68] reported enhanced spatial inhomogeneity of cardiac innervation in patients who have heart failure due to both ischemic and nonischemic heart disease, using immunohistochemical staining of ventricular tissues. The degree of heterogenating was associated with a history of ventricular arrhythmia and sudden cardiac death.

The precise relationship between arrhythmia and sympathetic nerve dysfunction in heart failure patients is still unclear. Enhanced beta-adrenoreceptor stimulation may represent a primary reason for lethal arrhythmias [69]. Reduced reuptake or increased release of norepinephrine, as indicated with MIBG or HED, lead to increased levels of local norepinephrine in the synaptic cleft. The down-regulation of beta-adrenoreceptors is associated with up-regulation of G-protein and subsequent activation of adenylyl cyclase, which lead to an increased level of intracellular cyclic adenosine monophosphate (cAMP). The cAMP will produce a rise in intracellular calcium ion levels via protein kinase A. Because the sympathetic innervation is heterogeneous in heart failure, heterogeneity of local calcium transients in the myocardium may occur and cause the triggering of the lethal arrhythmia by dispersion of repolarization. This concept may be supported indirectly by the fact that beta-blockers reduce sudden cardiac death in heart failure, because beta-blockers seem to inhibit this process [70].

Recent trials have demonstrated that the implantable cardioverter-defibrillator (ICD), which can convert episodes of ventricular fibrillation and tachycardia to sinus rhythm, improved survival in a population of subjects with heart failure by approximately 25% [71]. However, ICD implantation has drawbacks, such as the invasive nature of the procedure and higher costs compared with pharmacologic treatment. For this reason, risk stratification for sudden death in patients who have heart failure is necessary for selecting candidates for this therapy.

Evaluation of global and local sympathetic nerve function by imaging seems to have the potential to identify high risk for lethal arrhythmias. Unfortunately, most clinical studies assessing the prognostic value of imaging in heart failure did not distinguish between sudden cardiac death and pump failure in their data analysis. Therefore, the predictive value for prediction of lethal ventricular arrhythmias in heart failure patients is not defined. In a pilot study, Arora and colleagues [72] evaluated the possibility of autonomic nerve imaging using MIBG to select patients who would benefit from an ICD therapy. They studied 17 subjects with previous ICD implantation; 10 of them had at least one episode of discharge of ICD. The group with discharge showed significantly larger MIBG defects and lower uptake in the heart.

Further confirmation with a larger prospective study is required to determine if autonomic nerve imaging could be useful in selecting patients for ICD therapy.

Summary

The cardiac autonomic nervous system plays a pivotal role in heart failure patients. The pathophysiologic importance of alteration of the autonomic system has been well recognized. Pharmacologic intervention using beta-blockers, angiotensin-converting enzyme inhibitors, and angiotensin II type-1 receptor blockers, and nonpharmacologic therapy using ICD has improved mortality. The autonomic nervous dysfunction is related to the initiation and progression of the disease through direct effects on the myocardium and activation of other hormonal systems such as the rennin-angiotensin system.

Autonomic nerve imaging with SPECT and PET has contributed to the understanding of the role of the autonomic function in heart failure patients. Several studies using MIBG imaging have demonstrated a promising prognostic value. In addition, the value of imaging for predicting therapeutic efficacy is suggested. However, further confirmatory studies employing prospective randomized protocols are required to determine not only the incremental prognostic value, but also the cost efficacy of imaging procedures in the management of patients who have heart failure.

Acknowledgments

The authors thank Martha Bean and Gabriele Sonoda for their editorial assistance.

References

[1] Noble MI. Sympathetic activation in chronic heart failure. Int J Cardiol 2000;73(2):163–4.
[2] de Jong RM, Blanksma PK, van Waarde A, et al. Measurement of myocardial beta-adrenoceptor density in clinical studies: a role for positron emission tomography? Eur J Nucl Med Mol Imaging 2002;29(1): 88–97.
[3] Kaye D, Esler M. Sympathetic neuronal regulation of the heart in aging and heart failure. Cardiovasc Res 2005;66(2):256–64.
[4] Raffel DM, Wieland DM. Assessment of cardiac sympathetic nerve integrity with positron emission tomography. Nucl Med Biol 2001;28(5):541–59.
[5] Tseng H, Link JM, Stratton JR, et al. Cardiac receptor physiology and its application to clinical imaging: present and future. J Nucl Cardiol 2001;8(3):390–409.
[6] Foody JM, Farrell MH, Krumholz HM. beta-Blocker therapy in heart failure: scientific review. JAMA 2002; 287(7):883–9.
[7] Bristow MR, Saxon LA, Boehmer J, et al. Cardiac-resynchronization therapy with or without an implantable defibrillator in advanced chronic heart failure. N Engl J Med 2004;350(21):2140–50.
[8] Fukuda N, Granzier H. Role of the giant elastic protein titin in the Frank-Starling mechanism of the heart. Curr Vasc Pharmacol 2004;2(2):135–9.
[9] Sharma R, Anker SD, Immune and neurohormonal pathways in chronic heart failure. Congest Heart Fail 2002;8(1):23–8, 48.
[10] Goldstein DS, Brush Jr JE, Eisenhofer G, et al. In vivo measurement of neuronal uptake of norepinephrine in the human heart. Circulation 1988;78(1):41–8.
[11] Hein L, Altman JD, Kobilka BK. Two functionally distinct alpha2-adrenergic receptors regulate sympathetic neurotransmission. Nature 1999;402(6758): 181–4.
[12] Harvey RD, Belevych AE. Muscarinic regulation of cardiac ion channels. Br J Pharmacol 2003;139(6): 1074–84.
[13] Dae MW, De Marco T, Botvinick EH, et al. Scintigraphic assessment of MIBG uptake in globally denervated human and canine hearts–implications for clinical studies. J Nucl Med 1992;33(8):1444–50.
[14] Wieland DM, Brown LE, Rogers WL, et al. Myocardial imaging with a radioiodinated norepinephrine storage analog. J Nucl Med 1981;22(1):22–31.
[15] Nishimura T, Sugishita Y, Sasaki Y. [The results of questionnaire on quantitative assessment of 123I-metaiodobenzylguanidine myocardial scintigraphy in heart failure]. Kaku Igaku 1997;34(12):1139–48 [in Japanese].
[16] Bengel FM, Schwaiger M. Assessment of cardiac sympathetic neuronal function using PET imaging. J Nucl Cardiol 2004;11(5):603–16.
[17] Munch G, Nguyen NT, Nekolla S, et al. Evaluation of sympathetic nerve terminals with [(11)C]epinephrine and [(11)C]hydroxyephedrine and positron emission tomography. Circulation 2000;101(5):516–23.
[18] Law MP. Demonstration of the suitability of CGP 12177 for in vivo studies of beta-adrenoceptors. Br J Pharmacol 1993;109(4):1101–9.
[19] Delforge J, Mesangeau D, Dolle F, et al. In vivo quantification and parametric images of the cardiac beta-adrenergic receptor density. J Nucl Med 2002; 43(2):215–26.
[20] Elsinga PH, van Waarde A, Jaeggi KA, et al. Synthesis and evaluation of (S)-4-(3-(2′-[11C]isopropylamino)-2-hydroxypropoxy) -2H-benzimidazol -2-one ((S)-[11C] CGP 12388) and (S)-4-((3-(1′-[18F]-fluoroisopropyl) amino)-2-hydroxypropoxy) -2H- benzimidazol-2-one ((S)-[18F]fluoro-CGP 12388) for visualization of beta-adrenoceptors with positron emission tomography. J Med Chem 1997;40(23):3829–35.
[21] Momose M, Reder S, Raffel DM, et al. Evaluation of

cardiac beta-adrenoreceptors in the isolated perfused rat heart using (S)-11C–CGP12388. J Nucl Med 2004;45(3):471–7.

[22] DeGrado TR, Mulholland GK, Wieland DM, et al. Evaluation of (-)[18F]fluoroethoxybenzovesamicol as a new PET tracer of cholinergic neurons of the heart. Nucl Med Biol 1994;21(2):189–95.

[23] Kassiou M, Mardon K, Katsifis AG, et al. Radiosynthesis of [123I]N-methyl-4-iododexetimide and [123I] N-methyl-4-iodolevetimide: in vitro and in vivo characterisation of binding to muscarinic receptors in the rat heart. Nucl Med Biol 1996;23(2):147–53.

[24] Syrota A, Comar D, Paillotin G, et al. Muscarinic cholinergic receptor in the human heart evidenced under physiological conditions by positron emission tomography. Proc Natl Acad Sci USA 1985;82(2):584–8.

[25] Eisenhofer G, Friberg P, Rundqvist B, et al. Cardiac sympathetic nerve function in congestive heart failure. Circulation 1996;93(9):1667–76.

[26] Chua TP, Ponikowski P, Coats AJ. Chemoreflexes in heart failure. Circulation 1997;96(6):2090–1.

[27] Zucker IH, Schultz HD, Li YF, et al. The origin of sympathetic outflow in heart failure: the roles of angiotensin II and nitric oxide. Prog Biophys Mol Biol 2004;84(2–3):217–32.

[28] Kara T, Narkiewicz K, Somers VK. Chemoreflexes–physiology and clinical implications. Acta Physiol Scand 2003;177(3):377–84.

[29] Mansfield DR, Naughton MT. Sleep apnea and congestive heart failure. Minerva Med 2004;95(4):257–80.

[30] Malliani A. Cardiocardiac excitatory reflexes during myocardial ischemia. Basic Res Cardiol 1990;85(Suppl 1):243–52.

[31] Wang HJ, Zhang F, Zhang Y, et al. AT(1) receptor in paraventricular nucleus mediates the enhanced cardiac sympathetic afferent reflex in rats with chronic heart failure. Auton Neurosci 2005;121(1–2):56–63.

[32] Bristow MR. Myocardial beta-adrenergic receptor downregulation in heart failure. Int J Cardiol 1984;5(5):648–52.

[33] Choi DJ, Koch WJ, Hunter JJ, et al. Mechanism of beta-adrenergic receptor desensitization in cardiac hypertrophy is increased beta-adrenergic receptor kinase. J Biol Chem 1997;272(27):17223–9.

[34] Pitschner HF, Droege A, Mitze M, et al. Down-regulated beta-adrenoceptors in severely failing human ventricles: uniform regional distribution, but no increased internalization. Basic Res Cardiol 1993;88(2):179–91.

[35] Merlet P, Delforge J, Syrota A, et al. Positron emission tomography with 11C CGP-12177 to assess beta-adrenergic receptor concentration in idiopathic dilated cardiomyopathy. Circulation 1993;87(4):1169–78.

[36] Imamura Y, Ando H, Ashihara T, et al. Myocardial adrenergic nervous activity is intensified in patients with heart failure without left ventricular volume or pressure overload. J Am Coll Cardiol 1996;28(2):371–5.

[37] Sato M, Maehara K, Yaoita H, et al. Correlation between cardiac norepinephrine overflow during exercise and cardiac 123I-MIBG uptake in patients with chronic heart failure. J Nucl Med 2003;44(10):1618–24.

[38] Vesalainen RK, Pietila M, Tahvanainen KU, et al. Cardiac positron emission tomography imaging with [11C]hydroxyephedrine, a specific tracer for sympathetic nerve endings, and its functional correlates in congestive heart failure. Am J Cardiol 1999;84(5):568–74.

[39] Bengel FM, Permanetter B, Ungerer M, et al. Relationship between altered sympathetic innervation, oxidative metabolism and contractile function in the cardiomyopathic human heart; a non-invasive study using positron emission tomography. Eur Heart J 2001;22(17):1594–600.

[40] Hartmann F, Ziegler S, Nekolla S, et al. Regional patterns of myocardial sympathetic denervation in dilated cardiomyopathy: an analysis using carbon-11 hydroxyephedrine and positron emission tomography. Heart 1999;81(3):262–70.

[41] Ungerer M, Weig HJ, Kubert S, et al. Regional pre- and postsynaptic sympathetic system in the failing human heart–regulation of beta ARK-1. Eur J Heart Fail 2000;2(1):23–31.

[42] Link JM, Stratton JR, Levy W, et al. PET measures of pre- and post-synaptic cardiac beta adrenergic function. Nucl Med Biol 2003;30(8):795–803.

[43] Ungerer M, Hartmann F, Karoglan M, et al. Regional in vivo and in vitro characterization of autonomic innervation in cardiomyopathic human heart. Circulation 1998;97(2):174–80.

[44] Lee DS, Tu JV, Juurlink DN, et al. Risk-treatment mismatch in the pharmacotherapy of heart failure. JAMA 2005;294(10):1240–7.

[45] Francis GS, Cohn JN, Johnson G, et al. Plasma norepinephrine, plasma renin activity, and congestive heart failure. Relations to survival and the effects of therapy in V-HeFT II. The V-HeFT VA Cooperative Studies Group. Circulation 1993;87(6 Suppl):VI40–8.

[46] Cohn JN, Levine TB, Olivari MT, et al. Plasma norepinephrine as a guide to prognosis in patients with chronic congestive heart failure. N Engl J Med 1984;311(13):819–23.

[47] Cowie MR. BNP: soon to become a routine measure in the care of patients with heart failure? Heart 2000;83(6):617–8.

[48] Guzzetti S, Magatelli R, Borroni E, et al. Heart rate variability in chronic heart failure. Auton Neurosci 2001;90(1–2):102–5.

[49] Merlet P, Valette H, Dubois-Rande JL, et al. Prognostic value of cardiac metaiodobenzylguanidine imaging in patients with heart failure. J Nucl Med 1992;33(4):471–7.

[50] Nakata T, Miyamoto K, Doi A, et al. Cardiac death prediction and impaired cardiac sympathetic innervation assessed by MIBG in patients with failing and nonfailing hearts. J Nucl Cardiol 1998;5(6):579–90.

[51] Cohen-Solal A, Esanu Y, Logeart D, et al. Cardiac

metaiodobenzylguanidine uptake in patients with moderate chronic heart failure: relationship with peak oxygen uptake and prognosis. J Am Coll Cardiol 1999; 33(3):759–66.
[52] Momose M, Kobayashi H, Iguchi N, et al. Comparison of parameters of 123I-MIBG scintigraphy for predicting prognosis in patients with dilated cardiomyopathy. Nucl Med Commun 1999;20(6):529–35.
[53] Wakabayashi T, Nakata T, Hashimoto A, et al. Assessment of underlying etiology and cardiac sympathetic innervation to identify patients at high risk of cardiac death. J Nucl Med 2001;42(12):1757–67.
[54] Ogita H, Shimonagata T, Fukunami M, et al. Prognostic significance of cardiac (123)I metaiodoben zylguanidine imaging for mortality and morbidity in patients with chronic heart failure: a prospective study. Heart 2001;86(6):656–60.
[55] Imamura Y, Fukuyama T, Mochizuki T, et al. Prognostic value of iodine-123-metaiodobenzylguanidine imaging and cardiac natriuretic peptide levels in patients with left ventricular dysfunction resulting from cardiomyopathy. Jpn Circ J 2001;65(3):155–60.
[56] Matsui T, Tsutamoto T, Maeda K, et al. Prognostic value of repeated 123I-metaiodobenzylguanidine imaging in patients with dilated cardiomyopathy with congestive heart failure before and after optimized treatments–comparison with neurohumoral factors. Circ J 2002;66(6):537–43.
[57] Gerson MC, McGuire N, Wagoner LE. Sympathetic nervous system function as measured by I-123 metaiodobenzylguanidine predicts transplant-free survival in heart failure patients with idiopathic dilated cardiomyopathy. J Card Fail 2003;9(5):384–91.
[58] Yamada T, Shimonagata T, Fukunami M, et al. Comparison of the prognostic value of cardiac iodine-123 metaiodobenzylguanidine imaging and heart rate variability in patients with chronic heart failure: a prospective study. J Am Coll Cardiol 2003;41(2):231–8.
[59] Nakata T, Wakabayashi T, Kyuma M, et al. Prognostic implications of an initial loss of cardiac metaiodobenzylguanidine uptake and diabetes mellitus in patients with left ventricular dysfunction. J Card Fail 2003; 9(2):113–21.
[60] Kyuma M, Nakata T, Hashimoto A, et al. Incremental prognostic implications of brain natriuretic peptide, cardiac sympathetic nerve innervation, and noncardiac disorders in patients with heart failure. J Nucl Med 2004;45(2):155–63.
[61] Pietila M, Malminiemi K, Ukkonen H, et al. Reduced myocardial carbon-11 hydroxyephedrine retention is associated with poor prognosis in chronic heart failure. Eur J Nucl Med 2001;28(3):373–6.
[62] Suwa M, Otake Y, Moriguchi A, et al. Iodine-123 metaiodobenzylguanidine myocardial scintigraphy for prediction of response to beta-blocker therapy in patients with dilated cardiomyopathy. Am Heart J 1997; 133(3):353–8.
[63] Nakata T, Wakabayashi T, Kyuma M, et al. Cardiac metaiodobenzylguanidine activity can predict the long-term efficacy of angiotensin-converting enzyme inhibitors and/or beta-adrenoceptor blockers in patients with heart failure. Eur J Nucl Med Mol Imaging 2005;32(2):186–94.
[64] Solomon SD, Wang D, Finn P, et al. Effect of candesartan on cause-specific mortality in heart failure patients: the Candesartan in Heart failure Assessment of Reduction in Mortality and morbidity (CHARM) program. Circulation 2004;110(15):2180–3.
[65] Meredith IT, Broughton A, Jennings GL, et al. Evidence of a selective increase in cardiac sympathetic activity in patients with sustained ventricular arrhythmias. N Engl J Med 1991;325(9):618–24.
[66] Simmons WW, Freeman MR, Grima EA, et al. Abnormalities of cardiac sympathetic function in pacing-induced heart failure as assessed by [123I]metaiodobenzylguanidine scintigraphy. Circulation 1994;89(6): 2843–51.
[67] Lerch H, Bartenstein P, Wichter T, et al. Sympathetic innervation of the left ventricle is impaired in arrhythmogenic right ventricular disease. Eur J Nucl Med 1993;20(3):207–12.
[68] Cao JM, Fishbein MC, Han JB, et al. Relationship between regional cardiac hyperinnervation and ventricular arrhythmia. Circulation 2000;101(16):1960–9.
[69] Tomaselli GF, Zipes DP. What causes sudden death in heart failure? Circ Res 2004;95(8):754–63.
[70] CIVISIIinvestigators. The cardiac insufficiency bisoprolol study II (CIBIS-II): a randomised trial. Lancet 1999;353(9146):9–13.
[71] Corsello A. An implantable cardioverter-defibrillator but not amiodarone reduced risk for death in congestive heart failure. ACP J Club 2005;143(1):6.
[72] Arora R, Ferrick KJ, Nakata T, et al. I-123 MIBG imaging and heart rate variability analysis to predict the need for an implantable cardioverter defibrillator. J Nucl Cardiol 2003;10(2):121–31.

ELSEVIER
SAUNDERS

Heart Failure Clin 2 (2006) 205 – 214

HEART
FAILURE
CLINICS

Imaging to Differentiate Between Ischemic and Nonischemic Cardiomyopathy

Jeroen J. Bax, MD, PhD[a,*], Don Poldermans, MD, PhD[b], Joanne D. Schuijf, MSc[a], Arthur J.H.A. Scholte, MD[a], Abdou Elhendy, MD, PhD[b], Ernst E. van der Wall, MD, PhD[a]

[a]*Leiden University Medical Center, Leiden, The Netherlands*
[b]*Erasmus Medical Center, Rotterdam, The Netherlands*

Chronic heart failure is becoming the main problem in clinical cardiology in terms of the number of patients involved. Over the past decade, the number of patients affected with heart failure has increased dramatically, with recent estimations showing that 4.9 million patients in the United States have chronic heart failure, and 550.000 new patients are diagnosed annually, resulting in 970,000 hospitalizations [1]. The diagnostic and therapeutic costs involved with heart failure are estimated to be more than $11 billion per year [1]. The major part of costs appears related to the hospitalizations of these patients for decompensated heart failure. The major question that needs to be addressed is: what causes congestive heart failure?

To address this issue, Gheorghiade and Bonow [2] pooled data from 13 randomized multicenter heart failure drug trials (with more than 20,000 patients) conducted between 1986 and 1997. The authors concluded that coronary artery disease (CAD) was the underlying cause in almost 70% of the patients, and it is likely that this figure is even higher because many patients in these trials did not undergo coronary angiography. From these data, it can be concluded that the main cause of heart failure is therefore chronic CAD.

* Corresponding author. Department of Cardiology, Leiden University Medical Center, Albinusdreef 2, 2333 ZA, Leiden, The Netherlands.

E-mail address: jbax@knoware.nl (J.J. Bax).

The long-term prognosis of these patients remains poor, despite advances in different therapies. Data from the Framingham study demonstrated a 5-year mortality rate of 75% for men and 62% for women [3]. More recent data from Cowie and colleagues [4] showed a 12-month mortality rate of 38%, and the extrapolation of these data resulted in a comparable 5-year mortality rate found in the Framingham study [5].

What are the main therapeutic options for ischemic heart failure?

Presently, four main therapeutic options are available for heart failure, including medical treatment, heart transplantation, surgery, and cardiac resynchronization therapy (CRT).

Medical therapy

Medical therapy has changed substantially over the recent years, with the introduction of new medications. Angiotensin-converting enzyme (ACE) inhibitors have been demonstrated in large heart failure trials (SAVE, SOLVD) to improve survival [6,7]. Angiotensin II receptor blockers have also been evaluated in patients who have heart failure. In the ELITE II Trial [8], a direct comparison with ACE inhibitors was performed, showing a comparable reduction in mortality using either drug. Moreover, various trials

1551-7136/06/$ – see front matter
doi:10.1016/j.hfc.2006.01.003

with β-blockers have demonstrated a significant reduction in overall mortality [9], and more recently, spironolactone has been demonstrated to be useful in the treatment of heart failure [10], although the prescription of this drug may be somewhat limited by potential hyperkalemia [11]. Last, amiodarone has contributed to a reduction in sudden death in patients who have heart failure, as demonstrated in the CAMIAT Trial [12]. In patients who have ischemic as well as patients who have nonischemic cardiomyopathy (ICM and NICM, respectively), medical therapy remains the cornerstone of therapy.

Heart transplantation

Heart transplantation is another therapeutic option with an excellent long-term prognosis and can be used in patients who have ischemic and nonischemic heart failure. However, the limited number of donor hearts is exceeded largely by the demand [13], and many patients who have heart failure have significant comorbidity, excluding them as candidates for heart transplantation.

Surgery

Surgery is a third option in patients who have heart failure. Revascularization is indicated in patients who have ICM in the presence of ischemia or viability [14]. In some patients, revascularization is combined with mitral valve repair (in the presence of severe mitral regurgitation with left ventricular [LV] annular dilatation) or LV reconstruction (in the presence of severe LV aneurysm). In patients who have NICM, mitral valve repair can be performed in the presence of severe LV dilatation and functional mitral regurgitation [15]. Also, partial left ventriculectomy (left ventriculoplasty) has been performed successfully, with promising midterm results by partial exclusion of the anteroseptum. As shown in a study by Horii and colleagues [16], in 70 patients, a 23% to 33% improvement in LV ejection fraction was demonstrated at 2-year follow-up, with 1-year and 4-year survival rates of 75% and 69%, respectively.

Cardiac resynchronization therapy

Cardiac resynchronization therapy is the fourth therapy and includes simultaneous right and left ventricular pacing in heart failure patients. The underlying concept is that heart failure may be secondary to interventricular (right versus left ventricle) or intraventricular (within the left ventricle) dysynchrony, which may be corrected by CRT. Indeed, the initial results with CRT have shown improvement in heart failure symptoms, quality of life, exercise capacity, and systolic LV function [17]. Moreover, recent trials have also shown a significant reduction in the number of hospitalizations for heart failure and a reduction in mortality [18]. This therapy has been demonstrated to be effective in both patients who have ischemic and those who have nonischemic heart failure, although patients who have nonischemic heart failure may exhibit greater benefit [19].

To determine the optimal therapeutic option, the differentiation between ICM and NICM is needed. Invasive coronary angiography allows immediate discrimination between the two entities, based on the identification of CAD. However, with the introduction of various imaging modalities, early differentiation may now become possible in a noninvasive manner. This article discusses the potential role of the different imaging modalities for this purpose.

Noninvasive imaging techniques to differentiate ischemic from nonischemic cardiomyopathy

Several imaging techniques have been proposed to assess the underlying cause of heart failure (Box 1). These techniques rely on the assessment of the functional consequences of CAD, including ischemia

Box 1. Imaging techniques to assess the cause of heart failure in ischemic versus nonischemic cardiomyopathy

Visualization of consequences of coronary artery disease: infarction or ischemia

- PET and SPECT (assessment of function, perfusion, and metabolism
- Echocardiography (assessment of function and perfusion)
- MRI (assessment of function and perfusion)

Visualization of coronary arteries

- Electron beam-computed tomography (EBCT)
- Multislice-computed tomography (MSCT)
- MRI

and infarction. For this purpose, visualization of the perfusion, function, and metabolism have been used. Visualization can be obtained with echocardiography, nuclear imaging, and MRI. Alternatively, direct visualization of the coronary arteries in a noninvasive manner (with MRI or CT techniques) allows direct distinction between ICM and NICM.

Visualization of consequences of coronary artery disease: infarction or ischemia

Echocardiography

Resting two-dimensional (2-D) echocardiography provides the first clues to differentiating between heart failure patients who have and those who do not have CAD. Typically, heart failure patients who do not have CAD have a dilated left ventricle on 2-D echocardiography, with diffuse wall thinning and segmental hypokinesia to akinesia, with the exception of the basal segments. In contrast, patients who have ICM frequently have regional wall thinning or wall motion abnormalities in areas of previous infarction. In particular, the value of end-diastolic wall thickness has been used to identify regions with previous infarction. Schinkel and coworkers [20] have demonstrated that regions with an end-diastolic wall thickness <6 mm consisted predominantly of scar tissue. Still, resting wall motion abnormalities do not differentiate adequately between ICM and NICM; and various studies have demonstrated the occurrence of regional variations in wall motion in idiopathic dilated cardiomyopathy (secondary to differences in wall stress) on the one hand and the presence of diffuse wall motion abnormalities in patients who have ICM and multiple infarctions on the other hand.

With stress echocardiography, an integrated assessment of resting and stress-induced wall motion abnormalities is possible. In particular, the induction of regional wall motion abnormalities (reflecting ischemia) has been demonstrated to be highly accurate for the detection of CAD. A pooled analysis of 15 available studies (with 1849 patients) on the diagnostic accuracy of exercise echocardiography has shown a weighted mean sensitivity of 84% and specificity of 82% for the detection of CAD. Similarly, a pooled analysis of 28 studies (with 2246 patients) with dobutamine echocardiography has yielded a sensitivity and specificity of 80% and 84%, respectively [21]. Accordingly, the value of stress echocardiography for the differentiation between ICM and NICM was shown by Sharp and colleagues [22] who evaluated 70 patients who had cardiomyopathy using dobutamine stress echocardiography. The authors demonstrated that the induction of regional wall motion abnormalities was both a sensitive and specific marker of CAD, making the exclusion of NICM possible with high accuracy.

In addition to the evaluation of contractile function, myocardial perfusion can also be evaluated with echocardiography using intravenous contrast administration [23]. Recent contrast agents are composed of high-molecular weight inert gases, with micro-bubbles that stay in the vascular space. Because the micro-bubbles behave similarly to red blood cells in terms of rheology, contrast echocardiography allows the direct visualization of myocardial perfusion. Initial studies demonstrated good agreement between nuclear imaging and contrast echocardiography for assessing resting perfusion (and perfusion defects). In addition, the combination of contrast echocardiography with vasodilator stress allows accurate detection of coronary artery stenoses [24]; in particular, contrast echocardiography has been shown to correctly identify 97% of the territories supplied by significant coronary artery stenoses and 82% of the territories supplied by normal arteries. More recently, Senior and colleagues [25] used contrast echocardiography (at rest and after vasodilation) in patients presenting with acute heart failure to differentiate between ischemic and nonischemic heart failure. Using this approach, the sensitivity and specificity to detect CAD were found to be 82% and 97%, respectively. In addition, among the clinical and biochemical markers, ECG, and resting echocardiographic variables, contrast echocardiography was the only independent predictor of the presence or absence of CAD.

Echocardiography can even be used to noninvasively visualize the coronary arteries. In 1992, Sawada and colleagues [26] reported on the use of transthoracic echocardiography to visualize the coronary arteries in 59 patients who had cardiomyopathy (32 with ICM and 27 with NICM, assessed by coronary angiography). Visualization of the coronary arteries was feasible in 93% of patients, and the accuracy to assess or exclude CAD was 86%. Moreover, the coronary flow reserve can be assessed by contrast-enhanced transthoracic echocardiography. Caiati and colleagues [27] have demonstrated the feasibility of this approach in 56 patients with or without significant left anterior descending (LAD) stenosis. By the use of a second harmonic Doppler imaging method with contrast enhancement, the coronary flow was assessed at rest and during maximal hyperemia (after pharmacologic vasodilation), yielding the coronary flow reserve. In patients who had significant LAD stenosis, the flow reserve was significantly lower than in patients who did not have LAD stenosis (1.54 ± 0.7 versus 2.79 ± 0.9, $P<.001$). The method was further validated by showing good agreement between the echocardiographic approach and measurements with intracoronary Doppler flow wires [28]. Finally, this echocardiographic approach even allowed for the recovery of coronary flow reserve after percutaneous intervention [29].

Nuclear imaging

Nuclear imaging has also been used to assess the cause of heart failure. With stress-rest SPECT imaging, the hallmark of ischemia (indicating CAD) is reversibility of perfusion defects. In addition, fixed perfusion defects reflect scar formation, also indicating CAD. With the introduction of gated SPECT imaging, it is now possible to also assess the LV ejection fraction (EF), LV volumes, and regional wall motion during the same session. Indeed, SPECT myocardial perfusion imaging has a high accuracy for the diagnosis of CAD, with an average sensitivity and specificity of 86% and 74%, based on a pooled analysis of 79 studies with 8964 patients (Fig. 1) [21]. The lower specificity can be attributed to the post-test referral bias; a better parameter may be the normalcy rate, which was 89% in pooled data from 10 studies with 549 patients [21]. Also, the inclusion of LV function data obtained from the ECG-gated images has further increased the accuracy of SPECT [30].

An early study with thallium 201 imaging has demonstrated that patients who have ICM have extensive and diffuse defects in tracer uptake, whereas tracer uptake was mostly homogenous in patients who have NICM [31]. Danias and colleagues [32] reported initially on the feasibility of gated SPECT with technetium 99m sestamibi to discriminate between ICM and NICM. The authors evaluated 37 patients who had heart failure and demonstrated a significant difference in summed stress, rest, and reversibility scores (reflecting reversible and irreversible defects) between the two groups. The difference in summed stress scores was particularly dramatic: 6.9 ± 3.8 versus 32.9 ± 7.7 ($P<.001$, NICM versus ICM). Also, the variability in regional wall motion scores was larger in patients who had ICM, indicating more regional wall motion abnormalities (rather than diffusely reduced wall motion). In a subsequent study, Danias and colleagues [33] evaluated 164 patients (LVEF </=40%) with heart failure of unknown origins. The summed stress score had a sensitivity of 87%, with a specificity of 63% to detect CAD. The integration of wall motion information increased sensitivity to 94% but reduced specificity to 32%.

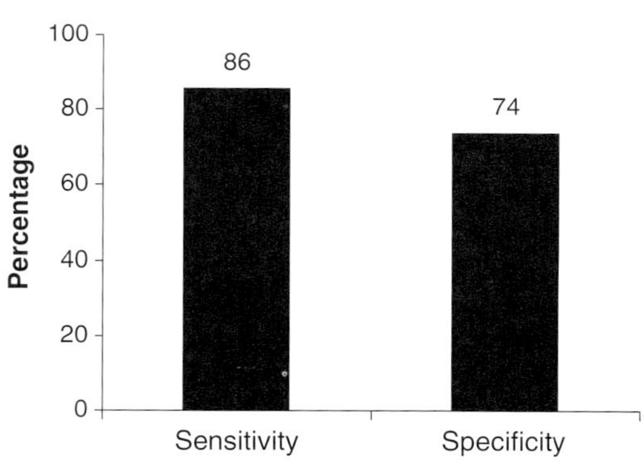

Fig. 1. Diagnostic accuracy of myocardial perfusion imaging with SPECT based on a pooled analysis of 79 studies with 8964 patients. (*From* Schuijf JD, Shaw LJ, Wijns W, et al. Cardiac imaging in coronary artery disease: differing modalities. Heart 2005;91:1111; with permission.)

Positron emission tomography (PET) also has been used in the diagnosis of the cause of heart failure. Various tracers have been used, and Eisenberg and colleagues [34] evaluated 20 patients using PET with radioactive carbon 11 (^{11}C)-palmitate. The majority (80%) of patients who have ICM had extensive areas of reduced accumulation of ^{11}C-palmitate, compared with none of the patients who had NICM. Mody and coworkers [35] used nitrogen 13 (^{13}N)-ammonia (to assess perfusion) and fluorine 18-fluorodeoxyglucose (^{F}18-FDG) (to assess glucose usage) to discriminate between patients who had ICM and those who had NICM. Both tracers showed significantly more defects in patients who had ICM, whereas the majority of patients who had NICM had homogenous uptake of both tracers. When quantitative analyses were applied, the sensitivity and specificity were 100% and 80%, respectively, to discriminate between the two groups. In a subsequent study, nine (four ICM, five NICM) patients were evaluated with ^{13}N-ammonia and FDG PET before undergoing heart transplantation [36]. Histologic results from the explanted hearts demonstrated a good correlation between the defects in ^{13}N-ammonia and FDG uptake on the one hand and the presence of infarcted tissue on the other hand in the patients who had ICM. In the patients who have NICM, the uptake of both tracers was homogeneous and histology did not reveal scar tissue. Despite the homogenous tracer uptake in patients who had NICM, PET studies with ^{11}C-acetate demonstrated reduced oxidative metabolism [37].

MRI

MRI is being used increasingly in clinical cardiology. The versatility of MRI permits the assessment of multiple aspects of CAD, and this technique can also be used in the noninvasive evaluation of patients who have heart failure. First, similar to echocardiography, a dilated LV with diffuse segmental hypokinesia is suspect for NICM. However, a more detailed analysis of segmental function reveals differences in contraction. With tagged MRI, heterogeneity in regional three-dimensional (3-D) displacements and strain has been demonstrated, with abnormalities located predominantly in the septum [38]. Still, outspoken regional contractile dysfunction and reduced end-diastolic wall thickness correlate well with regions of transmural infarction, which is indicative of CAD (Fig. 2).

With stress-rest MRI, both perfusion and function can be evaluated, and similar to stress echocardiography and SPECT imaging, it is possible to identify CAD with high accuracy. A pooled analysis of 17 reports (with 502 patients) using stress-rest MRI to assess perfusion revealed a weighted mean sensitivity and specificity of 84% and 85%, respectively, to detect CAD (Fig. 3) [21]. Also, a pooled analysis of 10 studies (with 654 patients) using the presence of wall motion abnormalities revealed a weighted mean sensitivity and specificity of 89% and 84%, respectively, to detect CAD (Fig. 4) [21]. However, stress-rest MRI has not yet been used to discriminate patients who have ICM and NICM.

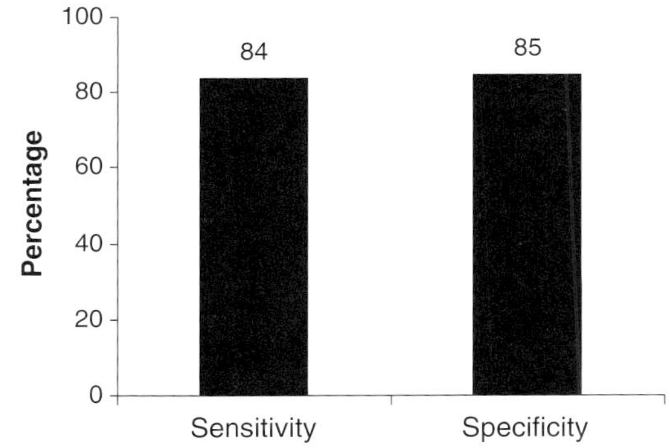

Fig. 3. Diagnostic accuracy of stress-rest perfusion imaging with MRI to detect significant CAD based on 17 studies with 502 patients. (*From* Schuijf JD, Shaw LJ, Wijns W, et al. Cardiac imaging in coronary artery disease: differing modalities. Heart 2005;91:1113; with permission.)

More recently, contrast-enhanced MRI has gained substantial popularity for the assessment of scar tissue. Contrast hyperenhancement on delayed resting MRI is defined as regions of increased signal intensity on T1-weighted images acquired more than 5 minutes after the intravenous administration of a contrast agent. The mechanism underlying the hyperenhancement appears to be related to the interstitial space between collagen fibers, which is larger in scar tissue compared with the densely packed myocytes in normal myocardium, and the contrast agent will be trapped in these areas in infarcted tissue. An excellent

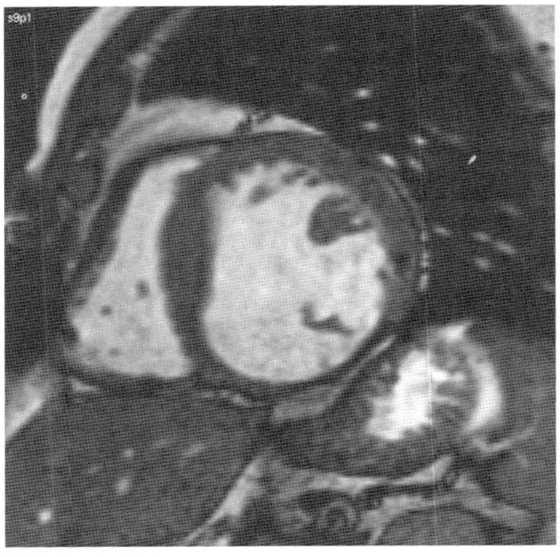

Fig. 2. Short-axis resting MRI of a patient who has an inferior infarction. The inferior wall shows severe thinning with an end-diastolic wall thickness <6 mm, indicating scar tissue.

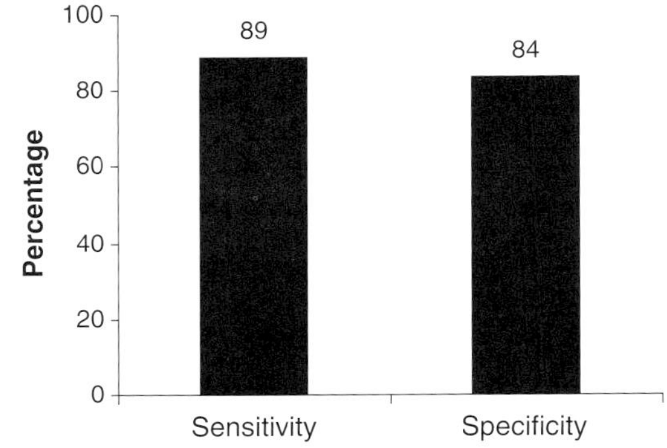

Fig. 4. Diagnostic accuracy of stress-rest wall motion imaging with MRI to detect significant CAD (data based on a pooled analysis of 10 studies with 654 patients). (*From* Schuijf JD, Shaw LJ, Wijns W, et al. Cardiac imaging in coronary artery disease: differing modalities. Heart 2005;91:1113; with permission.)

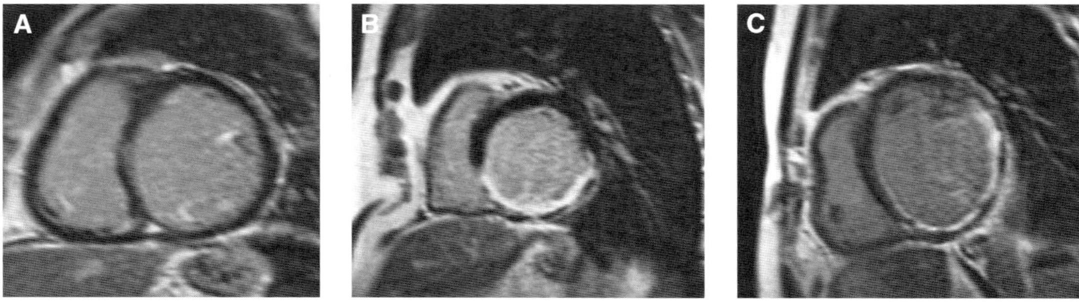

Fig. 5. MRI examples of patients with different cardiomyopathies. (*A*) Short-axis contrast-enhanced MRI of a patient who has severe heart failure and NICM. No hyperenhancement is visible, indicating no scar tissue. (*B*) Short-axis contrast-enhanced MRI study of a patient who has heart failure, ICM, and a previous inferior infarction. Transmural hyperenhancement (*white tissue*) is present in the inferior wall. (*C*) Short-axis contrast-enhanced MRI study of a heart failure patient who has ICM and extensive scar formation (*white tissue*).

correlation between hyperenhancement on MRI and histology has been demonstrated in animal experiments [39]. Moreover, the excellent spatial resolution of MRI allows the detection of minimal regions of scar tissue and the distinction between transmural and subendocardial infarction. Based on the presence and location of scar tissue on contrast-enhanced MRI, it is possible to differentiate between ICM and NICM. McCrohon and colleagues [40], who have extensively explored this concept, evaluated 90 consecutive patients who had heart failure, including 63 patients who had NICM and 27 who had ICM. All patients who had ICM had regions with hyperenhancement on MRI, ranging from subendocardial to transmural scar tissue. Notably, the subendocardium was always involved in the hyperenhanced region, which is compatible with the spatial progress of infarction. In patients who had NICM, three patterns were observed. In 59% of the patients, no hyperenhancement was present; in 28% of patients, patchy or longitudinal striae of midwall hyperenhancement were noted; and in 13% of patients, hyperenhancement extended from the subendocardium into the wall (indistinguishable from ICM). Thus, the majority of patients could be correctly classified according to the presence (or absence) and pattern of hyperenhancement on MRI. Examples of contrast-enhanced MRI in patients who have ICM and NICM are demonstrated in Fig. 5.

Of interest, contrast-enhanced MRI also has been used in patients who have heart failure secondary to myocarditis. In 32 patients diagnosed with myocarditis, 88% have shown regions of hyperenhancement, which are located mainly in the mid part of the lateral wall. In addition, the hyperenhanced regions correlated well with active inflammation on histologic analysis of biopsies.

Direct visualization of the coronary arteries

MRI

Various MRI techniques have been developed to visualize the coronary arteries, including 2-D and 3-D techniques. A pooled analysis of 28 studies (with 903 patients) comparing MRI with invasive angiography has shown a weighted mean sensitivity of 72% and a specificity of 87% to detect obstructive CAD

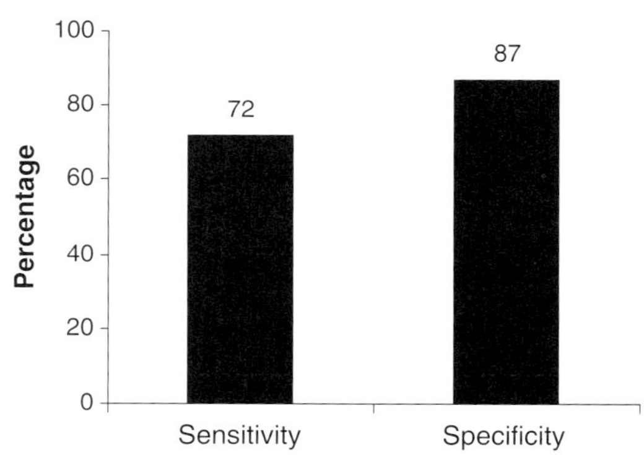

Fig. 6. Current diagnostic accuracy of noninvasive coronary angiography with MRI to detect significant CAD based on a pooled analysis of 28 studies with 903. (*From* Schuijf JD, Shaw LJ, Wijns W, et al. Cardiac imaging in coronary artery disease: differing modalities. Heart 2005;91:1115; with permission.)

(Fig. 6) [21]. In addition to the suboptimal diagnostic accuracy, the individual studies show a wide variation in diagnostic accuracy, and MRI techniques are still hampered by a relatively long acquisition time, with a substantial percentage of segments remaining uninterpretable. Some of these shortcomings may be overcome with the introduction of 3-Tesla systems and new contrast agents. Currently, large studies on the detection (or exclusion) of CAD to assess the cause of heart failure have not been performed.

CT techniques

Two CT techniques have been used for the noninvasive visualization of the coronary arteries, electron beam CT (EBCT) and multislice CT (MSCT). With EBCT, x-rays are created through an electron beam that is guided along a 210°-tungsten target ring in the gantry, and images are acquired with high temporal resolution (in the range of 50–100 ms) and 1.5- to 3.0-mm slice thickness. To cover the entire heart, 40 to 50 slices are necessary, typically requiring a breath hold of 30 to 40 seconds, depending on the heart rate. A pooled analysis of 10 studies (with 538 patients) comparing EBCT with invasive angiography has shown a weighted mean sensitivity and specificity of 87% and 91%, respectively, to detect CAD (Fig. 7) [21]. Limitations include the high percentage of uninterpretable segments (approximately 20%), overestimation of luminal narrowing by extensive coronary calcifications, and motion artifacts.

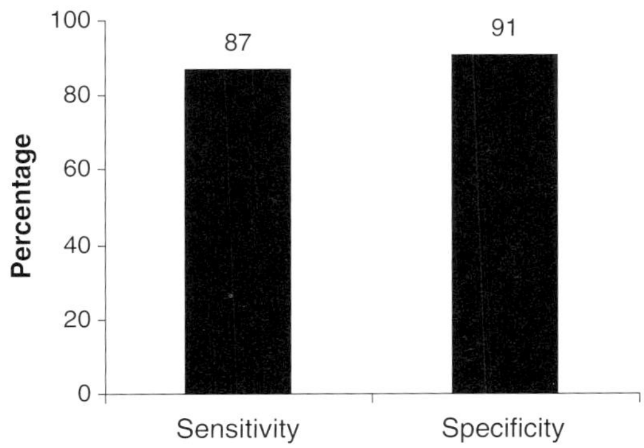

Fig. 7. Current diagnostic accuracy of noninvasive coronary angiography with EBCT to detect significant CAD based on a pooled analysis of 10 studies with 538 patients. (*From* Schuijf JD, Shaw LJ, Wijns W, et al. Cardiac imaging in coronary artery disease: differing modalities. Heart 2005;91:1116; with permission.)

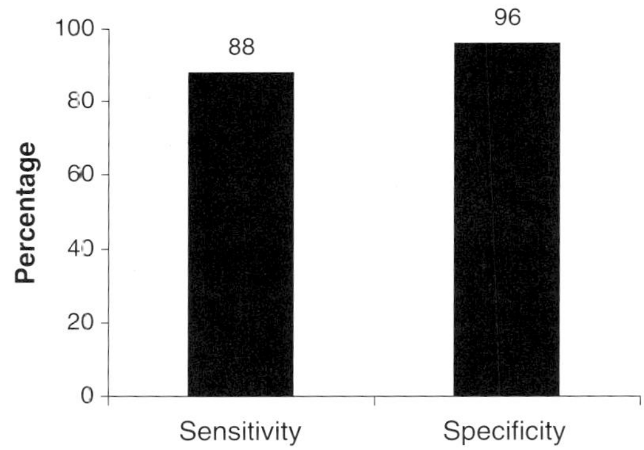

Fig. 8. Current diagnostic accuracy of noninvasive coronary angiography with 16-slice MSCT to detect significant CAD based on a pooled analysis of 11 studies with 681 patients. (*From* Schuijf JD, Shaw LJ, Wijns W, et al. Cardiac imaging in coronary artery disease: differing modalities. Heart 2005;91:1115; with permission.)

MSCT systems allow acquisition of multiple slices instead of one slice in a single gantry rotation, thereby enabling visualization of the coronary arteries. The initial studies with four-slice scanners had suboptimal accuracy for detecting CAD, and approximately 20% of segments were excluded for nondiagnostic quality [21]. The newer 16-slice scanners with submillimeter collimation and faster rotation times yield a higher diagnostic accuracy. Pooled data from 11 studies (with 681 patients) comparing 16-slice MSCT with invasive angiography have shown a weighted mean sensitivity and specificity of 88% and 96%, respectively (Fig. 8) [21]. The most recent results with the latest 64-slice scanners have revealed a sensitivity and specificity of 99% and 95%, respectively [41]. The limitations of this technique include the high radiation exposure (9–12 mSv), the need for low heart rates, and reduced image quality in patients who have severe coronary calcifications. Presently, coronary angiography with EBCT or MSCT to assess the cause of heart failure has not been studied extensively. Examples of MSCT in heart failure patients who have ICM and those who have NICM are shown in Fig. 9.

The CT techniques, however, also can be used for the assessment of coronary artery calcium rather than angiography. The exclusion of coronary artery calcium is likely to exclude CAD; this concept was evaluated in 125 heart failure patients who underwent EBCT and invasive coronary angiography [42]. Indeed, 71 of 72 patients who had ICM showed coronary artery calcium on EBCT, yielding a sensitivity of 99%; conversely, 44 of 53 patients who had NICM

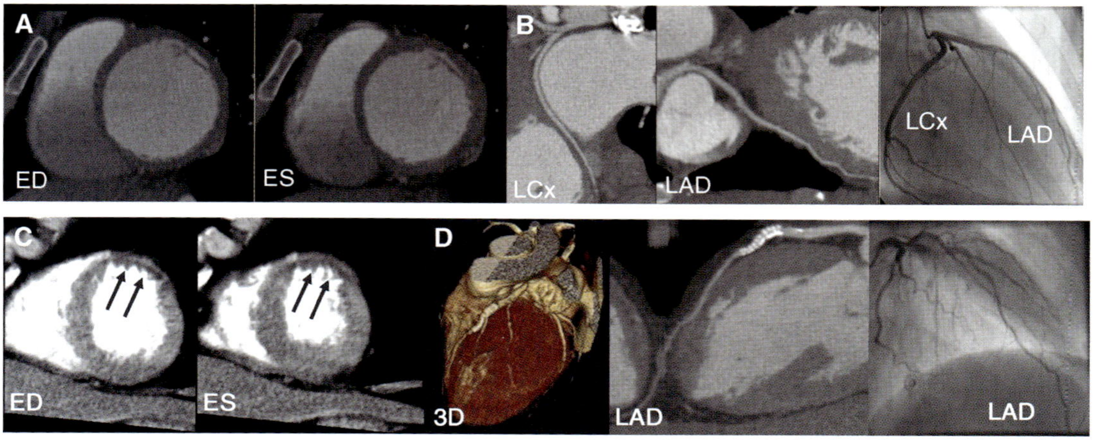

Fig. 9. Examples of MSCT imaging in patients with respectively nonischemic and ischemic heart failure. (*A* and *B*) Short-axis reconstructions are provided in end-diastole and end-systole, revealing severe reduced contractility (*A*). (*B*) Curved multiplanar reconstructions of LCx and LAD are provided, showing normal coronary arteries. To the right, the corresponding invasive coronary angiogram is provided, confirming the MSCT findings. (*C* and *D*) Examples of a patient with ischemic heart failure are shown. (*C*) Short-axis reconstructions are provided in end-diastole and end-systole, revealing reduced contractility in the anterior LV wall, corresponding to a region of previous infarction (*arrows*). (*D*) 3-D volume-rendered reconstruction is shown demonstrating the presence of diffuse irregularities in the coronary arteries. Also, calcifications proximal to the coronary stent can be observed in the curved multiplanar reconstruction of the LAD. To the right, the corresponding invasive coronary angiogram is shown. ED, end-diastole; ES, end-systole; LAD, left anterior descending; LCx, left circumflex.

(according to invasive angiography) did not have coronary artery calcium (specificity, 83%).

Clinical implications

Differentiating between ICM and NICM is important for determining the appropriate therapy. Invasive angiography allows direct detection or exclusion of CAD, but noninvasive imaging in patients who have heart failure may also provide this information. Presently, the imaging techniques can be divided into techniques that visualize ischemia and scar tissue as markers of CAD and techniques that permit noninvasive angiography. Most likely, these techniques will have complementary value in the evaluation of heart failure patients. Finally, in addition to their diagnostic value, imaging techniques also can provide prognostic information in patients who have heart failure and are useful in the assessment of response to therapy.

References

[1] American Heart Association. Heart disease and stroke statistics, 2005 update. Dallas (TX): American Heart Association; 2005.

[2] Gheorghiade M, Bonow RO. Chronic heart failure in the United States: a manifestation of coronary artery disease. Circulation 1998;97:282–9.

[3] Anderson KM, Kannel WB, Grossman W, et al. Survival after the onset of congestive heart failure in Framingham Heart Study subjects. Circulation 1993; 88:107–15.

[4] Cowie MR, Wood DA, Coats AJ, et al. Incidence and aetiology of heart failure: a population-based study. Eur Heart J 1999;20:421–8.

[5] Khand A, Gemmel I, Clark A, et al. Is the prognosis of heart failure improving? J Am Coll Cardiol 2000; 36:2284–6.

[6] Pfeffer MA, Braunwald E, Moye LA, et al. Effect of captopril on mortality and morbidity in patients with left ventricular dysfunction after myocardial infarction: results of the Survival and Ventricular Enlargement Trial. N Engl J Med 1992;327:669–77.

[7] The SOLVD investigators. Effect of enalapril on survival in patients with reduced left ventricular ejection fractions and congestive heart failure. N Engl J Med 1991;325:293–302.

[8] Pitt B, Poole-Wilson PA, Segal R, et al. Effect of losartan compared with captopril on mortality in patients with symptomatic heart failure: randomized trial–the Losartan Heart Failure Study ELITE II. Lancet 2000;355:1582–7.

[9] Braunwald E. Expanding indications for beta-blockers in heart failure. N Engl J Med 2001;344:1711–2.

[10] Pitt B, Zannad F, Remme WJ, et al. The effect of spironolactone on morbidity and mortality in patients

with severe heart failure. N Engl J Med 1999;341: 709–17.

[11] Juurlink DN, Mamdani MM, Lee DS, et al. Rates of hyperkalemia after publication of the Randomized Aldactone Evaluation Study. N Engl J Med 2004; 351:543–51.

[12] Caims JA, Connolly SJ, Roberts R, et al for the CAMIAT investigators. Randomized trial of outcome after myocardial infarction in patients with frequent or repetitive premature depolarizations. Lancet 1997; 349:675–82.

[13] Evans RW, Manninen DL, Garrison LP, et al. Donor availability as the primary determinant of the future of heart transplantation. JAMA 1986;255:1892–8.

[14] Rahimtoola SH. The hibernating myocardium. Am Heart J 1989;117:211–21.

[15] Romano MA, Bolling SF. Update on mitral repair in dilated cardiomyopathy. J Card Surg 2004;19: 396–400.

[16] Horii T, Isomura T, Komeda M, et al. Left ventriculoplasty for nonischemic dilated cardiomyopathy. J Card Surg 2003;18:121–4.

[17] Auricchio A, Abraham WT. Cardiac resynchronization therapy: current state of the art: cost versus benefit. Circulation 2004;109:300–7.

[18] Cleland JG, Daubert JC, Erdmann E, et al. The effect of cardiac resynchronization on morbidity and mortality in heart failure. N Engl J Med 2005;352:1539–49.

[19] Molhoek SG, Bax JJ, Van Erven L, et al. Comparison of benefits from cardiac resynchronization therapy in patients with ischemic cardiomyopathy versus idiopathic dilated cardiomyopathy. Am J Cardiol 2004; 93:860–3.

[20] Schinkel AF, Bax JJ, Boersma E, et al. Assessment of residual myocardial viability in regions with chronic electrocardiographic Q-wave infarction. Am Heart J 2002;144:865–9.

[21] Schuijf JD, Shaw LJ, Wijns W, et al. Cardiac imaging in coronary artery disease: differing modalities. Heart 2005;91:1110–7.

[22] Sharp SM, Sawada SG, Segar DS, et al. Dobutamine stress echocardiography: detection of coronary artery disease in patients with dilated cardiomyopathy. J Am Coll Cardiol 1994;24:934–9.

[23] Kaul S. Echocardiographic insights into regional flow-function relationships in coronary artery disease. J Nucl Cardiol 2005;12:216–26.

[24] Peltier M, Vancraeynest D, Pasquet A, et al. Assessment of the physiologic significance of coronary disease with dipyridamole real-time myocardial contrast echocardiography: comparison with technetium-99m sestamibi single-photon emission computed tomography and quantitative coronary angiography. J Am Coll Cardiol 2004;43:257–64.

[25] Senior R, Janardhanan R, Jeetley P, et al. Myocardial contrast echocardiography for distinguishing ischemic from nonischemic first-onset acute heart failure: insights into the mechanism of acute heart failure. Circulation 2005;112:1587–93.

[26] Sawada SG, Ryan T, Segar D, et al. Distinguishing ischemic cardiomyopathy from nonischemic dilated cardiomyopathy with coronary echocardiography. J Am Coll Cardiol 1992;19:1223–8.

[27] Caiati C, Montaldo C, Zedda N, et al. New noninvasive method for coronary flow reserve assessment: contrast-enhanced transthoracic second harmonic echo Doppler. Circulation 1999;99:771–8.

[28] Caiati C, Montaldo C, Zedda N, et al. Validation of a new noninvasive method (contrast-enhanced transthoracic second harmonic echo Doppler) for the evaluation of coronary flow reserve: comparison with intracoronary Doppler flow wire. J Am Coll Cardiol 1999;34:1193–200.

[29] Ruscazio M, Montisci R, Colonna P, et al. Detection of coronary restenosis after coronary angioplasty by contrast-enhanced transthoracic echocardiographic Doppler assessment of coronary flow velocity reserve. J Am Coll Cardiol 2002;40:896–903.

[30] Smanio PE, Watson DD, Segalla DL, et al. Value of gating of technetium-99m sestamibi single-photon emission computed tomographic imaging. J Am Coll Cardiol 1997;30:1687–92.

[31] Eichhorn EJ, Kosinski EJ, Lewis SM, et al. Usefulness of dipyridamole-thallium-201 perfusion scanning for distinguishing ischemic from nonischemic cardiomyopathy. Am J Cardiol 1988;62:945–51.

[32] Danias PG, Ahlberg AW, Clark III BA, et al. Combined assessment of myocardial perfusion and left ventricular function with exercise technetium-99m sestamibi gated single-photon emission computed tomography can differentiate between ischemic and nonischemic dilated cardiomyopathy. Am J Cardiol 1998; 82:1253–8.

[33] Danias PG, Papaioannou GI, Ahlberg AW, et al. Usefulness of electrocardiographic-gated stress technetium-99m sestamibi single-photon emission computed tomography to differentiate ischemic from nonischemic cardiomyopathy. Am J Cardiol 2004;94: 14–9.

[34] Eisenberg JD, Sobel BE, Geltman EM. Differentiation of ischemic from nonischemic cardiomyopathy with positron emission tomography. Am J Cardiol 1987;59: 1410–4.

[35] Mody FV, Brunken RC, Stevenson LW, et al. Differentiating cardiomyopathy of coronary artery disease from nonischemic dilated cardiomyopathy utilizing positron emission tomography. J Am Coll Cardiol 1991;17:373–83.

[36] Berry JJ, Hoffman JM, Steenbergen C, et al. Human pathologic correlation with PET in ischemic and nonischemic cardiomyopathy. J Nucl Med 1993;34: 39–47.

[37] Beanlands RS, Bach DS, Raylman R, et al. Acute effects of dobutamine on myocardial oxygen consumption and cardiac efficiency measured using carbon-11 acetate kinetics in patients with dilated cardiomyopathy. J Am Coll Cardiol 1993;22:1389–98.

[38] Young AA, Dokos S, Powell KA, et al. Regional

heterogeneity of function in nonischemic dilated cardiomyopathy. Cardiovasc Res 2001;49:308–18.
[39] Kim RJ, Fieno DS, Parrish TB, et al. Relationship of MRI delayed contrast enhancement to irreversible injury, infarct age, and contractile function. Circulation 1999;100:1992–2002.
[40] McCrohon JA, Moon JC, Prasad SK, et al. Differentiation of heart failure related to dilated cardiomyopathy and coronary artery disease using gadolinium-enhanced cardiovascular magnetic resonance. Circulation 2003;108:54–9.
[41] Mollet NR, Cademartiri F, Van Mieghem CA, et al. High-resolution spiral computed tomography coronary angiography in patients referred for diagnostic conventional coronary angiography. Circulation 2005;112:2318–23.
[42] Budoff MJ, Shavelle DM, Lamont DH, et al. Usefulness of electron beam computed tomography scanning for distinguishing ischemic from nonischemic cardiomyopathy. J Am Coll Cardiol 1998;32:1173–8.

ELSEVIER
SAUNDERS

Heart Failure Clin 2 (2006) 215 – 230

HEART
FAILURE
CLINICS

Review of Noninvasive Imaging for Hypertrophic Cardiac Syndromes and Restrictive Physiology

Steven J. Fowler, MD, Jagat Narula, MD, Swaminatha V. Gurudevan, MD*

University of California at Irvine, Orange, CA, USA

Restrictive cardiac pathophysiology is characterized by functional impairment of the left ventricular (LV) diastole with preservation of systolic function. Diastolic dysfunction manifests when a small increase in LV volume causes an abrupt rise in LV pressure, leading in turn to elevation in left atrial pressures and symptoms of congestive heart failure. Various degrees of restrictive pathophysiology may be seen in clinical conditions involving the pericardium, myocardium, or endocardium, making it a challenge to differentiate these conditions on clinical grounds alone. This article reviews the noninvasive imaging modalities and methodologies that have emerged to aid the clinician in the definitive diagnosis and differentiation of hypertrophic cardiac syndromes.

Classification

In the current World Health Organization/International Federation and Society of Cardiology classification, cardiomyopathies are categorized on the basis of their pathophysiologic features and constitute a group of disorders in which the primary feature is the involvement of the heart muscle itself [1]. Considerable overlap exists among cardiovascular disease states that share restrictive pathophysiology, especially those that manifest impairment in LV relaxation. Based on their pathology, clinical hypertrophic syndromes may be grossly divided into two main categories: first, an "intrinsic" phenotype of *primary* cardiomyopathies—clinical entities that arise from *direct* involvement of the myocardium in the absence of hemodynamic insult—and second, a "reactive" phenotype of *secondary* cardiomyopathies—clinical entities that arise from remodeling of the myocardium in response to chronic LV pressure overload (eg, hypertension, valvular heart disease). The anatomic and physiologic changes that occur in each group of conditions are similar: both groups manifest with hypertrophy of the ventricle involved, and both can lead to diastolic dysfunction.

Primary hypertrophic cardiac syndromes include hypertrophic cardiomyopathy (HCM) and restrictive cardiomyopathy (RCM). HCM is defined by left or right ventricular hypertrophy, often asymmetric, which usually involves the interventricular septum. It is now understood that mutations in genes that encode myocardial sarcoplasmic proteins cause the disease in many patients [2]. RCM involves a decrease in the compliance of either or both ventricles with normal or near-normal systolic function. It is further classified based on myocardial or endomyocardial involvement and may be associated with a number of systemic conditions that involve noninfiltrative, infiltrative, and storage diseases, as well as endomyocardial disease states [3,4]. The most common causative factors are systemic conditions that lead to infiltration of the myocardium: these include amyloidosis, hemochromatosis, sarcoidosis, and lymphoproliferative diseases.

* Corresponding author. Division of Cardiology, University of California at Irvine, Building 53, Route 81, Room 100, 101 The City Drive South, Orange, CA 9286.

E-mail address: guru@uci.edu (S.V. Gurudevan).

1551-7136/06/$ – see front matter
doi:10.1016/j.hfc.2006.04.001

Secondary hypertrophic cardiac syndromes that demonstrate restrictive pathophysiology include left ventricular hypertrophy, often symmetric, which may be attributed to hypertensive, congenital, or valvular disease. For the purpose of review, the authors focus primarily on hypertensive heart disease (HHD), because it is the archetypal entity in this class. Constrictive pericarditis is a syndrome that falls slightly outside the proposed classification schema but deserves mention, because it often involves systemic disease before clinical presentation and can demonstrate restrictive physiology. Disease processes that may affect the pericardium include chronic infectious, malignant, and collagen-vascular disease, as well as postradiation and postsurgical fibrotic disease. For HHD, HCM, and RCM, the restrictive pattern of impaired relaxation with preserved or enhanced contractile function serves as a characteristic feature until late in the course of the disease, when supervening systolic dysfunction may occur. The distinction between these major functional classes is not absolute: shared features of restrictive physiology make differentiation between these conditions an ongoing diagnostic challenge for the clinical cardiologist.

Clinical features

Hypertrophic cardiac syndromes, regardless of cause, manifest physiologic features of early restriction, related to the increased wall stiffness of the ventricle and the resultant impairment in diastolic filling. Often, clinical progression of the syndrome follows the time-frame of the underlying pathologic process; it is generally insidious, beginning with dyspnea and fatigue while other signs and symptoms of systemic disease (eg, amyloidosis, iron storage disease) become evident. Right-sided heart failure findings tend to predominate with elevated neck veins, peripheral edema, and ascites. If the LV is largely affected, mild to moderate cardiomegaly may ensue. Impairment of LV relaxation and a consequent shift to late diastolic LV filling can manifest as a fourth heart sound (S4), whereas elevation in LV pressures can manifest as a third heart sound (S3). Valvular insufficiency, mainly involving the mitral or tricuspid valves, often develops secondarily in RCMs. When obstructive in nature, the hypertrophic cardiac syndrome will demonstrate auscultatory variability and accentuation during physical maneuvers that diminish preload, such as squat-to-stand and Valsalva. Kussmaul's sign, reflecting an inspiratory increase in central venous pressure, can be a key clinical manifestation of pericardial constriction.

On chest roentgenogram, mild cardiomegaly and biatrial enlargement, along with pulmonary venous hypertension, may be noted. Electrocardiographic findings of restrictive cardiac pathology often vary, reflecting the underlying causative process affecting the myocardium [5]. Augmented P-wave amplitude and altered morphology demonstrate chronic right or left atrial hypertrophy or overload, often seen with chronically elevated LV pressures. Diffuse, low-voltage, atrioventricular or intraventricular conduction delays serve as markers of RCM, whereas LV hypertrophy, ST-segment or T-wave abnormalities, and abnormal Q waves reflect an HHD or HCM pattern. Atrial and ventricular dysrhythmias are also commonly associated with HCM.

Hemodynamics

Hemodynamic investigation of the hypertrophic cardiac syndromes and restrictive pathophysiology typically reveals preserved LV systolic function and diminished LV compliance. The most common hemodynamic finding is the impairment of diastolic filling with elevated filling pressures and fixed stroke volume [6]. In some patients a typical series of hemodynamic waveforms has been reported, involving a dip-and-plateau waveform that reflects a rapid fall in left atrial pressures in early diastole coupled with an equilibration of pressures in late diastole (the "square-root sign"). However, static hemodynamic criteria have limitations, especially in patients who have coexisting myopathic and pericardial involvement [7]. The complex nature of the physiologic interactions that exist in hypertrophic cardiac syndromes has been a driving force in the development of novel noninvasive imaging modalities to assist the clinician further in the diagnosis and treatment of these conditions [8–10].

Noninvasive imaging

The goal of all noninvasive cardiac imaging is qualitatively and quantitatively to evaluate the morphologic, functional, and hemodynamic parameters distorted by the hypertrophic disease process. Newer modalities that aim at visualizing the pathologic and pathophysiologic processes at the tissue level offer further insight into mechanisms, prognosis, and potential treatment throughout the course of the disease.

Echocardiography

Transthoracic echocardiography

Echocardiography remains the major noninvasive imaging modality employed in the initial assessment of hypertrophic cardiac syndromes. The rapidity and ease of the echocardiographic examination make it the best initial choice for the clinician in the evaluation of cardiomyopathies. In addition to the assessment of LV systolic function, diastolic filling patterns may be evaluated; these correlate well with left-sided and right-sided filling pressures and disease-related prognosis [11]. Standard echocardiographic techniques used to delineate pathophysiology include two-dimensional, M-mode, Doppler, and tissue Doppler imaging. Newer echo algorithms and technology permit improved visualization of the myocardium and its microcirculation, with renewed focus on the independent evaluation of ventricular physiology.

M-mode echocardiography provides the basic platform to assess cardiac structure, dimensional changes, and first derivates during diastolic filling. Increased LV wall thickness of greater than 11 mm defines myocardial hypertrophy and is seen in HHD, HCM, and RCM alike [12]. In HHD, the pattern of hypertrophy is concentric, as the remodeling responds to the global increase in LV pressure. In HCM, the pattern of hypertrophy is asymmetric, often involving the septum (septal thickness $\geq$13 to 15 mm and septal–posterior wall ratio $\geq$1.5:1), with some forms (primarily in Japanese populations) involving only the apex [13]. Particular attention is paid to the parasternal or apical long axis views, which afford the best view of the LV outflow tract (LVOT) and enable evaluation of dynamic LVOT obstruction. This effect may be appreciated on M-mode recordings that demonstrate systolic anterior motion of the anterior mitral leaflet in mid- to late systole. In RCM, the pattern of hypertrophy is also concentric; both ventricular cavities are typically small with a decreased volume and large atria (>45 mm, measured in the apical four-chamber view). The atrial septum and cardiac valves may be thickened as well. A characteristic "granular sparkling" pattern of myocardial texture on two-dimensional echocardiography was originally described by Bhandari and Nanda [14] in patients who had amyloidosis, before the era of harmonic and high-frequency imaging. The inferior vena cava is typically dilated and does not collapse with inspiration (plethoric), reflecting increased right atrial pressure.

Dysfunction of LV myocardial fibers oriented in the longitudinal direction that occurs in hypertrophic syndromes has led to an interest in echocardiographic assessment of the LV long axis. In particular, displacement of the atrioventricular plane toward the apex is a direct reflection of longitudinal fiber contraction, and its measurement by M-mode provides information regarding global and regional systolic and diastolic function. Delayed onset of myofiber lengthening can effectively suppress early diastolic transmitral flow, even though the minor axis increases and mitral cusps separate normally [15]. Color M-mode imaging provides a unique window into the fluid dynamics of transmitral flow. The speed of propagation (slope of the black to red transition at the leading edge of the E-wave) is enhanced with the rapid relaxation and LV suction that occur in normal individuals [16]. Measurement of the ratio of the forward transmitral E to the tissue velocity E' of the mitral annulus can offer insight into the elevation in LV filling pressures that occurs in patients with heart failure. In RCM, E' is usually less than 8 cm per second, and an E/E' ratio greater than 15 indicates elevated LV pressure [17].

Doppler echocardiography has emerged as the primary clinical tool providing reliable data on diastolic performance [18]. Approaches routinely used in the assessment of diastolic dysfunction are measurements of transmitral and pulmonary venous flow and intraventricular filling patterns (Doppler flow propagation) [16]. The transmitral velocity pattern is easy to acquire and can rapidly categorize patients with normal or abnormal diastolic function based on E/A ratio (early to late filling velocity) [19,20]. Normal diastolic mitral inflow is biphasic, with early velocity generated by ventricular relaxation (E) exceeding later velocities generated by atrial contraction (A), and E/A ratio is greater than or equal to 1.2. (Fig. 1). Reduced diastolic compliance seen in HHD, HCM, and RCM reflects a steeper pressure–volume relationship of the hypertrophied LV. As LV volume rises in diastole, pressure rises rapidly, resulting in an initial high left atrial to left ventricular pressure gradient, with a rapid decrease in the filling gradient during early diastole. With various degrees of diastolic dysfunction, there are predictable changes in the mitral inflow pattern. Impaired relaxation is characterized by reversal of the normal transmitral E and A filling parameters. Doppler tissue imaging of the mitral annulus reveals a similar early (E_m) and late (A_m) patterning, opposite in direction to mitral inflow. A pathologic increase in LV stiffness results in decreased mitral annular velocities and subsequent reversal of E_m and A_m pattern with velocities less than the normal −8.0 cm per second.

The examination then focuses on pulsed Doppler recordings of pulmonary vein systolic (S), diastolic

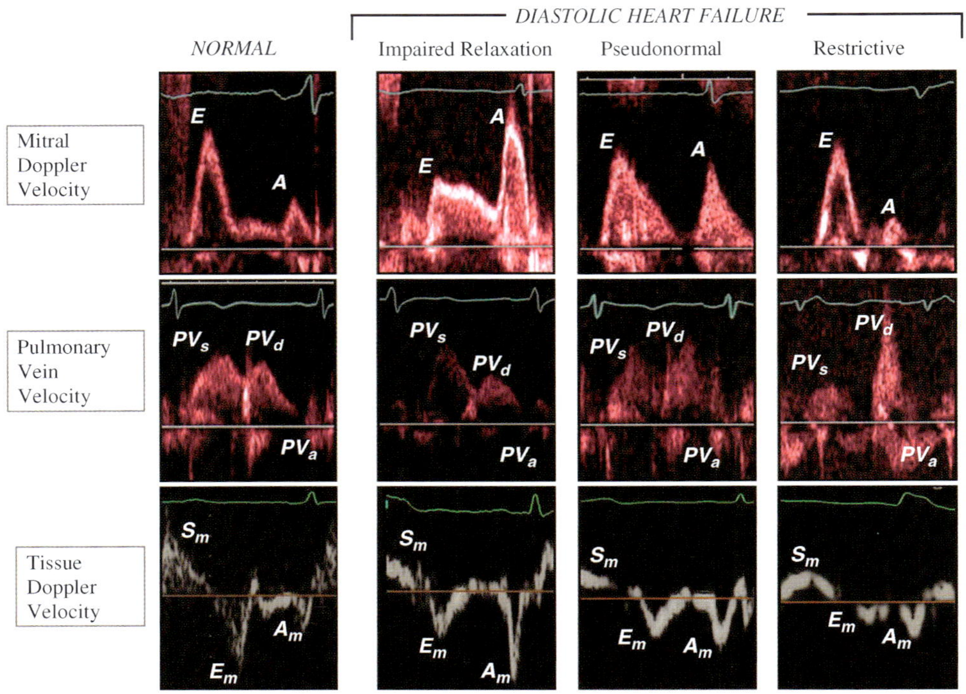

Fig. 1. Changes in Doppler echocardiographic profiles of patients who have different degrees of diastolic heart failure. As diastolic dysfunction worsens, *E/A* ratio initially declines; then the stage of pseudonormalization occurs. As filling pressures continue to rise, a restrictive filling pattern is seen. D, diastolic; m, mital annular; PV, pulmonary vein; S, systolic. (*Adapted from* Zile MR BD. New concepts in diastolic dysfunction and diastolic heart failure. Part I: diagnosis, prognosis, and measurements of diastolic function. Circulation 2002;105:1387–93.)

(*D*), and atrial reversal (*AR*) waves and the corresponding right-sided tricuspid inflow and hepatic vein flow waves [21]. Disease-free pulmonary vein flow is multiphasic, with *S*-predominant forward flow and relatively low retrograde *AR*. Progressive impairment in diastolic function leads to a *D*-predominant pulmonary venous flow pattern with both increased amplitude and prolongation of the *AR* velocity. Using these parameters, four stages of diastolic dysfunction may be determined: (1) impaired relaxation, (2) pseudonormalization, (3) restrictive, reversible diastolic dysfunction, and (4) restrictive, irreversible diastolic dysfunction [17,22]. Measurements of deceleration time and isovolumic relaxation time (IVRT) serve as continuous variables that are altered with progressive LV diastolic impairment. It is important to remember that these measurements assume the patient's sinus rhythm and are dependent on loading conditions [22]. Echocardiographic parameters serve to assess the properties of LV relaxation, which are best characterized invasively by measuring the time constant of LV relaxation tau (τ). τ describes the rate of LV pressure decay in an exponential equation [23]. It is an independent measure of the rate of ventricular relaxation, with a normal value of 33 $\pm$ 6 milliseconds. Along with responses to physiologic maneuvers such as Valsalva, these surrogate echocardiographic markers of relaxation can provide definitive information about the elevation of LV filling pressures and impairment in LV compliance that occur in conditions with restrictive cardiac physiology.

Doppler tissue imaging (DTI) measures the speed of motion of the interrogated myocardial tissue; a low-pass filter is used to identify low-frequency signals from tissue and exclude high-frequency signals from moving blood. To date, DTI is the best-studied and experimentally proven echocardiographic technique that helps differentiate between hypertrophic cardiac syndromes. Reduced myocardial velocity profiles have been shown to predict subclinical ventricular dysfunction in patients who have hypertrophic cardiac syndromes before and independently of the degree of LV hypertrophy [24–27]. Tissue velocity signals are also less load-sensitive than blood velocity signals. Compared with transmitral flow velocity, myocardial velocity gradient (MVG), defined as the slope of the regression line for the transmural velocity profile between the endocardium and epicardium across the myocardial wall, was less affected by changes in preload. MVG may also help determine the cause of LV hypertrophy. In one study by Kato and colleagues [28], a peak negative MVG of 3.2 per second was shown to separate those who had HCM from those who had HHD (Fig. 2). The reduced peak negative MVG reflects both prolonged relaxation and elevated LV end diastolic pressure characteristic of both conditions. Overall, RCM has been shown to have the lowest MVG among the hypertrophic cardiac syndromes, showing that Doppler tissue-derived myocardial velocity profiles can be used successfully to differentiate the hypertrophic cardiac syndromes [29–31].

Limitations of conventional echocardiography include its reliance on geometric assumptions for quantification of functional measures. The overall quality of echocardiographic results depends on the ultrasound window of the patient as well as on the experience of the investigator [32]. Thus, the standard transthoracic approach may suffer from significant interstudy and intraobserver variability, which limits its usefulness for accurate visualization of cardiomyopathic features and observation of changes during follow-up [33–35].

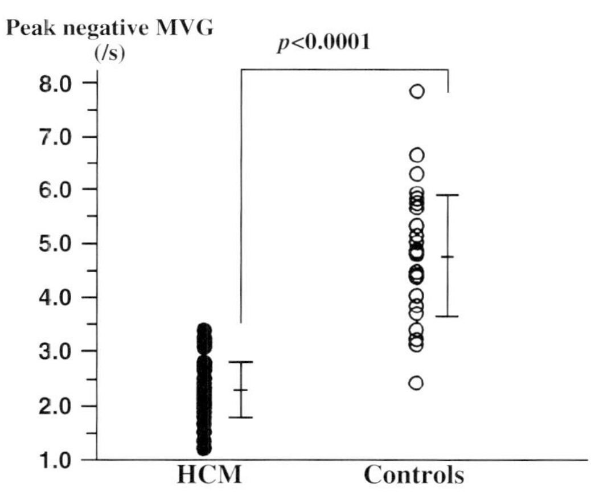

Fig. 2. Peak negative myocardial velocity gradient in normal controls and its change in hypertrophic cardiomyopathy. (*From* Kato TS, et al. Myocardial velocity gradient as a noninvasively determined index of left ventricular diastolic dysfunction in patients with hypertrophic cardiomyopathy. J Am Coll Cardiol 2003;42:278–85; with permission.)

Transesophageal echocardiography

Transesophageal echocardiography (TEE) affords a unique physical perspective on the LV. The superior imaging quality and ease with which pulmonary veins may be interrogated lend themselves well to the study of hypertrophic cardiac syndromes. Moreover, the direct visualization of the pericardium and potential pericardial pathology in the transgastric view may aid in diagnosis of constriction rather than restriction [36]. Investigators have persistently built on pioneering work by Schiavone and colleagues [37] noting the respiratory variation in the pulmonary venous flow using TEE. Focusing primarily on loading conditions, numerous studies have been done to "unmask" the occult changes in pulmonary vein flow seen in restrictive causative patterns. The volume entering the LV cavity is influenced by many factors, including the pressure gradient between the pulmonary veins and LV, continued myocardial relaxation, elastic recoil (ventricular suction), and stiffness properties of the myocardium. Volume expansion has been found to be safe and effective in augmenting the diastolic impairment of restrictive physiology, increasing the likelihood of a positive diagnosis by TEE [38]. The invasive nature of the procedure and logistical challenges limit the routine use of TEE. However, in combination with newer imaging algorithms and processing, TEE offers the potential for optimal echocardiographic windows in all patient types.

Strain and strain rate imaging

The term strain (ε) represents the relative deformation of myocardium, and strain rate represents the speed of deformation of myocardium [39]. Strain is a dimensionless quantity and is produced by application of stress. It represents the fractional or percentage change from the original or unstressed dimension and includes both lengthening, or expansion (positive strain), and shortening, or compression (negative strain) (Fig. 3). Myocardial strain rates reflect the speed with which regional myocardial shortening or lengthening occurs; they are calculated by integrating myocardial Doppler velocities measured at two locations separated by a given distance. Strain and strain rate may be derived from myocardial tissue velocities either off-line or in real time, using DTI. These parameters are relatively homogeneous throughout the myocardium and, compared with DTI, are less influenced by cardiac motion. Myocardial function may be more accurately assessed with strain and strain rate imaging, despite generally showing more background noise [40]. Because it is based on DTI, strain rate

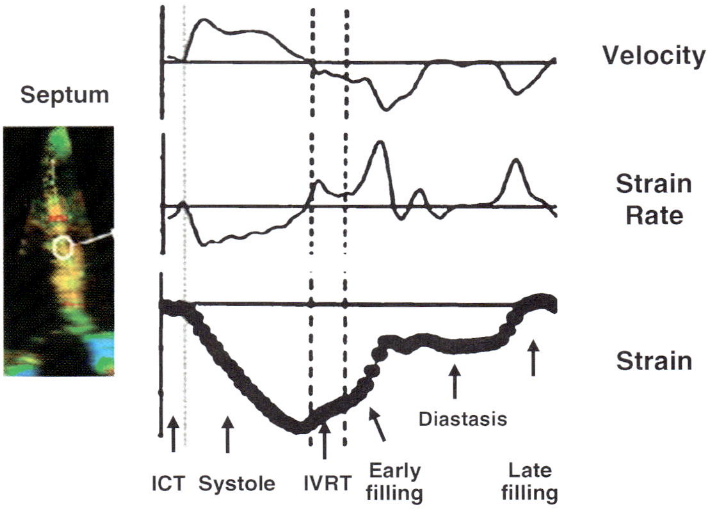

Fig. 3. Myocardial velocity and peak strain along with strain rate and its relationship to IVRT, ICT, and systolic intervals. ICT, isovolumic contraction time; IVRT, isovolumic relaxation time. (*From* Sutherland GR, et al. Strain and strain rate imaging: a new clinical approach to quantifying regional myocardial function. Review. J Am Soc Echocardiogr 2004;17:788–802; with permission.)

imaging is sensitive to misalignment between the cardiac axis and the ultrasound beam. Hence, the smallest possible sector should be used and a single wall recorded at a time.

Strain rate imaging has demonstrated a 96% diagnostic accuracy in differentiating HCM from HHD, using an ε(sys) cutoff of −10.6% [40]. The ε(sys) parameter significantly correlated with both pulmonary arterial wedge pressure and LV end-diastolic pressure and its derivatives, providing an excellent means of using functional lusitropic parameters to distinguish restrictive processes [41]. Strain and strain rate imaging has been shown to augment the sensitivity of DTI, providing further resolution to the diagnosis of hypertrophic cardiac syndromes [41].

Myocardial contrast echocardiography

Myocardial contrast echocardiography is another promising development in cardiac imaging that may aid in the diagnosis of restrictive physiology and various myopathic states. The technique involves the infusion of gas-filled microbubbles that improve echocardiographic resolution and provide the real-time assessment of myocardial blood flow. Characterization of the contrast echo, differentiated from that of myocardial tissue, improves the sensitivity of contrast ultrasound and is the basis for new contrast-specific imaging modes [42]. Harmonic imaging greatly improves sensitivity to contrast and enables excellent LV cavity opacification, which in turn improves endocardial border detection and enhances Doppler assessment of LV function. Applied in apical hypertrophies, this can increase diagnostic accuracy to 91%, comparable to that of cardiac MRI [43]. This technique may also be adapted to assess myocardial perfusion and viability, as the microbubbles infiltrate the microcirculation of the myocardium. When compared with PET, it has additional advantages in that it directly reflects capillary blood volume and replacement kinetics [44]. As applied to cardiomyopathic states, this technology aids in the definitive diagnosis by differentiating the microcirculatory uptake of contrast in the areas of disease. To date, published literature is available primarily for HCM and subsequent alcohol septal ablation [45,46]; however, ongoing study is extending the application to other hypertrophic and restrictive states.

Live three-dimensional echocardiography

Advances in computer processing and transducer technologies have allowed three-dimensional (3D) echocardiography to join the mainstream of cardiac imaging. Currently, live 3D echo is available on certain echocardiographic instruments, and, with it, software has been developed to help analyze LV structure and function in real time [47]. The images obtained are less dependent on the traditional geometric assumptions used by conventional two-dimensional echocardiography. Several published studies have now shown high concordance between 3D echo calculations of LV volume and ejection fraction and the "gold standard" of cardiac magnetic resonance imaging [48]. These studies have also demonstrated the superior accuracy and reproducibility of live 3D over conventional two-dimensional echocardiography methods. Additionally, real-time 3D echocardiography has shown considerable promise as a tool for detecting and quantifying LV intraventricular dyssynchrony [49,50]. Although in its infancy, this technique is of interest in identifying global or regional abnormalities seen in hypertrophic cardiac syndromes. Thus far, studies with 3D echocardiography have demonstrated the impact of hypertrophic ventricular geometry and real-time LV outflow obstruction in HCM, before and after surgical ablation [51,52].

Velocity vector imaging

Because of the helical architecture of the myofibers that compose the LV [53], myocardial motion is a complex amalgam of radial, longitudinal, and

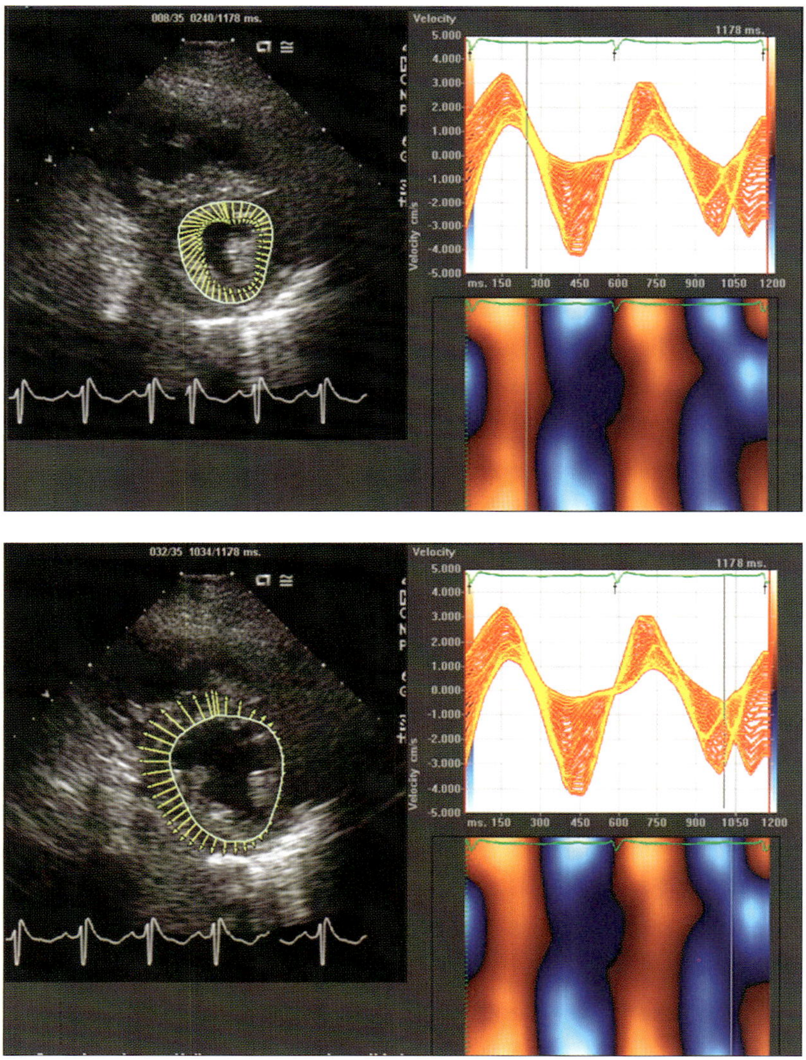

Fig. 4. Velocity vector imaging of a patient who has HHD in systole (*top*) and diastole (*bottom*). Each arrow represents the velocity of a specific point along the radial axis of the left ventricle.

circumferential torsion, which is not easily measured with current technology. LV torsion is due to opposingly directed apical and basal rotation throughout the cardiac cycle and has been proposed as a sensitive marker of LV function [54,55]. DTI investigations have shown that patients who had HCM had reduced myocardial shortening on a regional basis; however, LV torsion was *increased* [56].

New methods that do not rely on Doppler but instead track ultrasonic speckle have the advantage of directionally unconstrained imaging of myocardial motion [57]. Velocity vector imaging– is a new technique developed to eliminate the inherent angle dependency of conventional echocardiography. It uses an advanced tracking algorithm to estimate myocardial velocity at a set of points on a contour in a two-dimensional sequence of B-mode images [58,59]. The velocity is displayed as a vector overlaid on the B-mode image, where the length of the vector indicates the magnitude of the tissue velocity and the direction of the vector indicates the direction in which the tissue is moving (Fig. 4). New applications of this technology have been shown to elucidate subtle LV dyssynchrony and torsional mechanics not appreciated by other applications [60]. In patients who have HHD and impaired relaxation, subendocardial fibers demonstrate slower times for detorsion in early diastole, despite exaggerated twist and faster torsion in systole. This novel application will play a role in future evaluation of hypertrophic cardiac syndromes and restrictive physiology; it is currently under further investigation.

Cardiac magnetic resonance imaging

Cardiac magnetic resonance

Cardiac magnetic resonance imaging (CMR) has made great strides in becoming the imaging modality of choice for LV structure and function. It is the currently accepted gold-standard modality for evaluating LV mass and volumes. CMR visualizes left and right ventricular morphology and function with a high degree of accuracy and reproducibility [61]. CMR is geometrically unconstrained; it is able freely to image and reconstruct the heart in multiple planar views and to perform the full panoply of novel diagnostic algorithms—from strain and strain rate imaging to DTI and flow velocities—making it an ideal modality for evaluating hypertrophic cardiac syndromes and restrictive physiology.

CMR evaluates all myocardial segments with equal accuracy and can reveal unusual forms of hypertrophy that are difficult to assess with echocardiography, such as apical hypertrophies. A multislice and multiphase gradient echo sequence in the short axis plane provides for accurate measurement of the septum and the free wall of the left and right ventricle, which is needed to ascertain the presence, distribution, and severity of the hypertrophic process. Conventional echo may underestimate this measure by some 20% to 30% [62]. Cine-MR sequences in the horizontal and vertical long axis planes of the LV afford a precise view of the apex and make possible uncompromised evaluation of potential hypertrophy. CMR has been established as an accurate method for quantifying LV myocardial mass; it has been shown in HCM patients that the 3D CMR method based on Simpson's rule is the best way to quantify myocardial mass [63].

With regard to myocardial functional parameters, velocity-encoded cine-CMR imaging may also be used to quantify and monitor the restrictive filling pattern of the ventricles in patients who have hypertrophic syndrome by measuring the diastolic flow across the mitral and tricuspid valves [64]. Newer "real-time," fast-imaging cine-CMR sequences have used the visualization of septal flattening during early inspiration effectively to endorse ventricular coupling and thus rule out restrictive pathophysiology [65]. Other functional changes in patients who have hypertrophy that may be detected using myocardial tagging include complex and diffuse alteration of myocardial contraction [66]. The evaluation of the complex torsional mechanics of the LV quantified by tagged CMR has been further verified against DTI [67].

Gadolinium-enhanced CMR is useful in the differentiation of normal from disorganized myocardial tissue in patients who have hypertrophic cardiac syndromes. Delayed signal enhancement (DE) after the administration of gadolinium-diethylenetriaminepentaacetic acid on T1-weighted spin-echo images has been found in the most hypertrophied myocardium, presumably attributable to regional myocardial ischemia and fibrosis or myocardial degeneration and necrosis. As the integrity of the cell membrane breaks down, gadolinium contrast diffuses into and is retained in the intracellular space and may be seen approximately 10 to 15 minutes after the initial pulse sequences [68]. This late myocardial enhancement in the hypertrophic areas of HCM has been reported using T1-weighted sequences with an inversion pulse to suppress the signal of normal myocardium [69]. In the reports on CMR findings in RCM, specifically in infiltrative diseases, the signal intensity of the myocardium has been found to be low on T1- and

T2-weighted images in comparison with the intensity observed in images from patients who have HCM, and it tends to involve the lateral wall. DE-CMR patterns for infiltrative processes manifesting as RCM have been demonstrated using numerous case series and vary according to the entity involved [70]. In HCM, contrast enhancement patterns are patchy and found in the midwall of the ventricle at points in the anterior and posterior septum, inconsistent with a distinct coronary distribution. In sarcoidosis, nodules of high signal intensity on T2 fat-suppression sequences are noted primarily on the lateral wall. However, in amyloidosis, the DE-CMR, using various inversion recovery times, reveals a diffuse patterning. In cardiac iron overload, the ferromagnetic properties of the infiltrated areas leave a characteristic epicardial signal void on T2 gradient echo sequencing. In myocarditis with endocardial fibrosis, areas of edema and scar are noted by intense hyperenhancement along the endocardium; this then shifts to a midwall pattern as the myocardium heals. Using these patterns and novel CMR sequences can be technically challenging, not to mention the ease of confusion with focal areas of ischemia. However, as CMR comes into more regular use in the clinical evaluation of cardiomyopathies, the diagnostic specificity of delayed hyperenhancement patterns should improve with experience (Fig. 5).

The restrictive diastolic features caused by impaired filling of the ventricles are common to the hypertrophic cardiomyopathies and are well visualized using CMR. New, fast spin-echo sequences allow for reduced breath-hold time and fewer artifacts [71]. Flow studies allow for interrogation of all pertinent cardiovascular filling hemodynamics.

Magnetic resonance spectroscopy

MRI can also provide qualitative information on metabolic issues at the tissue level, aside from those inferred from gadolinium enhancement. Cardiac energy use has been investigated using radiolabeled phosphate and hydrogen magnetic resonance spectroscopy (MRS) [72,73]. This novel method of CMR imaging allows researchers to image the level of phosphate metabolism to determine disease activity in ailing areas of myocardium. MRS studies with both ^{31}P and ^{1}H have demonstrated that the myocardial phosphocreatine-to-ATP ratio correlated with the degree of failure in diseased human hearts (Fig. 6) [74,75]. Moreover, the depletion of myocyte creatine could be reliably followed throughout the patho-

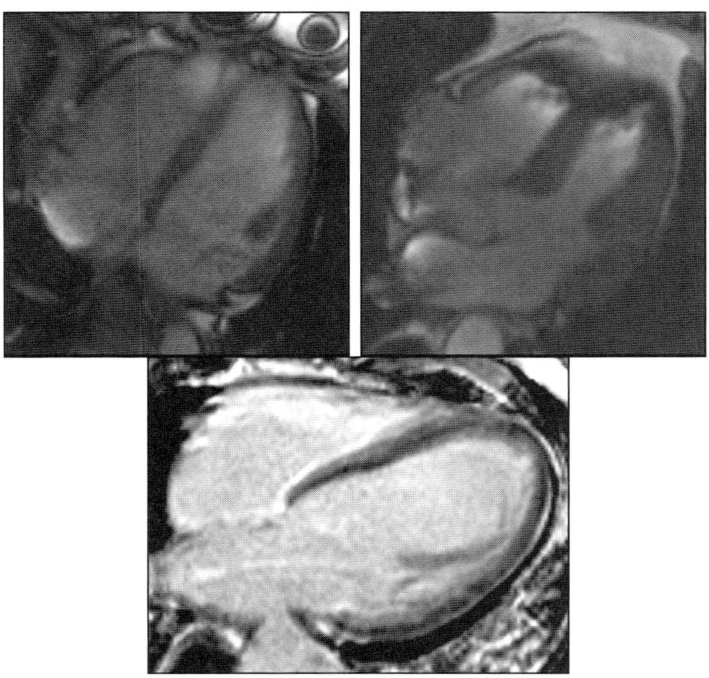

Fig. 5. CMR images of a normal patient (*top left*), a patient who has HHD (*top right*), and a patient who has dilated cardiomyopathy associated with mixed connective tissue disease (*bottom*).

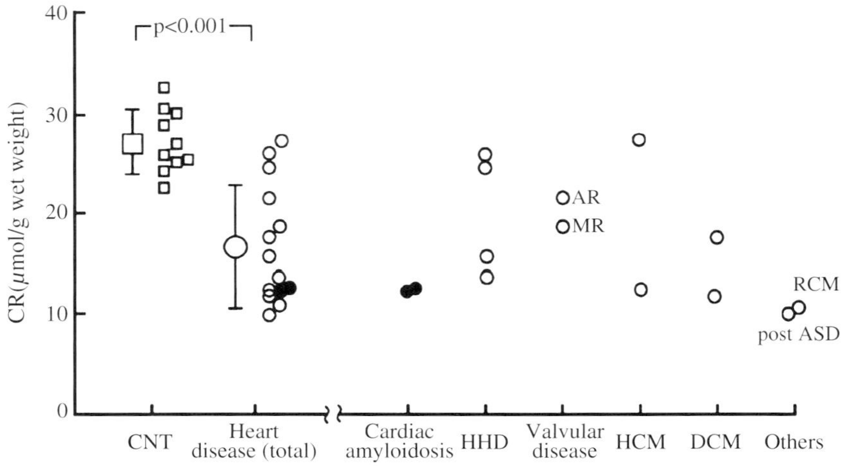

Fig. 6. Magnetic resonance spectroscopy and measurement of phosphocreatine in patients who have various cardiac conditions. The cause may be differentiated based on the relative degree of phosphocreatine. AR, aortic regurgitation; ASD, atrial septal defect; CNT, controls; CR, total creatine; DCM, dilated cardiomyopathy; MR, mitral regurgitation. (*From* Nakae I, Mitsunami K, Matsuo S, et al. Myocardial creatine concentration in various nonischemic heart diseases assessed by 1H magnetic resonance spectroscopy. Circ J 2005;69(6):711–6; with permission.)

physiologic process of advanced heart failure [76]. The early energetic derangement seen in diastolic dysfunction has been demonstrated in normotensive diabetic patients [77] and could easily be extended to study the metabolism of restrictive physiology. Although MRS is still considered a research tool and primarily found in specialized centers, more recent studies are identifying new scan algorithms to integrate it into the routine noninvasive CMR evaluation of cardiomyopathies [78].

CT

Since the advent of multidetector ultrafast CT technology applied to the noninvasive imaging of the heart and vasculature, new potential has emerged from this modality. Advances in software and multidetector algorithms have enabled the cardiac CT to achieve isotropic submillimeter spatial resolution, superior to that of any modality available today. Retrospective data selection allows for motion-free

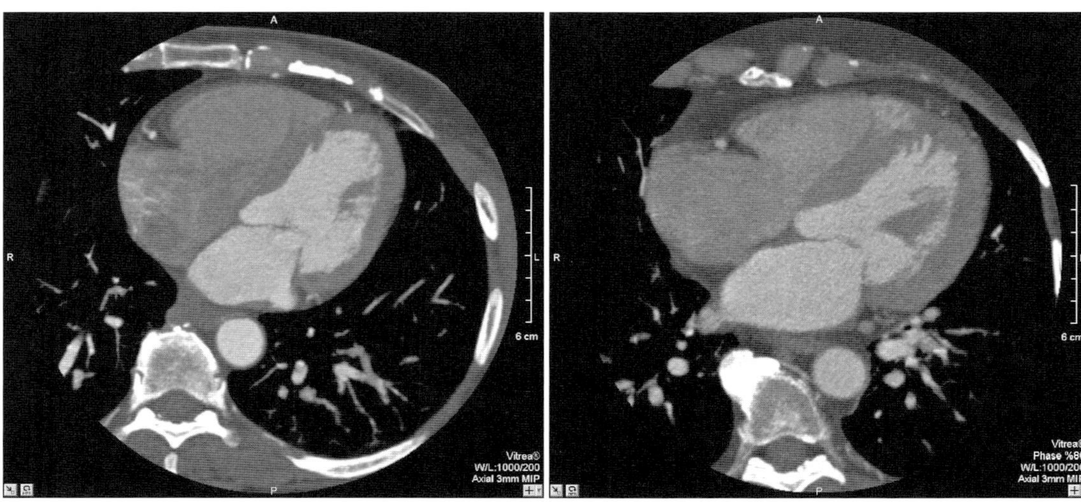

Fig. 7. Sixty-four–slice multidetector CT axial images of a normal patient (*left*) and one who has HHD and mild concentric LV hypertrophy (*right*). Increased wall thickness and decreased chamber size in diastole may be appreciated.

images and concise temporal review of the pertinent data collected. Furthermore, like CMR, CT has the capacity to provide multiplanar images and reconstructions without geometric constraint, providing unlimited imaging of the entire heart, regardless of patient body type. Although drawbacks include the use of potentially nephrotoxic contrast agents and exposure to significant ionizing radiation, cardiac CT is poised to become one of the first-line imaging modalities in the evaluation of cardiac structure and function. Limited data are available, mostly consisting of case reports of various clinical entities related to the hypertrophic cardiac syndromes. Research is ongoing, and promising leaps are being made as multidetector CT develops (Fig. 7) [79].

Nuclear medicine

Noninvasive nuclear modalities provide important information about the derangements in myocardial perfusion and metabolism that occur in patients who have hypertrophic cardiac syndromes. Single photon emission tomography (SPECT) serves as the primary imaging modality for the assessment of myocardial perfusion, whereas positron emission tomography (PET) focuses on myocardial metabolism. These imaging modalities have served as the foundation for early investigations into the pathophysiology of cardiomyopathic processes [80].

Single photon emission tomography

SPECT is a valuable imaging technique for visualizing myocardial ischemia associated with hypertrophic cardiac syndromes. SPECT can detect decreased perfusion and myocardial viability using radiolabeled thallium-201 (^{201}Tl) and technetium-99 (^{99}Tc) sestamibi or tetrofosmin [80–83]. Both sestamibi and tetrofosmin are retained within the mitochondria, making possible the assessment of intact mitochondrial function.

Subendocardial ischemia is known to occur in patients who have HCM, and several studies have documented the ability of SPECT to identify these ischemic regions in such patients [84]. Data from Dilsizian and colleagues [85] have shown that defects on thallium scan correlate with tachycardia-induced ST segment depression, suggesting an ischemic mechanism of syncope, cardiac arrest, and sudden cardiac death that often accompanies HCM. The link between thallium defects and myocardial ischemia in patients who have HCM is further supported by evidence for abnormal lactate metabolism during rapid atrial pacing in the same patients [86]. Patients who have the apical variant of hypertrophic cardiomyopathy also demonstrate perfusion deficits on thallium scintigraphy, but these have not been associated with adverse clinical outcomes [87].

The mainstay of medical therapy of HCM consists of beta-adrenergic blocking drugs and calcium-channel blockers. The mechanisms responsible for the beneficial effects of these drugs may relate to the inhibition of sympathetic stimulation of the heart and the reduction of myocardial oxygen requirements by reducing heart rate, LV contractility, outflow tract obstruction, and myocardial wall stress during exercise [88]. Verapamil has also been shown to improve indices of LV relaxation and rapid diastolic filling [89–91] and has been associated with both improved exercise performance and reduced symptomatology in patients who have HCM [90]. Verapamil also has the capacity to dilate small arteries, an action potentially valuable in HCM patients, who have been shown to have both anatomic and functional abnormalities of the small coronary arteries [92,93]. Further evidence for the efficacy of medical therapy is the improvement in exercise-induced thallium abnormalities that is seen in patients who have HCM following verapamil therapy [94] or surgical relief of LV outflow obstruction [95].

Investigation of the contribution of the sympathetic nervous system to the pathology of hypertrophic cardiac syndromes is also possible using ^{123}I metaiodobenzylguanidine SPECT. Findings suggest that sympathetic activity in the septum varies among types of hypertrophic syndromes, being higher in HCM than in HHD; these data further elucidate potential pathologic mechanisms and means of distinctly diagnosing this group of disorders [96–98].

Positron emission tomography

PET is a well-established noninvasive method of evaluating myocardial perfusion and metabolism [99]. PET imaging differs from conventional radionuclide imaging in that it uses radionuclides that decay with positron emission; this technique has the advantage of being able to assess perfusion and metabolism simultaneously. PET is most commonly used in patients who have ischemic heart disease [100]; its application in the diagnosis and management of hypertrophic cardiac syndromes has not yet approached the routine clinical arena but is an area of ongoing investigation.

When PET is applied in the clinical diagnosis of hypertrophic cardiac syndromes, Knaapen and col-

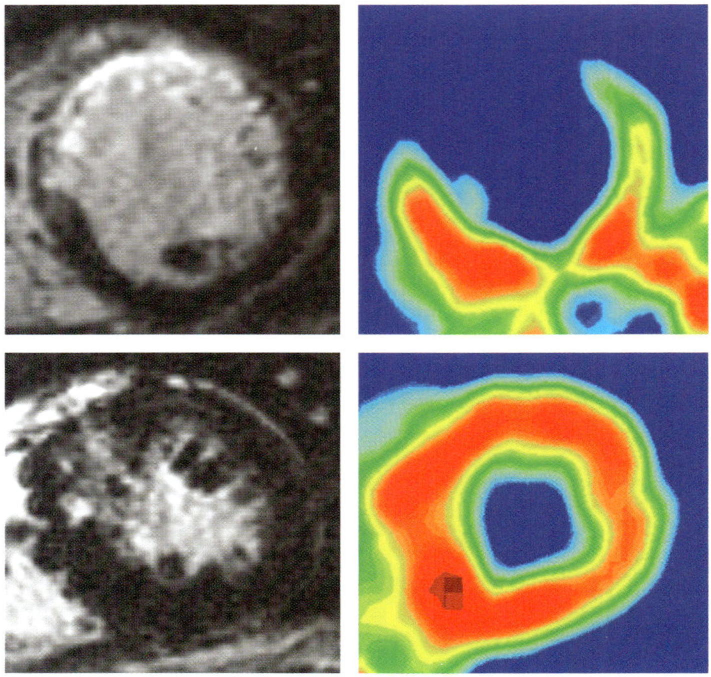

Fig. 8. Midventricular short axis view of patient who has anterior MI (*top*) and patient who has HCM (*bottom*). Left panels demonstrate CMR images, and right panels demonstrate anatomic tissue fraction PET images. (*From* Knaapen P, van Dockum WG, Bondarenko O, et al. Delayed contrast enhancement and perfusable table index in hypertrophic cardiomyopathy: comparison between cardiac MRI and PET. J Nucl Med 2005; 46(6):923–9; with permission.)

leagues [101] have shown that the perfusable tissue index (PTI) obtained with PET using ^{15}O-labeled water and carbon monoxide reflects the fraction of the myocardium that is able to exchange water rapidly (Fig. 8). Differentiation between fibrosis and myocardium may be made on the basis of this principle. It has been shown that the PTI is reduced in patients who have an advanced stage of idiopathic dilated cardiomyopathy, possibly because of increased interstitial and perivascular fibrosis [102]. More recent matched measurements of DE CMR and PET PTI have found a preservation of tissue perfusion in the areas of hypertrophy in patients who have HCM, similar to the SPECT findings. These results suggest that delayed hyperenhancement in the hypertrophied septum in HCM by CMR is not caused *solely* by fibrotic replacement scarring [103]. The use of this novel method is ongoing: it will continue to provide important noninvasive evidence of "micro-infarct" in areas of diseased myocardium, allowing insight into the possible pathophysiology of the hypertrophic cardiac syndromes.

Summary

Noninvasive imaging plays a crucial role in the diagnosis of hypertrophic cardiac syndromes and restrictive pathophysiology. Newer imaging modalities are becoming accepted as advances in instrument technology and computer processing make possible their transformation from time-consuming research tools into powerful clinical techniques that can provide qualitative and quantitative evaluation of the morphologic, functional, and hemodynamic parameters distorted by the hypertrophic disease process. Methods of noninvasive visualization of the pathologic and pathophysiologic processes at the tissue level are readily increasing, offering further insight into mechanisms, prognosis, and potential treatment through the course of these often confusing diseases. Further promise in the effort to provide a complete, noninvasive picture of the cardiomyopathies lies in the combination of modalities that allows for optimal spatial and temporal resolution, with concomitant metabolic information.

References

[1] Zipes DP, Libby P, Bonow RO, et al. Braunwald's heart disease: a textbook of cardiovascular medicine. 7th edition. 2005.

[2] Maron B. Hypertrophic cardiomyopathy: a systematic review. JAMA 2002;287:1308–20.

[3] Artz GWJ. Restrictive cardiomyopathy. Curr Treat Options Cardiovasc Med 2000;2:431.

[4] Kushwaha SS, Fallon JT, Fuster V. Medical progress: restrictive cardiomyopathy. N Engl J Med 1997; 336:267–76.

[5] Hancock EW. Cardiomyopathy: differential diagnosis of restrictive cardiomyopathy and constrictive pericarditis. Heart 2001;86:343–9.

[6] Kern M. Hemodynamic rounds: interpretation of cardiac pathophysiology from pressure waveform analysis. 2nd edition. Wiley-Liss; 1999.

[7] Vaitkus PT, Kussmaul WG. Constrictive pericarditis versus restrictive cardiomyopathy: a reappraisal and update of diagnostic criteria. Am Heart J 1991;122: 1431–41.

[8] Sagristà-Sauleda JA, Angel J, Sánchez A, et al. Effusive-constrictive pericarditis. N Engl J Med 2004;350:469–75.

[9] Eltzschig HK. Effusive-constrictive pericarditis [correspondence]. N Engl J Med 2004;350:2310–2.

[10] Chinnaiyan KM, Leff CB, Marsalese DL. Constrictive pericarditis versus restrictive cardiomyopathy: challenges in diagnosis and management. Cardiol Rev 2004;12:314–20.

[11] Asher CR, Klein AL. Diastolic heart failure: restrictive cardiomyopathy, constrictive pericarditis, and cardiac tamponade: clinical and echocardiographic evaluation. Cardiol Rev 2002;10:218–29.

[12] Otto CM. Textbook of clinical echocardiography. 2nd edition. 2000.

[13] Sakamoto T. Apical hypertrophic cardiomyopathy (apical hypertrophy): an overview. J Cardiol 2001; 37:161–78.

[14] Bhandari AKNN. Myocardial texture characterization by two-dimensional echocardiography. Am J Cardiol 1983;51:817–25.

[15] Henein MYGD. Suppression of left ventricular early diastolic filling by long axis asynchrony. Br Heart J 1995;73:151–7.

[16] Rakowski H, Appleton CP, Chan KL, et al. Canadian consensus recommendations for the measurement and reporting of diastolic dysfunction by echocardiography: from the Investigators of Consensus on Diastolic Dysfunction by Echocardiography. J Am Soc Echocardiogr 1996;9:736–60.

[17] Garcia M, Thomas JD, Klein A. New Doppler echocardiographic applications for the study of diastolic function. J Am Coll Cardiol 1998;32:865–75.

[18] Oh J, Appleton CP, Hatle L, et al. The noninvasive assessment of left ventricular diastolic function with two-dimensional and Doppler echocardiography. J Am Soc Echocardiogr 1997;10:246–70.

[19] Giannuzzi P, Imparato A, Temporelli PL, et al. Doppler-derived mitral deceleration time of early filling as a strong predictor of pulmonary capillary wedge pressure in postinfarction patients with left ventricular systolic dysfunction. J Am Coll Cardiol 1994;23:1630–7.

[20] Appleton CP, Hatle LK, Popp RL. Relation of transmitral flow velocity patterns to left ventricular diastolic function: new insights from a combined hemodynamic and Doppler echocardiographic study. J Am Coll Cardiol 1988;12:426–40.

[21] Appleton CP, Jensen JL, Hatle LK, et al. Doppler evaluation of left and right ventricular diastolic function: a technical guide for obtaining optimal flow velocity recordings. J Am Soc Echocardiogr 1997; 10:271–92.

[22] Zile MR, Brutsaert D. New concepts in diastolic dysfunction and diastolic heart failure. Part I: diagnosis, prognosis, and measurements of diastolic function. Circulation 2002;105:1387–93.

[23] Tei C. New noninvasive index for combined systolic and diastolic ventricular function. J Cardiol 1995; 26:135–6.

[24] Nageuh SF, Backinski LL, Meyer D, et al. Tissue Doppler imaging consistently detects myocardial abnormalities in patients with hypertrophic cardiomyopathy and provides a novel means for an early diagnosis before and independently of hypertrophy. Circulation 2001;104:128–30.

[25] Nunez J, Zamorano JL, Perez de Isla L, et al. Differences in regional systolic and diastolic function by Doppler tissue imaging in patients with hypertrophic cardiomyopathy and hypertrophy caused by hypertension. J Am Soc Echocardiogr 2004;17: 717–22.

[26] Cardim N, Oliveira AG, Longo S, et al. Doppler tissue imaging: regional myocardial function in hypertrophic cardiomyopathy and in athlete's heart. J Am Soc Echocardiogr 2003;16:223–32.

[27] Nagueh SF, McFalls J, Meyer D, et al. Tissue Doppler imaging predicts the development of hypertrophic cardiomyopathy in subjects with subclinical disease. Circulation 2003;108:395–8.

[28] Kato TS, Noda A, Izawa H, et al. Myocardial velocity gradient as a noninvasively determined index of left ventricular diastolic dysfunction in patients with hypertrophic cardiomyopathy. J Am Coll Cardiol 2003;42:278–85.

[29] Oki T, Tanaka H, Yamada H, et al. Diagnosis of cardiac amyloidosis based on the myocardial velocity profile in the hypertrophied left ventricular wall. Am J Cardiol 2004;93:864–9.

[30] De Backer J, Matthys D, Gillebert TC, et al. The use of tissue Doppler imaging for the assessment of changes in myocardial structure and function in inherited cardiomyopathies. Eur J Echocardiogr 2005;6:243–50.

[31] D'Andrea A, D'Andrea L, Caso P, et al. The usefulness of Doppler myocardial imaging in the

study of the athlete's heart and in the differential diagnosis between physiological and pathological ventricular hypertrophy. Echocardiography 2006; 23:149–57.

[32] Cheitlin MD, Armstrong WF, Aurigemma GP, et al. ACC/AHA guidelines for the clinical application of echocardiography. Circulation 1997;95:1686–744.

[33] Germain P, Roul G, Kastler B, et al. Inter-study variability in left ventricular mass measurement: comparison between M-mode echocardiography and MRI. Eur Heart J 1992;13:1011–9.

[34] Otterstad JE, Froeland G, St-John Sutton M, et al. Accuracy and reproducibility of biplane two-dimensional echocardiographic measurements of left ventricular dimensions and function [see comments]. Eur Heart J 1997;18:507–13.

[35] van Royen N, Jaffe CC, Krumholz H, et al. Comparison and reproducibility of visual echocardiographic and quantitative radionuclide imaging for measuring left ventricular ejection fraction. Am J Cardiol 1996;77:843–50.

[36] Izumi C, Iga K, Sekiguchi K, et al. Usefulness of the transgastric view by transesophageal echocardiography in evaluating thickened pericardium in patients with constrictive pericarditis. J Am Soc Echocardiogr 2002;15:1004–8.

[37] Schiavone WA, Calafiore PA, Salcedo EE. Transesophageal Doppler echocardiographic demonstration of pulmonary venous flow velocity in restrictive cardiomyopathy and constrictive pericarditis. Am J Cardiol 1989;63:1286–8.

[38] Abdalla IA, Murray RD, Lee JC, et al. Does rapid volume loading during transesophageal echocardiography differentiate constrictive pericarditis from restrictive cardiomyopathy? Echocardiography 2002; 19:125–34.

[39] Sutherland GR, DiSalvo G, Herbats L, et al. Strain and strain rate imaging: a new clinical approach to quantifying regional myocardial function. Review. J Am Soc Echocardiogr 2004;17:788–802.

[40] Kato TS, Noda A, Izawa H, et al. Discrimination of nonobstructive hypertrophic cardiomyopathy from hypertensive left ventricular hypertrophy on the basis of strain rate imaging by tissue Doppler ultrasonography. Circulation 2004;110:3808–14.

[41] Koyama J, Davidoff R, Falk RH. Longitudinal myocardial function assessed by tissue velocity, strain, and strain rate tissue Doppler echocardiography in patients with AL (primary) cardiac amyloidosis. Circulation 2003;107:2446–52.

[42] Villanueva FS, Wagner WR, Vannan MA, et al. Targeted ultrasound imaging using microbubbles. Cardiol Clin 2004;22:283–98.

[43] Monakier D, Woo A, Vannan MA, et al. Myocardial contrast echocardiography in chronic ischemic and nonischemic cardiomyopathies. Cardiol Clin 2004; 22:269–82.

[44] Van Camp G, Ay T, Pasquet A, et al. Quantification of myocardial blood flow and assessment of its transmural distribution with real-time power modulation myocardial contrast echocardiography. J Am Soc Echocardiogr 2003;16:263–70.

[45] Faber L. Targeting percutaneous transluminal septal ablation for hypertrophic obstructive cardiomyopathy by intraprocedural echocardiographic monitoring. J Am Soc Echocardiogr 2000;13:1074–9.

[46] Faber L, Seggewiss H, Gleichmann U. Percutaneous transluminal septal myocardial ablation in hypertrophic obstructive cardiomyopathy: results with respect to intraprocedural myocardial contrast echocardiography. Circulation 1998;98:2415–21.

[47] Monaghan MJ. Role of real time 3D echocardiography in evaluating the left ventricle. Heart 2006;92: 131–6.

[48] Jenkins C, Bricknell K, Hanekom L, et al. Reproducibility and accuracy of echocardiographic measurements of left ventricular parameters using realtime three-dimensional echocardiography. J Am Coll Cardiol 2004;44:878–86.

[49] Kapetanakis S, Kearney MT, Siva A, et al. Real-time three-dimensional echocardiography. A novel technique to quantify global left ventricular mechanical dyssynchrony. Circulation 2005;112:992–1000.

[50] Zhang X, Ramachandra I, Liu Z, et al. Noninvasive three-dimensional electrocardiographic imaging of ventricular activation sequence. Am J Physiol Heart Circ Physiol 2005;298:2724–32.

[51] Qin JX, Shiota T, Lever HM, et al. Impact of left ventricular outflow tract area on systolic outflow velocity in hypertrophic cardiomyopathy: a real-time three-dimensional echocardiographic study. J Am Coll Cardiol 2002;39:308–14.

[52] Sitges M, Qin JX, Lever HM, et al. Evaluation of left ventricular outflow tract area after septal reduction in obstructive hypertrophic cardiomyopathy: a real-time 3-dimensional echocardiographic study. Am Heart J 2005;150:852–8.

[53] Streeter Jr DD, Sponitz HM, Patel DP, et al. Fiber orientation in the canine left ventricle during diastole and systole. Circ Res 1969;24:339–47.

[54] Hansen DE, Daughters II GT, Alderman EL. Effect of volume loading, pressure loading, and inotropic stimulation on left ventricular torsion in humans. Circulation 1991;83:1315–26.

[55] Yun KL, Niczyporuk MA, Daughters II GT, et al. Alterations in left ventricular diastolic twist mechanics during acute human cardiac allograft rejection. Circulation 1991;83:962–73.

[56] Young AA, Kramer CM, Ferrari VA, et al. Three-dimensional left ventricular deformation in hypertrophic cardiomyopathy. Circulation 1994;90:854–67.

[57] Bohs LN, Geiman BJ, Anderson ME, et al. Speckle tracking for multi-dimensional flow estimation. Ultrasonics 2000;38:369–75.

[58] Notomi Y, Lysyansky P, Setser RM, et al. Measurement of ventricular torsion by two-dimensional ultrasound speckle tracking imaging. J Am Coll Cardiol 2005;45:2034–41.

[59] Helle-Valle T, Crosby J, Edvardsen T, et al. New noninvasive method for assessment of left ventricular rotation: speckle tracking echocardiography. Circulation 2005;112:3149–56.

[60] Vannan MA, Pedrizzetti G, Li P, et al. Effect of cardiac resynchronization therapy on longitudinal and circumferential left ventricular mechanics by velocity vector imaging: description and initial clinical application of a novel method using high-frame rate B-mode echocardiographic images. Echocardiography 2005;22:826–30.

[61] Benjelloun H, Cranney GB, Kirk KA, et al. Interstudy reproducibility of biplane cine nuclear magnetic resonance measurements of left ventricular function. Am J Cardiol 1991;67:1413–20.

[62] Rickers C, Wilke NM, Jerosch-Herold M, et al. Utility of cardiac magnetic resonance imaging in the diagnosis of hypertrophic cardiomyopathy. Circulation 2005;112:855–61.

[63] Suzuki J, Shimamoto R, Nishikawa J, et al. Morphological onset and early diagnosis in apical hypertrophic cardiomyopathy: a long term analysis with nuclear magnetic resonance imaging. J Am Coll Cardiol 1999;33:146–51.

[64] Spirito P, Seidman CE, McKenna WJ, et al. The management of hypertrophic cardiomyopathy. N Engl J Med 1997;336:775–85 [see comments].

[65] Francone M, Dymarkowski S, Kalantzi M, et al. Real-time cine MRI of ventricular septal motion: a novel approach to assess ventricular coupling. J Magn Reson Imaging 2005;21:305–9.

[66] Petitjean C, Rougon N, Cluzel P, et al. Quantification of myocardial function using tagged MR and cine MR images. Int J Cardiovasc Imaging 2004;20:497–508.

[67] Notomi Y, Setser RM, Shiota T, et al. Assessment of left ventricular torsional deformation by Doppler tissue imaging: validation study with tagged magnetic resonance imaging. Circulation 2005;111:1141–7.

[68] Kim RJ, Choi KM, Judd RM, et al. Assessment of myocardial viability by contrast enhancement. Philadelphia: Lippincott Williams and Wilkins; 2003.

[69] Bogaert J, Goldstein M, Tannouri F, et al. Late myocardial enhancement in hypertrophic cardiomyopathy with contrast-enhanced MR imaging. Am J Roentgenol 2003;180:981–5.

[70] Mahrholdt H, Wagner A, Judd RM, et al. Delayed enhancement cardiovascular magnetic resonance assessment of non-ischaemic cardiomyopathies. Eur Heart J 2005;26:1461–74.

[71] Shah DJ, Judd RM, Kim RJ. Technology insight: MRI of the myocardium. Nat Clin Pract Cardiovasc Med 2005;2:597–605.

[72] Schaefer S. Magnetic resonance spectroscopy in human cardiomyopathies. J Cardiovasc Magn Reson 2000;2:151–7.

[73] Nakae I, Mitsunami K, Matsuo S, et al. Myocardial creatine concentration in various nonischemic heart diseases assessed by 1H magnetic resonance spectroscopy. Circ J 2005;69:711–6.

[74] Neubauer S, Krahe T, Schindler R, et al. 31P magnetic resonance spectroscopy in dilated cardiomyopathy and coronary artery disease: altered cardiac high-energy phosphate metabolism in heart failure. Circulation 1992;86:1810–8.

[75] Neubauer S, Horn M, Pabst T, et al. Contributions of 31P–magnetic resonance spectroscopy to the understanding of dilated heart muscle disease. Eur Heart J 1995;16:115–8.

[76] Nakae I, Mitsunami K, Omura T, et al. Proton magnetic resonance spectroscopy can detect creatine depletion associated with the progression of heart failure in cardiomyopathy. J Am Coll Cardiol 2003; 42:1587–93.

[77] Diamant M, Lamb HJ, Groeneveld Y, et al. Diastolic dysfunction is associated with altered myocardial metabolism in asymptomatic normotensive patients with well-controlled type 2 diabetes mellitus. J Am Coll Cardiol 2003;42:328–35.

[78] Chida K, Otani H, Saito H, et al. Feasibility of rapid-sequence 31P magnetic resonance spectroscopy in cardiac patients. Acta Radiol 2005;46:386–90.

[79] Kondo C, Mori S, Endo M, et al. Real-time volumetric imaging of human heart without electrocardiographic gating by 256-detector row computed tomography: initial experience. J Comput Assist Tomogr 2005;29:694–8.

[80] Udelson JE, Bonow RO, Dilsizian V. The historical and conceptual evolution of radionuclide assessment of myocardial viability. J Nucl Cardiol 2004; 11:318–34.

[81] Dilsizian V, Rocco TP, Strauss HW, et al. Technetium-99m isonitrile myocardial uptake at rest. I. Relation to severity of coronary artery stenosis. J Am Coll Cardiol 1989;14:1673–7.

[82] Dilsizian V, Rocco TP, Freedman NM, et al. Enhanced detection of ischemic but viable myocardium by the reinjection of thallium after stress-redistribution imaging. N Engl J Med 1990;323: 141–6.

[83] Bonow RO, Dilsizian V. Thallium 201 for assessment of myocardial viability. Semin Nucl Med 1991;21: 230–41.

[84] Perrone-Filardi P, Bacharach SL, Dilsizian V, et al. Regional systolic function, myocardial blood flow and glucose uptake at rest in hypertrophic cardiomyopathy. Am J Cardiol 1993;72:199–204.

[85] Dilsizian V, Bonow RO, Epstein SE, et al. Myocardial ischemia detected by thallium scintigraphy is frequently related to cardiac arrest and syncope in young patients with hypertrophic cardiomyopathy. J Am Coll Cardiol 1993;22:796–804.

[86] Cannon 3rd RO, Dilsizian V, O'Gara PT, et al. Myocardial metabolic, hemodynamic, and electrocardiographic significance of reversible thallium-201 abnormalities in hypertrophic cardiomyopathy. Circulation 1991;83:1660–7.

[87] Lee KH, Jang HJ, Lee SC, et al. Myocardial thallium defects in apical hypertrophic cardiomyopathy are

associated with a benign prognosis. Thallium defects in apical hypertrophy. Int J Cardiovasc Imaging 2003;19:381–8.

[88] Thompson DS, Naqvi N, Juul SM, et al. Effects of propranolol on myocardial oxygen consumption, substrate extraction, and haemodynamics in hypertrophic obstructive cardiomyopathy. Br Heart J 1980; 44:488–98.

[89] Alvares RF, Shaver JA, Gamble WH, et al. Isovolumic relaxation period in hypertrophic cardiomyopathy. J Am Coll Cardiol 1984;3:71–81.

[90] Bonow RO, Dilsizian V, Rosing DR, et al. Verapamil-induced improvement in left ventricular diastolic filling and increased exercise tolerance in patients with hypertrophic cardiomyopathy: short- and long-term effects. Circulation 1985;72:853–64.

[91] Bonow RO, Rosing DR, Bacharach SL, et al. Effects of verapamil on left ventricular systolic function and diastolic filling in patients with hypertrophic cardiomyopathy. Circulation 1981;64:787–96.

[92] Cannon 3rd RO, Rosing DR, Maron BJ, et al. Myocardial ischemia in patients with hypertrophic cardiomyopathy: contribution of inadequate vasodilator reserve and elevated left ventricular filling pressures. Circulation 1985;71:234–43.

[93] Maron BJ, Wolfson JK, Epstein SE, et al. Intramural ("small vessel") coronary artery disease in hypertrophic cardiomyopathy. J Am Coll Cardiol 1986;8: 545–57.

[94] Udelson JE, Bonow RO, O'Gara PT, et al. Verapamil prevents silent myocardial perfusion abnormalities during exercise in asymptomatic patients with hypertrophic cardiomyopathy. Circulation 1989;79: 1052–60.

[95] Cannon 3rd RO, Dilsizian V, O'Gara PT, et al. Impact of surgical relief of outflow obstruction on thallium perfusion abnormalities in hypertrophic cardiomyopathy. Circulation 1992;85:1039–45.

[96] Shimizu M, Ino H, Okeie K, et al. Cardiac sympathetic activity in the asymmetrically hypertrophied septum in patients with hypertension or hypertrophic cardiomyopathy. Clin Cardiol 2000;23:365–70.

[97] Li ST, Tack CJ, Fananapazir L, et al. Myocardial perfusion and sympathetic innervation in patients with hypertrophic cardiomyopathy. J Am Coll Cardiol 2000;35:1867–73.

[98] Sipola P, Vanninen E, Aronen HJ, et al. Cardiac adrenergic activity is associated with left ventricular hypertrophy in genetically homogeneous subjects with hypertrophic cardiomyopathy. J Nucl Med 2003;44:487–93.

[99] Schelbert H. Metabolic imaging to assess myocardial viability. J Nucl Med 1994;35:8S–14S.

[100] Marin-Neto JA, Dilsizian V, Arrighi JA, et al. Thallium scintigraphy compared with 18F-fluorodeoxyglucose positron emission tomography for assessing myocardial viability in patients with moderate versus severe left ventricular dysfunction. Am J Cardiol 1998;82:1001–7.

[101] Knaapen P, Boellaard R, Gotte MJ, et al. The perfusable tissue index: a marker of myocardial viability. J Nucl Cardiol 2003;10:684–91.

[102] Knaapen P, Boellaard R, Gotte MJ, et al. Perfusable tissue index as a potential marker of fibrosis in patients with idiopathic dilated cardiomyopathy. J Nucl Med 2004;45:1299–304.

[103] Knaapen P, van Dockum WG, Bondarenko O, et al. Delayed contrast enhancement and perfusable tissue index in hypertrophic cardiomyopathy. Comparison between cardiac MRI and PET. J Nucl Med 2005; 46:923–9.

ELSEVIER
SAUNDERS

Heart Failure Clin 2 (2006) 231 – 247

HEART
FAILURE
CLINICS

Novel Imaging Strategies for Predicting Remodeling and Evolution of Heart Failure: Targeting the Renin-angiotensin System

Jamshid Shirani, MD[a,*], Jagat Narula, MD[b], William C. Eckelman, PhD[c], Vasken Dilsizian, MD[d]

[a]*Geisinger Medical Center, Danville, PA, USA*
[b]*University of California at Irvine, Irvine, CA, USA*
[c]*Molecular Tracer, LLC, Bethesda, MD, USA*
[d]*University of Maryland Medical Center, Baltimore, MD, USA*

Left ventricular (LV) remodeling constitutes the final common pathway for the progression of systolic dysfunction to end-stage heart failure (HF) [1,2]. The renin–angiotensin system (RAS), particularly its autocrine and paracrine components within the tissues, occupies a central place in the pathogenesis and progression of LV remodeling [3,4]. Pharmacologic strategies that are aimed at blockade of the RAS, including angiotensin-converting enzyme (ACE) inhibitors, angiotensin II (AII) type 1 receptor blockers, and aldosterone antagonists, have been used successfully in preventing and retarding ventricular remodeling in patients who are at risk for or who have established systolic dysfunction [5–9]. Many questions, however, remain unanswered regarding the timing of initiation, optimal dosage, and proper monitoring of antiangiotensin therapy in individual patients. Additionally, significant variation has been noted in individual response to renin–angiotensin blockade as a result of background genetic differences. Finally, the more important tissue component of the RAS is not directly accessible in clinical practice and the circulating neurohormonal levels are correlated poorly to their upregulation at the tissue level. Pharmacogenomics and molecular imaging are two rapidly advancing fields that promise to provide a better understanding of the pathophysiology of the RAS in health and disease. This article briefly reviews the potential evaluation of tissue expression of angiotensin in HF and presents data on initial attempts to target the RAS system by using novel imaging strategies.

Left ventricular remodeling

The clinical syndrome of systolic HF is regarded as a progressive disorder that begins with an acute or chronic, anatomic or functional loss of cardiac myocytes that results in a decrease in LV pump function. This is followed by activation of a series of compensatory mechanisms, including the neurohormonal systems that aim to restore cardiac function [10]. Although these compensatory mechanisms may contribute favorably to cardiac function in the short term, their sustained activation eventually results in further myocyte loss and cardiac decompensation, in a process that is referred to as ventricular remodeling [11]. Once this cascade of events has been initiated, LV remodeling becomes an independent contributor to the progression of HF [12]. Principal among the changes that promote ventricular remodeling are LV dilation, wall thinning, increased end-diastolic wall

* Corresponding author. Department of Cardiology, Geisinger Medical Center, 100 North Academy Avenue, Danville, PA 17822-2160.

E-mail address: jshirani1@geisinger.edu (J. Shirani).

doi:10.1016/j.hfc.2006.05.002

stress, and altered geometry from a normal prolate ellipse to a more spherical chamber. The end result of these morphologic changes is a functional afterload mismatch that may, in turn, lead to a decrement in forward cardiac output, subendocardial ischemia, and increased oxidative stress [13–19]. Development of functional mitral regurgitation often is an additional adverse hemodynamic burden on the remodeling LV [20].

At the cellular level, the cardiac myocytes in the remodeled ventricles exhibit decreased expression of α-myosin heavy chain gene, increased expression of β-myosin heavy chain [21,22], progressive loss of contractile proteins [23], excitation contraction coupling [24], as well as decreased responsiveness to β-adrenergic stimulation [25]. The unfavorable structural changes in cardiac myocytes is compounded by continued muscle cell loss through necrotic [26] and apoptotic pathways [27,28], as well as changes in the composition and volume of the extracellular matrix (Fig. 1) [29]. The latter is manifested as interstitial, perivascular, and replacement fibrosis and may contribute to impaired diastolic function, reduced coronary flow reserve, and progressive contractile dysfunction (Fig. 2) [30,31]. Myocardial fibrosis in chronic HF is a dynamic process that is determined by a balance between collagen synthesis and its degradation by matrix metalloproteinases (MMPs) [32]. The activity of MMPs is regulated by another group of glycoproteins, called tissue inhibitors of MMP, which bind to and inactivate these enzymes [33]. The dynamic nature of the structural changes in the ventricular remodeling is emphasized by their reversibility in response to appropriate therapy, such as coronary revascularization (in chronic ischemic heart disease), antiangiotensin therapy, or β-blockers

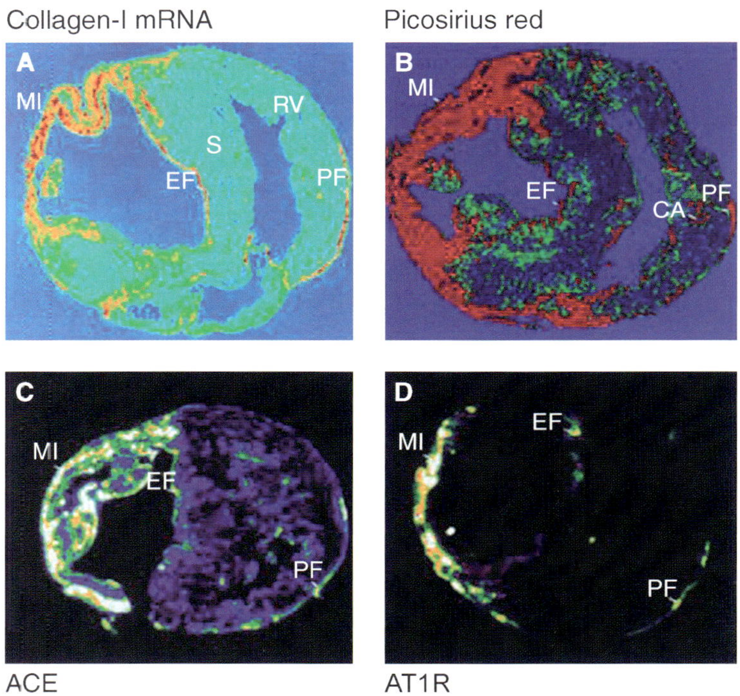

Fig. 1. Tissue repair in infarcted rat heart induced by permanent left coronary artery ligation. Data are presented for week 4 after myocardial infarction. (*A*) In situ hybridization for type I collagen mRNA expression. Increased expression of type I collagen mRNA (yellow and red) is seen at the site of transmural left ventricular MI. Same is true at remote sites that include interventricular septum (S) and right ventricle (RV). This involves endocardial fibrosis (EF) of S, a perivascular fibrosis and microscopic scarring of S and RV, and fibrosis of visceral pericardium (PF). (*B*) Picrosirius red collagen-specific staining demonstrates fibrillar collagen accumulation at site of MI, EF, perivascular fibrosis of intramural vessels (CA), and PF. (*C*) Autoradiographic detection of ACE-binding density. High-density ACE binding (white, red, and yellow) is seen at site of MI, EF, and PF. (*D*) Autoradiographic detection of angiotensin II receptor binding. High-density angiotensin II receptor binding is anatomically coincident with high-density ACE binding and sites of type I collagen mRNA expression and fibrous tissue formation. (*Adapted from* Weber KT. Extracellular matrix remodeling in heart failure: a role for de novo angiotensin II generation. Circulation 1997;96:4068; with permission.)

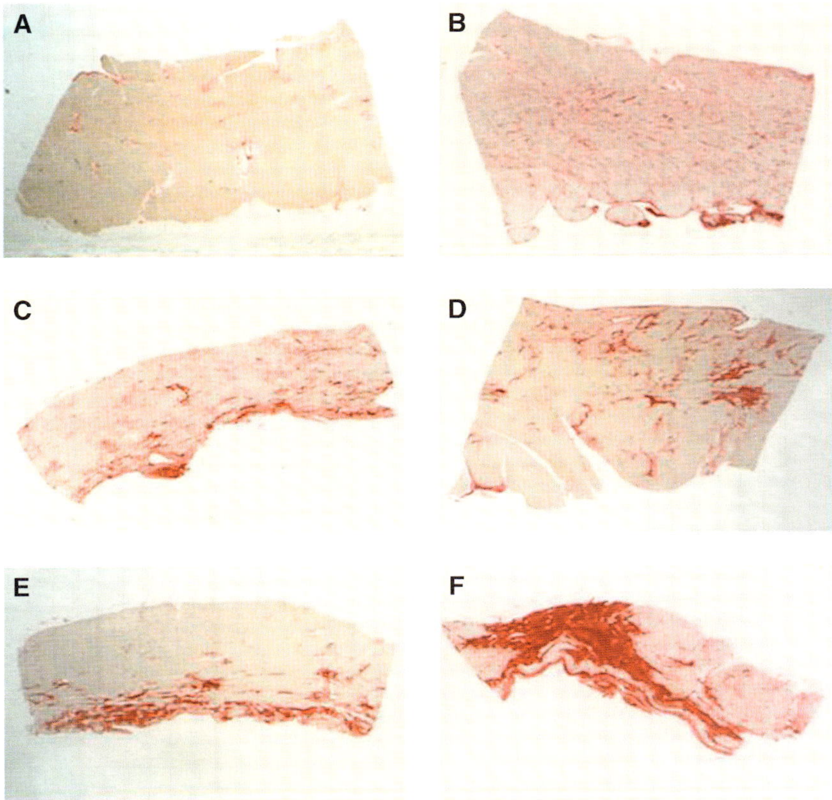

Fig. 2. Significant variations exist in collagen content and distribution of transmural left ventricular sections in ischemic cardiomyopathy. Photomicrographs of left ventricular myocardium stained with Picrosirius red demonstrating normal (*A*), patchy, scattered areas of replacement fibrosis (*B–D*), nontransmural infarct (*E*), and transmural infarct (*F*) from patients who had stable chronic ischemic heart disease and severe left ventricular dysfunction who underwent orthotopic cardiac transplantation.

[34,35]. Patients who had HF and gained objective benefit from β-blockers (increased LV ejection fraction) also demonstrated increased sarcoplasmic reticulum calcium ATPase mRNA and α-myosin heavy chain mRNA and decreased β-myosin heavy chain mRNA in their right ventricular endomyocardial biopsy specimens [35].

Neurohormonal activation

The evidence for the role of neurohormonal upregulation in the progression of LV dysfunction comes primarily from experimental and clinical trials that consistently demonstrated a beneficial effect on the natural history of the disease [8,36–42]. The favorable effect of ACE inhibitors and β-adrenergic blocking agents on LV remodeling has led to the development of the neurohormonal model of HF in which persistent overexpression of biologically active molecules results in irreversible damage to cardiac myocytes [43]. The neurohormonal model also explains common clinical manifestations of HF in patients with different etiologies of HF. The adrenergic nervous system and RAS are the best-studied compensatory mechanisms and are activated early in the course of systolic HF. These neurohormonal systems along with other molecular and cellular adaptive changes are responsible for the transition from compensated, asymptomatic LV systolic dysfunction to symptomatic HF.

The renin-angiotensin system

Circulating renin-angiotensin system

Systemic RAS is an endocrine system that is initiated by the release of renin from the kidney and acts to provide homeostasis to the cardiovascular and renal systems. Renin acts in circulating blood on angiotensinogen (Ao) of hepatic origin to produce angiotensin I (AI), which, in turn, is modified to AII through enzymatic action of the ACE predominantly in the pulmonary circulation. The endocrine RAS acts to protect against volume depletion and electrolyte imbalance through prompt production of AII; however, sustained activation of systemic RAS provides hemodynamic stimulus for cardiac and vascular hypertrophy. Other cardiac effects of AII are mediated through its direct mitogenic, inflammatory, and profibrotic properties [44–46]. Most of these actions are attributed to interaction of AII with the AII type 1 plasma membrane receptor (AT_1R) that mediates vasoconstriction, aldosterone secretion, renal sodium reabsorption, as well as dipsogenic and tachycardic responses [47]. The vasoconstrictive effect of AII is potentiated by the metabolism of bradykinin, a vasodilator, through the action of ACE.

Within the systemic RAS, a series of counter-regulatory processes is in place to mitigate the effects of AII [48–51]. This effector hormone also interacts with AII type 2 plasma membrane receptor (AT_2R) that has multiple cardioprotective effects. Following production, AII is degraded rapidly by angiotensinases—mainly to angiotensin-(1–7) and angiotensin-(3–8), now designated AIII and AIV, respectively. Both of these fragments have vasodilatory properties. The conversion of AII to its vasodilatory fragments occurs with the action of a newly discovered ACE homolog, ACE2. Unlike ACE, ACE2 does not convert AI to AII and is not inhibited by ACE inhibitors, and thus, ACE2 increase circulating levels of angiotensin-(1–7). Additionally, ACE2 inhibits the formation of AII by providing an alternative pathway for AI degradation.

Cardiac tissue renin-angiotensin system

A significant proportion of the cellular changes that take place in response to AII likely is dependent on locally produced hormone and these effects are largely independent of the hemodynamic effects of the systemic AII [4]. Among other organs, the heart expresses all components of RAS [46,52]. The intracellular AII is derived from the internalization of AT_1R–AII receptor complex or made in situ through the action of intracellular renin [53]. Nuclear and chromatin AT_1R-like AII binding sites have been identified and shown to be involved in upregulation of renin and Ao; this indicates the presence of a functional intracellular receptor pathway [54]. Experiments using ^{125}I-labeled AI and AII infusions showed that more than 90% of cardiac tissue AI and more than 75% of cardiac tissue AII is synthesized at the cardiac tissue site and is not derived from circulation [55]. In addition to AII, prorenin is shown to internalize by way of specific receptors with subsequent intracellular activation [56]. The internalized and activated renin can generate AII inside the cell [57]. The locally synthesized AII induces vasoconstriction and exerts direct inotropic and chronotropic influence, in part by increasing sympathetic tone and releasing arginine vasopressin. In addition, AII induces mitogenic, inflammatory, profibrotic, and apoptotic effects on the heart directly and indirectly through its interaction with endothelin, transforming growth factor–β, oxidative stress, and cytokines [58,59]. The cardiac RAS is under control of tissue-specific regulatory influences that are activated by biomechanical stress, such as acute myocardial infarction (Fig. 3) [60]. Glucocorticoids, estrogen, thyroid hormone, and atrial natriuretic peptide upstage cardiac RAS. Finally, mechanical stretch results in prominent induction of RAS and plays a crucial role in the process of LV remodeling remotely after initial myocardial injury.

In addition to generating AII within the cell, prorenin and renin also may exert independent pathologic effects inside the cell after binding to specific cell surface receptors or after internalization. Therefore, renin may not only be a protease but also acts as a hormone with specific cellular actions. Although, for the most part, renin that is localized to the cardiovascular system is derived from circulation, and thus, is of renal origin, other tissue sources of renin have been reported and may provide alternative means of activation of RAS at local tissue level.

Aldosterone, a steroid hormone, is secreted from adrenal cortex in response to AII or other stimuli, such as potassium, and acts to prevent water and sodium loss. Aldosterone also is made locally in various tissues, including the myocardium, as well as the endothelial and vascular smooth muscle cells in intramyocardial coronary arteries [61–63]. Mineralocorticoid receptors that are activated by aldosterone also are widespread, including expression in the myocardium. The presence of immunoreactivity in the heart and blood vessels was demonstrated by using monoclonal anti-idiotypic antibody (H10E), which interacts with the steroid-binding domain of mineralocorticoid receptors [63]. Local tissue synthesis of aldosterone seems to be driven mainly by AII and may participate in a positive feedback loop, because aldosterone upregulates the AT_1R and ACE expression in cardiac cells.

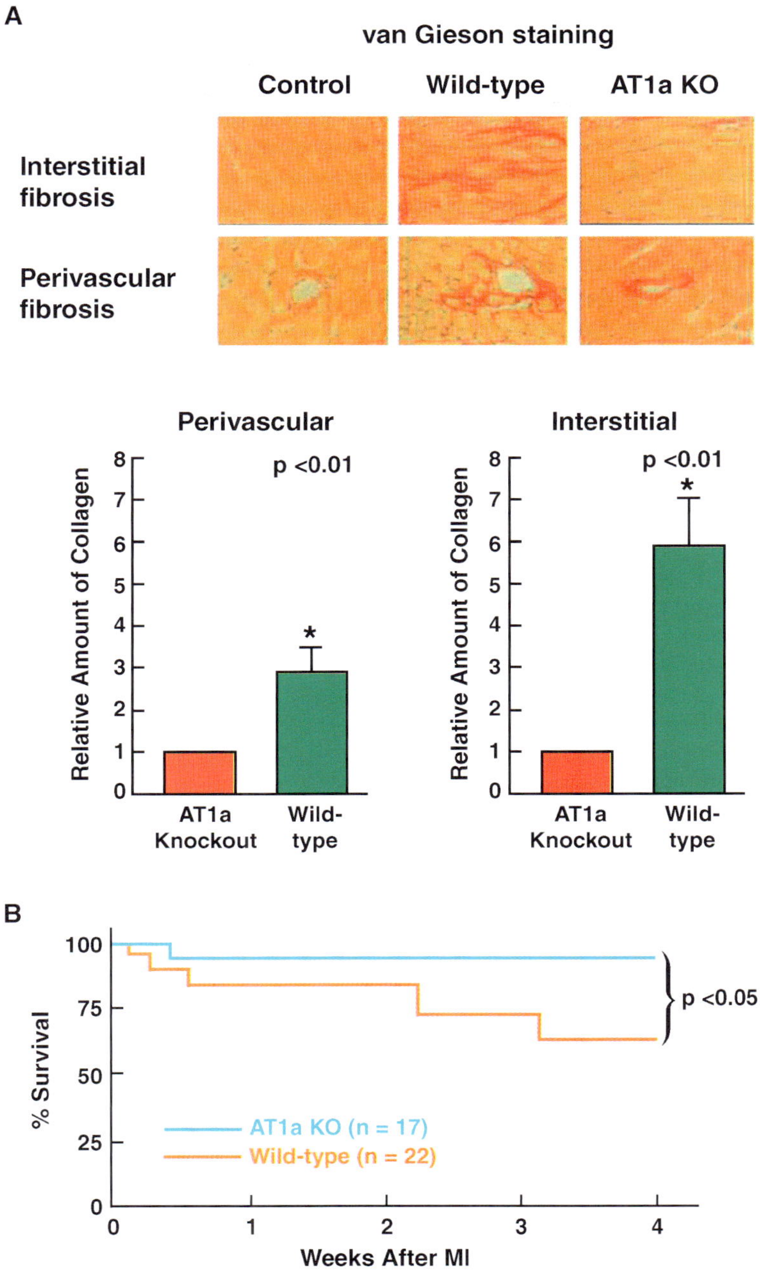

Fig. 3. The role of angiotensin II type 1A (AT1a) receptor in reactive fibrosis and remodeling in noninfarcted myocardium. The extent of interstitial fibrosis and perivascular fibrosis are shown in AT1a receptor knockout (KO) mice and wild-type mice at 1 and 4 weeks after large acute myocardial infarction (*A*). At 4 weeks after infarction, control mice showed more marked left ventricular remodeling and fibrosis than did AT1a KO mice. Additionally, despite producing similar initial infarct size, the cumulative 4-week mortality was reduced from 22.7% to 5.9% in AT1a KO mice compared with controls (*B*). These findings indicate that AT1a receptors play a pivotal role in the progression of left ventricular remodeling after myocardial infarction. (*Adapted from* Harada K, Sugaya T, Murakami K, et al. Angiotensin II type 1A receptor knockout mice display less left ventricular remodeling and improved survival after myocardial infarction. Circulation 1999;100:2093–9; with permission.)

Renin-angiotensin system in heart failure

The failing human heart shows increased levels of prorenin, renin, and ACE compared with nonfailing hearts [64,65]. Cardiac AII formation also increases early and progresses throughout the course of HF [66]; however, AII receptor density remains unchanged during the course of mild to moderate HF [66,67]. In vitro and in vivo evidence support the role of AII as the primary modulator of cardiac remodeling that occurs in response to pressure or volume overload or ischemic damage. Activation of the RAS results in growth (myocyte hypertrophy, interstitial and perivascular collagen deposition, and remodeling of the coronary arterial system) and apoptosis. These adverse effects are mediated primarily through the AT_1R that activates the mitogen-activated protein kinases, which contain components that promote growth and apoptosis [68–71]. Pressure overload and mechanical stretch increase the expression of these receptors on cardiac myocytes and fibroblasts and lead to the rapid release of AII from myocardial cells (Fig. 4) [72]. AII also induces the generation of reactive oxygen species in cardiac myocytes that is implicated in cellular hypertrophy, systolic dysfunction, and programmed cell death. Other molecules that are involved in the process of cardiac remodeling often potentiate or ameliorate the effects of AII on the cardiovascular system. For example, cardiotrophin-1 directly potentiates the effects of AII on myocyte hypertrophy, whereas bradykinin produces the opposite effect [73]. Myocyte hypertrophy that is induced by the activation of RAS is associated with specific changes in the expression of different isoforms of contractile proteins, myocardial enzymes, and secretory products [74]. AII also induces programmed cell death, and therefore, contributes further to LV systolic dysfunction by reducing the total number of functional cardiac myocytes [75,76]. The remaining hypertrophied myocytes exhibit abnormal intracellular calcium handling that is manifest as reduced capacity for calcium sequestration and impaired diastolic relaxation [77].

Elevated plasma aldosterone levels correlate with mortality in patients who have HF and directly mediate cardiac hypertrophy, fibrosis, and inflammation. The locally produced aldosterone also acts on local receptors. During early phases of LV remodeling, aldosterone alters transmembrane ion currents and predisposes to cardiac arrhythmias. Subsequently, aldosterone—independently or in conjunction with AII—produces vascular endothelial dysfunction, inflammation, and widespread tissue injury, including myocardial fibrosis [78]. Increased myocardial expression of aldosterone synthase, the enzyme that catalyzes the final step of aldosterone production, has been found in the failing myocardium, and a positive correlation between the level of aldosterone synthase and the degree of myocardial fibrosis has been observed [78–80]. These adverse tissue effects of aldosterone may be independent of blood pressure and AII levels and mediated through an increase in oxidative stress [80,81]. Also, acting through mineralocorticoid receptors, aldosterone further participates in the process of LV remodeling by inducing myocyte apoptosis and activating MMP, both of which are related intimately to LV remodeling [82,83].

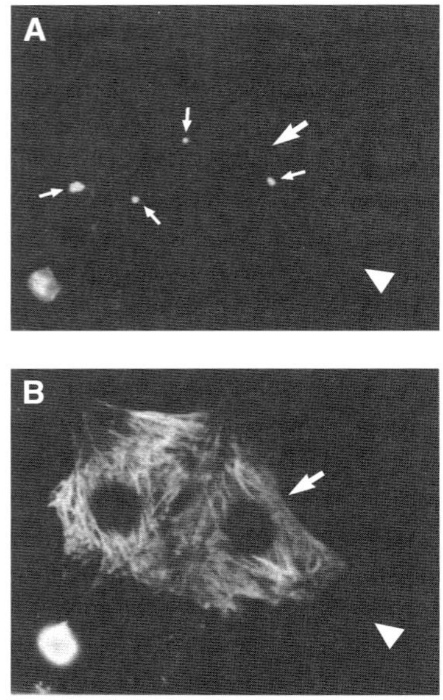

Fig. 4. Evidence for tissue angiotensin II in the cardiac myocyte. (*A*) Fluorescence staining of a rat ventricular myocyte with an antibody directed against angiotensin II. The focal areas of staining (*small arrows*) within the cell indicate the presence of angiotensin II. (*B*) The same cell (*larger arrow*) stains avidly with an antisarcomeric myosin antibody, which indicates that it is a myocyte. (*Adapted from* Sadoshima J-I, Xu Y, Slayter HS, et al. Autocrine release of angiotensin II mediates stretch-induced hypertrophy of cardiac myocytes *in vitro*. Cell 1993;75: 977–84; with permission).

The interstitial cells are increased substantially during the remodeling process. In acute myocardial infarction, AT_1R levels on cardiac myofibroblasts are increased substantially. AT_1R activation in cardiac fibroblasts results in proliferation, migration, and synthesis of extracellular matrix proteins. Several profibrotic messengers, including transforming growth factor-β1, are involved in this process [84]. Collagen, primarily types I and III, is deposited abundantly in the myocardium and may contribute to the impairment of LV relaxation, a reduction in diastolic coronary perfusion pressure, an increase in perfusion distance, and a decrease in microvascular dilatory function [85,86]. Alterations in infarcted and noninfarcted areas of LV myocardium eventually influence the size and shape of cardiac chambers as well as LV function. Once collagen is formed, the progression from hypertrophied to dilated LV involves the degradation of collagen cross-links that is mediated by MMP [87]. Cardiac RAS directly activates MMP, and thus, participates in the process of LV dilation [88].

Coronary arterial remodeling involves endothelial dysfunction, increased medial thickness, increased wall/lumen ratio, perivascular fibrosis, and decreased numbers of arterioles [89,90]. This results in reduced coronary flow reserve. AI and AII also exert a direct coronary vasoconstrictive effect in isolated heart preparation and in humans [91,92]. AII was shown to promote endothelial dysfunction that is mediated through AT_1R [93].

An additional effect of RAS activation in HF may be related to altered substrate use by myocytes as proposed by ^{123}I-β-methyl-iodophenylpentadecanoic acid (BMIPP) kinetics in patients who have HF using dynamic single-photon emission CT (SPECT) before and after treatment with an AT_1R blocker. BMIPP washout was enhanced at baseline and it improved significantly after treatment, which suggested that the improvement in fatty acid metabolism might represent a new mechanism for beneficial effects of AT_1R blockers [94].

Renin-angiotensin–aldosterone blockade in heart failure

Numerous clinical trials have established a direct beneficial effect of RAS blockade on outcome in patients who are susceptible to the development of HF and those who have varying degrees of manifest HF [3]. ACE inhibitors, AT_1R blockers, and aldosterone antagonists have been used successfully to prevent or retard LV remodeling, protect the vasculature, and reduce hospitalization and mortality in patients who have systolic dysfunction [5–9]. Additionally, treatment with ACE inhibitors causes significant reductions in myocardial infarction and nonsignificant reductions in strokes and other thromboembolic events [95]. ACE inhibitors also may improve symptoms and exercise capacity in patients who have HF. Although these statements effectively summarize the overall influence of RAS blockade in HF, there are multiple questions that have been raised in recent years.

Clinical heterogeneity in neurohormonal activation

After the initial myocardial injury, the rate of progression to symptomatic HF is substantially variable among individuals. The extent of myocardial injury in the index event and the magnitude of systemic response seem to be the predominant determinants of the rate of this progression. The impact of the individual variation in such a response to the overall rate of progression of LV remodeling is becoming increasingly evident.

There have been significant differences in the clinical response to RAS blockade in various subpopulations of patients. In part, this may relate to the genetic determinants of the individual response to RAS blockade. Polymorphisms in various components of RAS have been implicated in varying rates of disease progression and response to therapy in patients who have HF, which may explain inexorable progression of HF in a subset of patients despite adequate neurohormonal blockade. This also may be relevant in understanding the gender and racial differences in response to RAS blockade. Most patients in the large randomized clinical trials that established the benefit of ACE inhibitors in LV systolic dysfunction were white men. ACE inhibitors exert a lesser effect on blood pressure in black hypertensive patients compared with non-black hypertensive patients, and retrospective analyses suggested that ACE inhibitors may not be as effective in black patients who suffer from HF [96,97]. Similarly, men and women may respond differently to such interventions [98]. Further, not all patients who have enrolled in ACE inhibitor or aldosterone blocker studies derived clinical benefits; some experienced serious adverse drug reactions. In the Studies of Left Ventricular Dysfunction trial, nearly 5% of patients discontinued ACE inhibitor treatment because of worsening symptoms and an additional 8% had to discontinue the study drug because of adverse effects [5–7].

Altered response to renin-angiotensin system blockade during the course of heart failure

RAS is activated early in patients who have HF and there is a substantial incremental change in circulating renin, AII, and aldosterone with progression of disease. RAS, however, is a dynamic system, and blockade at a single step within the RAS cascade may result in activation of AII and aldosterone receptors through detour or escape mechanisms. Because of the lack of clinical access to tissue RAS, the current approach to this phenomenon involves empiric titration of drugs that act at diverse steps to achieve the desired effect. This approach may add to the risk for adverse reactions, especially in genetically susceptible individuals, and fail to offer advantage in others.

ACE inhibition is less effective in some patients who have HF. This is explained, at least in part, by the fact that AII also may be produced by ACE-independent mechanisms [99,100]. Thus, despite initial reductions in plasma aldosterone and serum AII levels following ACE inhibitor treatment, levels may increase slowly in some patients. This escape phenomenon has been the basis for therapy using direct AT_1R blockers and selective aldosterone antagonists [101].

Chymase, a mast cell enzyme, provides an alternative pathway for the production of AII. Upregulation of ACE and increased numbers of mast cells have been found in HF. There is a significant increase in the number of mast cells in the myocardium of patients who have ischemic cardiomyopathy, especially in the remote, noninfarct regions of the LV [102]. Conversely, ACE immunoreactivity is higher in the peri-infarct myocardium compared with remote myocardium and is lowest in regions with the highest numbers of mast cells. The distribution of AII, however, seems to be similar in the peri-infarct and remote regions of the LV in ischemic cardiomyopathy [103]. This observation raises the interesting question of whether AII may be produced by different mechanisms in various regions of the LV in ischemic cardiomyopathy. These observations also may explain why the addition of AT_1R blockers to ACE inhibitors and aldosterone antagonists is beneficial in HF. It also is likely that the significance of the neurohormonal factors decreases steadily during the course of progressive LV remodeling and is replaced by the morphologic features that independently determine the worsening of cardiac function.

The systemic renin-angiotensin system versus the tissue renin–angiotensin system

It has been suggested that ACE inhibitors differ in their ability to inhibit tissue ACE; however, no trial has shown an advantage for so-called "tissue-specific" ACE inhibitors in HF. Many important questions are relevant to clinical practice in HF, including the timing of initiation, optimal dosage, and the need for combination therapy, and necessitate a better understanding of the tissue RAS activity. Measurement of systemic RAS activity has been used to help predict the response of patients to RAS blockade; however, these measurements are difficult to make and generally lack accuracy. No consistent relationship has been found between the sustained increase in plasma renin activity and aldosterone after myocardial infarction and the risk for symptomatic HF. Also, circulating levels of RAS components are not predictive of future HF or its complications independent of other circulating neurohormones, such as natriuretic peptides and norepinephrine. In patients who had asymptomatic LV dysfunction, the long-term treatment with enalapril lowered plasma norepinephrine only in those subjects with elevated levels at baseline [104]. In contrast, in another large trial, captopril increased plasma renin activity and decreased serum aldosterone without altering the levels of plasma norepinephrine or natriuretic peptide [105]. In yet another study, ramipril administration after myocardial infarction decreased LV mass and plasma AII but did not affect the levels of plasma norepinephrine [106]. Further, although neurohormonal antagonists are beneficial, their salutary effects are not related directly to changes in circulating neurohormones [107]. Therefore, it is conceivable that a strategy that is aimed at assessment of tissue ACE upregulation should allow an optimal intervention with antiangiotensin agents and should minimize the likelihood of adverse reactions.

Suboptimal use of renin-angiotensin system blockade

Initial surveys have revealed the significant underuse and the use of smaller than recommended doses of RAS-blocking medications by physicians who treat patients who have HF. Primarily, this is due to a concern for potential adverse drug effects, especially in the elderly and in patients who have borderline systemic blood pressure or renal insufficiency. The underdosing and underuse of ACE inhibitors and perhaps other members of the RAS-blocking family may be resolved by objective measures that can guide the effective pharmacologic treatment of HF.

Personalized treatment of heart failure

Large clinical trials have regarded all individuals who are enrolled in the study as equals by design, and thus, ignore significant individual, often genetically based, differences in response to a given intervention. There is a clear need for an understanding of the genetic contribution to individual variability in drug efficacy and toxicity. Significant interindividual variability in response to RAS blockade has been recognized in patients who have HF. Although some patients may gain significant clinical benefit, others may show no therapeutic benefit, and yet others may experience serious adverse reactions. Factors, such as age, sex, race, comorbid conditions, concomitant medications, and renal and liver functions, are important determinants of individual response to RAS blockade; however, it is increasingly evident that genetic variability plays a central role in individual response to this group of agents. There is no reliable tool to predict the response of an individual patient to RAS blockade. Pharmacogenomics and molecular imaging have the potential to provide significant insight in this regard, especially when used in the context of large clinical trials. When patients are predefined by their genetic makeup and the activity of RAS, then sophisticated pharmacologic approaches can be undertaken to maximize the benefit and minimize the risk for toxicity.

Genetic polymorphism in renin-angiotensisn system components

Molecular variants of individual components of RAS have been believed to contribute to the inherited predisposition toward cardiovascular disease and their response to RAS blockade. The ACE deletion/insertion (DI) biallelic polymorphism of intron 16 is the most extensively studied cardiovascular polymorphism [108]. Although the clinical implications of this polymorphism have remained controversial, its physiologic association with enzymatic activity has been consistent. Thus, the D allele is linked to increased ACE activity and higher AII levels [109]. Subjects with the DD genotype have the highest levels of AII levels; DI heterozygotes have intermediate levels of AII, and those with the II genotype have the lowest levels of AII [109]. In patients who have HF, the DD genotype, as a genetic modifier, is associated with adverse disease progression and higher mortality. Patients who have HF and the DD genotype show significant resistance to the blood pressure lowering effect of ACE inhibitors and a higher prevalence of "aldosterone escape" while on an ACE inhibitor therapy [110]. The effect of spironolactone on LV remodeling also is diminished in the ACE DD subset compared with the ID and II subsets, similar to their diminished clinical response to ACE inhibitors [111].

In addition to the ACE gene, polymorphisms in the genes of renin, Ao, AT_1R, AT_2R, aldosterone synthase, and other RAS components have been demonstrated [112]. The association of renin and Ao gene polymorphisms with essential hypertension has been reported [113]. Polymorphisms in the Ao gene also have been linked to response to antihypertensive drugs. At least 25 different polymorphisms have been described in the AT_1R gene, and some have been associated with severe systemic hypertension, renal dysfunction, arterial stiffness, hemodynamic response to therapy with AT_1R blockers, and phenotypic expression of hypertrophic cardiomyopathy [114]. AT_2R gene polymorphism has been described and was correlated with LV mass in women who had hypertrophic cardiomyopathy [115]. The evaluation of the individual differences in the various genetic components of the RAS is expanding rapidly. Large studies are needed to investigate complex relationships between these genetic variants and predisposition to, progression of, and response to treatment in patients who have HF.

Cardiovascular molecular imaging

Molecular imaging is a rapidly developing field with the promise to provide highly individualized, noninvasive molecular and anatomic information within the context of a systemic or organ system disease. Such information may allow better disease definition, more intelligent choice of therapeutic intervention, and monitoring of response to treatment [116]. Nuclear imaging techniques, especially SPECT and positron emission tomography (PET), are well suited for cardiac molecular imaging because of the large number of potentially available molecular targets, high intrinsic sensitivity, and excellent depth penetration. PET is especially advantageous because it is quantitative and provides high spatial resolution. When combined with CT, PET-CT is especially suited to molecular imaging because it provides high-resolution anatomic information in addition to the molecular imaging. Cardiac MRI, myocardial contrast echocardiography, and optical imaging also techniques for molecular imaging that are developing rapidly. Regardless of the imaging strategies, the targeting agents may remain common and should be available for labeling with appropriate tracers. In the field of nuclear cardiology, molecular targets have been used for many years to detect myocardial necrosis or inflammation, intracardiac thrombi, and autonomic innervation.

Molecular targets of the renin-angiotensin system

The complex nature of the RAS has made it difficult to develop a comprehensive approach to study and monitor the various components of this system in vivo; however, at the same time it has provided a large number of targets for nuclear imaging using radiolabeled ligands. The ACE and the AT_1R are the two targets within the RAS that have received the most attention. The following summarizes the efforts that have been made in recent years to develop radioligands that are suitable for in vivo nuclear imaging; it should be noted that these attempts are only at the early stages of development.

^{18}F-labeled captopril

The initial attempts to develop specific ACE-binding radiotracers were made using ^{18}F-labeled captopril, an ACE inhibitor. Radiolabeled captopril was prepared to evaluate the feasibility of probing the distribution of ACE in vivo using PET. 4-cis-[^{18}F]fluorocaptopril (^{18}FCAP) was prepared by the reaction of the corresponding triflate with ^{18}F/Kryptofix 222 in acentonitrile followed by hydrolysis (2 N NaOH). The synthesis time was 1 hour with an average radiochemical yield (end of synthesis) of 12% and a specific activity of greater than 300 Ci (11,100 GBq)/mmol. In vivo biodistribution in rats at 30 minutes after administration showed high uptakes in organs that are known to have high ACE activity (eg, lungs, kidneys, aorta). The clearance of ^{18}FCAP is faster for lungs and kidneys, compared with the aorta. When different amounts of unlabeled 4-cis-fluorocaptopril (SQ 25,750) were coinjected in rats at a dose of greater than 5 μg/kg, the lung uptake decreased by one half, whereas only 1 μg/kg was needed to decrease the kidney uptake by one half. In general, the binding in the four tissues studied was saturable with the expected capacity. ^{18}FCAP was administered to a human and displaceable uptake was observed in the lung and kidney. The results demonstrated the feasibility of probing ACE in vivo using PET. This was the first demonstration that radiolabeled ACE inhibitors could be used in vivo (in rats and humans) to monitor ACE; however, FCAP had several shortcomings (eg, possession of a sulfhydryl group that formed captopril disulfide dimer and mixed with endogenous sulfhydryl compounds, including cysteine, glutathione, and proteins). This made determination of the input function (the amount of unbound FCAP available to bind to the enzyme) difficult because of the possible equilibrium involved and—from a technical point of view—carrying out the chromatography without artifacts. Also, it has been suggested that isomeric conversion of cis and trans isomers of FCAP may occur in the plasma [117,118]. Additionally, captopril is believed to have a higher affinity for vascular ACE than for the tissue ACE, and thus, is less suited to examine the tissue ACE activity in particular. In this regard the higher tissue affinity of lisinopril and zofenopril as compared with captopril was shown in an experimental study using quantitative in vitro autoradiography and enzymatic assay [119]. Although ACE activity in all regions of the heart, kidney, and serum was reduced markedly 4 hours after oral administration of lisinopril and zofenopril, it was inhibited only partially at the tissue level after captopril treatment [119].

^{18}F-labeled lisinopril

It has been known from the early development of ACE inhibitors that the normalized oral doses of most inhibitors had equivalent effects on serum ACE, but had differential effects in tissue, as distinguished by the magnitude and duration of their effects [120]. This effect may be explained by the structure of one of the two catalytic domains of ACE in complex with an inhibitor [121]. The carbonyl adjacent to the prolyl nitrogen atom of lisinopril provides a coordinating ligand to the zinc ion, whereas the carboxylate in the midportion of the inhibitor molecule forms a hydrogen bond with the glutamate in ACE. The C-terminal carboxylate of lisinopril binds to a lysine and a tyrosine rather than an arginine. There are two active sites on the somatic ACE. One may be in a more lipophilic pocket, which would explain the differential binding in tissue but not in plasma where proteolytic cleavage takes place. ACE in plasma is produced by proteolytic cleavage of the membrane-bound ACE, and therefore, both binding sites are available [122]. For all of these reasons, it seemed more reasonable to use ACE inhibitors with higher tissue affinity, such as lisinopril, to study the tissue distribution of ACE. This was especially true because the higher affinity of lisinopril, or other ACE inhibitors with a high affinity for tissue ACE, would result in higher resolution during in vitro autoradiography when compared with labeled captopril [123]. In addition, previous studies had shown that the lisinopril molecule could be modified significantly during the labeling process without compromising its affinity for tissue ACE. For example, tyrosine moiety could be reacted with the lysine in lisinopril to form a molecule that can be iodinated easily and has a high affinity for ACE ($K_D = 2$ nM), comparable to that for lisinopril ($K_D = 0.13$ nM) and higher than the affinity for captopril ($K_D = 22$ nM).

Other analogs of lisinopril, with larger substitutes on the ε-amino group of lysine, also have been reported. These studies collectively suggested that ^{18}F-labeled analogs of lisinopril could be prepared while maintaining its high affinity for ACE.

As a first step toward demonstrating the role of AII and ACE in directly regulating cardiac function in HF, the authors synthesized a new radiotracer [^{18}F]fluorobenzoyl-lisinopril by radiolabeling benzoic acid active ester with ^{18}F and reacting with the ϵ-amino group of lisinopril (Fig. 5) [124]. The presence and distribution of ACE activity and AII receptors were examined in relation to various forms of pathologic fibrosis and expansion of matrix and perivascular collagen in explanted hearts from patients who had HF [125]. Five- to 10-μm contiguous short-axis slices of explanted hearts from patients who had ischemic cardiomyopathy were incubated in vitro with [^{18}F]fluorobenzoyl-lisinopril, with and without 10^{-6} M lisinopril. Tissues were placed on a BAS5000 phosphorimager plate (Berthold Australia Pty Ltd., Bundoora, Australia) and the radioactivity was recorded as a function of position in photostimulating luminescence units (PSL). Picrosirius red, a collagen-specific stain, was used to define infarct (n=28, collagen volume fraction 63% ± 15%), peri-infarct (n=39, collagen volume fraction 14% ± 5%), and remote, noninfarct areas (n=11, collagen volume fraction 11% ± 3%) of LV myocardium. Mean [^{18}F]fluorobenzoyl-lisinopril binding was 6.5 ± 4.5 PSL/mm^2 in infarct, 7.6 ± 4.7 PSL/mm^2 in peri-infarct, and 5.0 ± 1.0 PSL/mm^2 in remote, noninfarct segments. The difference in mean [^{18}F]fluorobenzoyl-lisinopril binding was significant between remote, noninfarct, and peri-infarct segments ($P < .02$) segments. These preliminary data suggested that [^{18}F]fluorobenzoyl-lisinopril binds specifically to ACE; the binding is nonuniform in infarct, peri-infarct, and remote, noninfarct segments; and there is apparent increased ACE activity in the juxtaposed areas of replacement fibrosis. The increased ACE in the juxtaposed areas of replacement fibrosis may be a stimulus for collagen replacement and remodeling. The authors applied immunohistochemical staining method to verify the distribution and cellular localization of ACE. Using a mouse monoclonal antibody against ACE (Immuno-Biological Laboratories, Inc., Minneapolis, Minnesota), a similar distribution of ACE to autoradiographic [^{18}F]fluorobenzoyl-lisinopril binding was demonstrated. ACE immunoreactivity was localized primarily to myocytes and the media of small arteries. Some activity also was noted in endocardial cells and endothelial cells of intramyocardial arteries.

Similarly, the authors applied the peroxidase method to examine histochemically the distribution

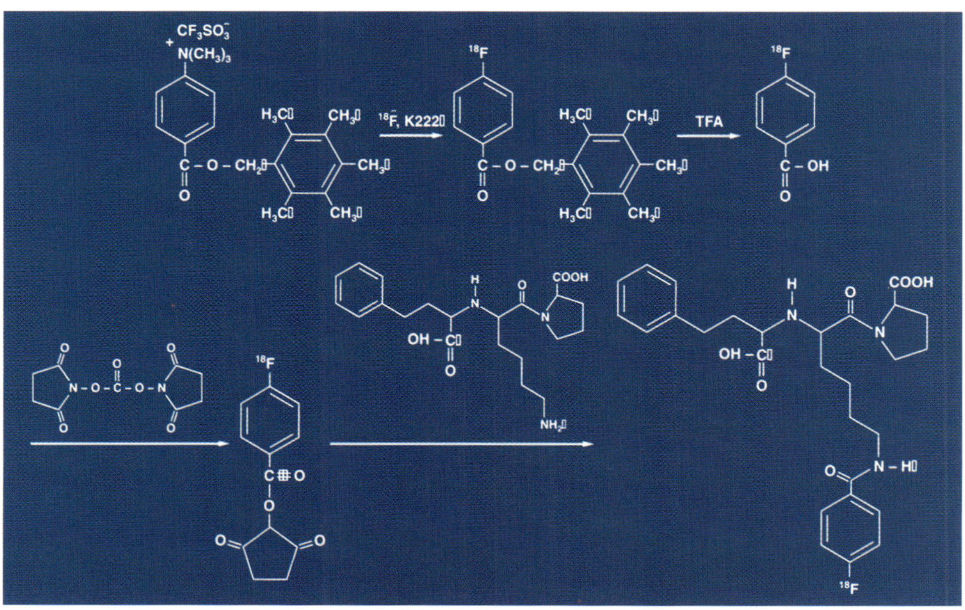

Fig. 5. Synthetic scheme for [^{18}F]fluorobenzoyl-lisinopril.

of AII receptors in remote, noninfarct, infarct and peri-infarct myocardium. A polyclonal antibody against the human AT$_1$R (Santa Cruz Biotechnology, Inc., Santa Cruz, California) was used (1:100 dilution) in conjunction with the Vectastain Elite ABC kit. For antigen retrieval, 5- to 10-mm thick sections were immersed in a 0.4% pepsin solution in 0.1 N HCl for 10 min at 37°C, followed by blocking with 2% bovine serum albumin and 10% normal goat serum. The sections were incubated overnight with AT$_1$R antibody. Bronchial and vascular smooth muscle cells from lung tissue of patients without pulmonary disease served as positive controls. In noninfarct myocardium, AT$_1$R immunoreactivity was confined to smooth muscle and endothelium and myocytes were nonreactive. In contrast, in peri-infarct myocardium, there was increased immunoreactivity for AT$_1$R, which was localized to the myocytes. Although some AT$_1$R immunoreactivity also was seen in infarct myocardium, it was localized predominantly in fibroblasts or within islands of surviving myocytes. These data confirmed the authors' previous quantitative autoradiographic observations concerning [^{18}F]fluorobenzoyl-lisinopril binding in normal, infarct, and peri-infarct myocardium. The immunoreactivity for AT$_1$R in the peri-infarct and infarct myocardium suggests a role for AII in LV remodeling and fibrosis in chronic ischemic cardiomyopathy.

Radioligands for imaging the angiotensin type 1 plasma membrane receptor distribution

The first PET radiotracer for the AT$_1$R was [^{11}C] MK-996 [126]. This compound, however, was difficult to synthesize and the same group developed its methoxy analog, L-159884 [127]. The latter was useful for PET imaging in the canine model [128]; however, unpublished human studies showed rapid metabolism of this compound, which made it unsuitable for use as a clinical imaging tool [129]. The same laboratory examined another class of nonpeptide AT$_1$R-selective antagonists based on the structure of SK-1080 [129]. An analog of the latter that contains an alkyl methoxy group, KR31173, has been developed and tested ex vivo after labeling the compound with ^{11}C for PET imaging. It was shown that [^{11}C] KR31173 binds selectively to AT$_1$R in various tissues, including the heart, and that the binding is inhibited by other selective AT$_1$R blockers. Several laboratories continue the search for an ideal AT$_1$R-specific radiotracer. No data have been reported for the use of these radiotracers in humans.

One laboratory has used a fluorescent and a Tc-99m–labeled AT$_1$R ligand peptide in a postmyocardial infarction murine model for assessment of the remodeling process [130]. Fluoresceinated AT$_1$R ligand (0.05 mg) was administered intravenously in 19 mice with 0- to 12-week-old myocardial infarction (MI) and persistently occluded infarct-related artery, followed by in vivo optical imaging by real-time fluorescence microscopy of the beating mouse heart. No uptake of the peptide was observed in the infarct on day 0 (n=3) and 1 (n=3), similar to control animals (n=3). Distinct dense uptake was observed in the infarct area at 1 (n=3), 3 (n=3), and 6 (n=3) weeks after infarction; the uptake was reduced markedly at 12 weeks (n=1) in the infarct zone, but extended in the peri-infarct region. Echo studies demonstrated significant LV remodeling and reduced LV ejection fraction. Histologic, immunohistochemical, and two-photon microscopy confirmed the localization of tracer within the myofibroblasts that produced collagen fibers identified by second harmonic generation. Surprisingly, no AT$_1$R uptake was seen in myocytes. Noninvasive nuclear imaging in 3 mice after MI and in 3 controls using a microSPECT-CT showed a threefold greater uptake of peptide in the infarct region as compared with remote regions. The noninvasive imaging of neurohumoral upregulation in remodeled myocardium offers the proof of concept that an appropriate imaging strategy can be developed that may allow AT$_1$R imaging and help predict the rate of remodeling and likelihood of development of HF.

Summary

The recent recommendations of the American College of Cardiology/American Heart Association [131] emphasize the development of management strategies that will prevent evolution of HF in those who are susceptible or suffer from LV dysfunction. The assessment of neurohumoral upregulation by appropriate molecular imaging should be able to identify the likelihood of adverse cardiac remodeling and rate of progression of the disease. This assessment should allow a more judicious use of neurohumoral antagonists especially in the subjects who do not suffer from manifest HF. The increasing life expectancy in the Western world and constant advances in the management of other cardiovascular diseases threaten to add tremendously to the burden of HF and a preventive rather than reactive approach would become a necessity. Targeting of RAS will help the understanding of an important aspect of this preventive strategy.

References

[1] Cohn JN, Ferrari R, Sharpe N. Cardiac remodeling–concepts and clinical implications: a consensus paper from an international forum on cardiac remodeling. On behalf of an International Forum on Cardiac Remodeling. J Am Coll Cardiol 2000; 35(3):569–82.

[2] Sutton MG, Sharpe N. Left ventricular remodeling after myocardial infarction: pathophysiology and therapy. Circulation 2000;101(25):2981–8.

[3] Brunner-La Rocca HP, Vaddadi G, Esler MD. Recent insight into therapy of congestive heart failure: focus on ACE inhibition and angiotensin-II antagonism. J Am Coll Cardiol 1999;33:1163–73.

[4] Re R. The clinical implication of tissue renin angiotensin system. Curr Opin Cardiol 2001;6:317–27.

[5] Konstam MA, Rousseau MF, Kronenberg MW, et al. Effects of the angiotensin converting enzyme inhibitor enalapril on the long-term progression of left ventricular dysfunction in patients with heart failure. SOLVD Investigators. Circulation 1992;86:431–8.

[6] Konstam MA, Kronenberg MW, Rousseau MF, et al. Effects of the angiotensin converting enzyme inhibitor enalapril on the long-term progression of left ventricular dilatation in patients with asymptomatic systolic dysfunction. SOLVD (Studies of Left Ventricular Dysfunction) Investigators. Circulation 1993; 88:2277–83.

[7] Greenberg B, Quinones MA, Koilpillai C, et al. Effects of long-term enalapril therapy on cardiac structure and function in patients with left ventricular dysfunction. Results of the SOLVD echocardiography substudy. Circulation 1995;91:2573–81.

[8] Pitt B, Zannad F, Remme WJ, et al. The effect of spironolactone on morbidity and mortality in patients with severe heart failure. Randomized Aldactone Evaluation Study Investigators. N Engl J Med 1999; 341:709–17.

[9] Pitt B, White H, Nicolau J, et al. Eplerenone reduces mortality 30 days after randomization following acute myocardial infarction in patients with left ventricular systolic dysfunction and heart failure. J Am Coll Cardiol 2005;46:425–31.

[10] Bristow MR. β-Adrenergic receptor blockade in chronic heart failure. Circulation 2000;101:558–69.

[11] Bristow MR. The adrenergic nervous system in heart failure. N Engl J Med 1984;311:850–1.

[12] Mann DL. Mechanisms and models in heart failure: a combinatorial approach. Circulation 1999;100: 999–1088.

[13] Cohn JN. Structural basis for heart failure: ventricular remodeling and its pharmacological inhibition. Circulation 1995;91:2504–7.

[14] Douglas PS, Morrow R, Ioli A, et al. Left ventricular shape, afterload, and survival in idiopathic dilated cardiomyopathy. J Am Coll Cardiol 1989;13:311–5.

[15] Vasan RS, Larson MG, Benjamin EJ, et al. Left ventricular dilation and the risk of congestive heart failure in people without myocardial infarction. N Engl J Med 1997;336:1350–5.

[16] Ross Jr J. Afterload mismatch in aortic and mitral valve disease: implications for surgical therapy. J Am Coll Cardiol 1985;5:811–26.

[17] Vatner SF. Reduced subendocardial myocardial perfusion as one mechanism for congestive heart failure. Am J Cardiol 1988;62:94E–8E.

[18] Shannon RP, Komamura K, Shen YT, et al. Impaired regional subendocardial coronary flow reserve in conscious dogs with pacing-induced heart failure. Am J Physiol 1993;265:H801–9.

[19] LeGrice IJ, Takayama Y, Holmes JW, et al. Impaired subendocardial function in tachycardia-induced cardiac failure. Am J Physiol 1995;268:H1788–94.

[20] Grigioni F, Detaint D, Avierinos J-F, et al. Contribution of ischemic mitral regurgitation to congestive heart failure after myocardial infarction. J Am Coll Cardiol 2005;45:260–7.

[21] Lowes BD, Minobe W, Abraham WT, et al. Changes in gene expression in the intact human heart: downregulation of α-myosin heavy chain in hypertrophied, failing ventricular myocardium. J Clin Invest 1997; 100:2315–24.

[22] Nakao K, Minobe W, Roden R, et al. Myosin heavy chain gene expression in human heart failure. J Clin Invest 1997;100:2362–70.

[23] Schaper J, Froede R, Hein ST, et al. Impairment of the myocardial ultrastructure and changes of the cytoskeleton in dilated cardiomyopathy. Circulation 199[illegible]; 83:504–14.

[24] Beuckelmann DJ, Nabauer M, Erdmann E. Intracellular calcium handling in isolated ventricular myocytes from patients with terminal heart failure. Circulation 1992;85:1046–55.

[25] Bristow MR, Ginsburg R, Minobe W, et al. Decreased catecholamine sensitivity and β-adrenergic-receptor density in failing human hearts. N Engl J Med 198[illegible]; 307:205–11.

[26] Mann DL, Kent RL, Parsons B, et al. Adrenergic effects on the biology of the adult mammalian cardiocyte. Circulation 1992;85:790–804.

[27] Narula J, Haider N, Virmani R, et al. Apoptosis in myocytes in end-stage heart failure. N Engl J Med 1996;335:1182–9.

[28] Olivetti G, Abbi R, Quaini F, et al. Apoptosis in the failing human heart. N Engl J Med 1997;336: 1131–41.

[29] Weber KT. Extracellular matrix remodeling in heart failure: a role for de novo angiotensin II generation. Circulation 1997;96:4065–82.

[30] Weber KT, Brilla CG, Janicki JS. Myocardial fibrosis: functional significance and regulatory factors. Cardiovasc Res 1993;27:341–8.

[31] Weber KT, Sun Y, Guarda E. Structural remodeling in hypertensive heart disease and the role of hormones. Hypertension 1994;23:869–77.

[32] Thomas CV, Coker ML, Zellner JL, et al. Increased matrix metalloproteinase activity and selective up-

regulation in LV myocardium from patients with end-stage heart failure. Circulation 1998;97:1708–15.
[33] Li YY, Feldman AM, Sun Y, et al. Differential expression of tissue inhibitors of metalloproteinases in the failing human heart. Circulation 1998;98:1728–34.
[34] Tsutsui H, Spinale FG, Nagatsu M, et al. Effects of chronic beta-adrenergic blockade on the left ventricular and cardiocyte abnormalities of chronic canine mitral regurgitation. J Clin Invest 1994;93: 2639–48.
[35] Lowes BD, Gilbert EM, Abraham WT, et al. Myocardial gene expression in dilated cardiomyopathy treated with beta-blocking agents. N Engl J Med 2002;346:1357–65.
[36] Cohn JN, Johnson G, Ziesche S, et al. A comparison of enalapril with hydralazine-isosorbide dinitrate in the treatment of chronic congestive heart failure. N Engl J Med 1991;325:303–10.
[37] The SOLVD Investigators. Effect of enalapril on survival in patients with reduced left ventricular ejection fractions and congestive heart failure. N Engl J Med 1991;325:293–302.
[38] The SOLVD Investigators. Effect of enalapril on mortality and the development of heart failure in asymptomatic patients with reduced left ventricular ejection fraction. N Engl J Med 1992;327:685–91.
[39] Bristow MR, Gilbert EM, Abraham WT, et al. Carvedilol produces dose-related improvements in left ventricular function and survival in subjects with chronic heart failure. Circulation 1996;94:2807–16.
[40] Packer M, Bristow MR, Cohn JN, et al, for the US Carvedilol Heart Failure Study Group. The effect of carvedilol on morbidity and mortality in patients with chronic heart failure. N Engl J Med 1996;334:1350–5.
[41] MERIT-HF Study Group. Effect of metoprolol CR/XL in chronic heart failure: Metoprolol CR/XL Randomised Intervention Trial in Congestive Heart Failure (MERIT-HF). Lancet 1999;353:2001–7.
[42] Pfeffer MA, Swedberg K, Granger CB, et al. Effects of candesartan on mortality and morbidity in patients with chronic heart failure: the CHARM-Overall programme. Lancet 2003;362:759–66.
[43] Packer M. The neurohormonal hypothesis: a theory to explain the mechanism of disease progression in heart failure. J Am Coll Cardiol 1992;20:248–54.
[44] Booz GW, Baker KM. The role of renin-angiotensin system in the pathophysiology of cardiac remodeling. Blood Press 1996;5(Suppl 2):10–8.
[45] Booz GW, Baker KM. Actions of angiotensin II on isolated cardiac myocytes. Heart Fail Rev 1998;3: 125–30.
[46] Bader M. Role of the local renin-angiotensin system in cardiac damage: a minireview focusing on transgenic animal models. J Mol Cell Cardiol 2002;34: 1455–62.
[47] Berry C, Touyz R, Dominiczak AF, et al. Angiotensin receptors: signaling, vascular pathophysiology, and interactions with ceramide. Am J Physiol 2001;281: H2337–65.
[48] Murphy TJ, Alexander RW, Griendling KK, et al. Isolation of a cDNA encoding the vascular type-1 angiotensin II receptor. Nature 1991;351:233–6.
[49] Sasaki K, Yamano Y, Bardhan S, et al. Cloning and expression of a complementary DNA encoding a bovine adrenal angiotensin II type-1 receptor. Nature 1991;351:230–2.
[50] Kambayashi Y, Bardhan S, Takahashi K, et al. Molecular cloning of a novel angiotensin II receptor isoform involved in phosphotyrosine phosphatase inhibition. J Biol Chem 1993;268:24543–6.
[51] Mukoyama M, Nakajima M, Horiuchi M, et al. Expression cloning of type 2 angiotensin II receptor reveals a unique class of seven-transmembrane receptors. J Biol Chem 1993;268:24539–42.
[52] Bader M. Role of the local renin-angiotensin system in cardiac damage: a minireview focusing on transgenic animal models. J Mol Cell Cardiol 2002;34: 1455–62.
[53] Nguyen G, Delarue F, Burckle C, et al. Pivotal role of the renin/prorenin receptor in angiotensin II production and cellular response to renin. J Clin Invest 2002; 109:1417–27.
[54] Re RN. The intracrine hypothesis and intracellular peptide hormone action. Bioessays 2003;25:401–9.
[55] De Mello WC, Jan Dancer AH. Angiotensin II and the heart. On the intracrine renin-angiotensin system. Hypertens 2000;35:1183–8.
[56] Saris JJ, van den Eijnden MM, Lamers JM, et al. Prorenin-induced myocyte proliferation. No role for intracellular angiotensin. Hypertension 2002;39:573–7.
[57] Peters J, Farrenkopf R, Clausmeyer S, et al. Functional significance of prorenin internalization in the rat heart. Circ Res 2002;90:1135–41.
[58] Gray MO, Long CS, Kalinyak JE, et al. Angiotensin II stimulates cardiomyocyte hypertrophy via paracrine release of TGF-beta 1 and endothelin-1 from fibroblasts. Cardiovasc Res 1998;40:352–63.
[59] Griendling KK, Ushio-Fukai M. Reactive oxygen species as mediators of angiotensin II signaling. Regul Pept 2000;91:21–7.
[60] Harada K, Sugaya T, Murakami K, et al. Angiotensin II type 1A receptor knockout mice display less left ventricular remodeling and improved survival after myocardial infarction. Circulation 1999;100:2093–9.
[61] Struthers AD. Aldosterone blockade in cardiovascular disease. Heart 2004;90:1229–34.
[62] Slight SH, Joseph J, Ganjam VK, et al. Extra-adrenal mineralocorticoids and cardiovascular tissue. J Mol Cell Cardiol 1999;31:1175–84.
[63] Lombes M, Oblin M-E, Gasc J-M, et al. Immunohistochemical and biochemical evidence for a cardiovascular mineralocorticoid receptor. Circ Res 1992;71:503–10.
[64] Studer R, Reinecke H, Muller B, et al. Increased angiotensin-I converting enzyme gene expression in the failing human heart: quantification by competitive RNA polymerase chain reaction. J Clin Invest 1994; 94:301–10.

[65] Danser AHJ, van Kesteren CAM, Bax WA, et al. Prorenin, renin, angiotensin and angiotensin converting enzyme in normal and failing hearts: evidence for renin binding. Circulation 1997;96:220–6.

[66] Neri Serneri GG, Boddi M, Cecioni I, et al. Cardiac angiotensin II formation in the clinical course of heart failure and its relationship with left ventricular function. Circ Res 2001;88:961–71.

[67] Regitz-Zagrosek V, Friedel N, Heymann A, et al. Regulation, chamber localization, and subtype distribution of angiotensin II receptors in human hearts. Circulation 1995;91:1461–71.

[68] Baker KM, Chernin MI, Wixson SK, et al. Renin-angiotensin system involvement in pressure-overload cardiac hypertrophy in rats. Am J Physiol 1990; 259:H324–32.

[69] Miyata S, Haneda T. Hypertrophic growth of cultured neonatal rat heart cells mediated by type 1 angiotensin II receptor. Am J Physiol 1994;266: H2443–51.

[70] Kudoh S, Komuro I, Mizuno T, et al. Angiotensin II stimulates c-Jun NH2-terminal kinase in cultured cardiac myocytes of neonatal rats. Circ Res 1997; 80:139–46.

[71] Pan J, Fukuda K, Kodama H, et al. Role of angiotensin II in activation of the JAK/STAT pathway induced by acute pressure overload in the rat heart. Circ Res 1997;81:611–7.

[72] Sadoshima J-I, Xu Y, Slayter HS, et al. Autocrine release of angiotensin II mediates stretch-induced hypertrophy of cardiac myocytes *in vitro*. Cell 1993; 75:977–84.

[73] Sato M. Myocardial protection by preconditioning of heart with losartan, an angiotensin II type 1-receptor blocker. Implication of bradykinin-dependent and bradykinin-independent mechanisms. Circulation 2000;102(Suppl III):III-346–51.

[74] Swynghedauw B. Molecular mechanisms of myocardial remodeling. Physiol Rev 1999;79:215–62.

[75] Fortuno MA, Ravassa S, Fortuno A, et al. Cardiomyocyte apoptotic cell death in arterial hypertension: mechanisms and potential management. Hypertens 2001;38:1406–12.

[76] Fortuno MA, Lopez N, Gonzalez A, et al. Involvement of cardiomyocyte survival-apoptosis balance in hypertensive cardiac remodeling. Expert Rev Cardiovasc Ther 2003;1:293–307.

[77] Rothermund L, Pinto YM, Vetter R, et al. Effects of angiotensin II subtype 1 receptor blockade on cardiac fibrosis and sarcoplasmic reticulum Ca2+ handling in hypertensive transgenic rats overexpressing the Ren2 gene. J Hypertens 2001;19:1465–72.

[78] Brilla CG, Zhou G, Matsubara L, et al. Collagen metabolism in cultured adult rat cardiac fibroblasts: response to angiotensin II and aldosterone. J Mol Cell Cardiol 1994;26:809–20.

[79] Takeda Y, Yoneda T, Demura M, et al. Calcineurin inhibition attenuates mineralocorticoid-induced cardiac hypertrophy. Circulation 2002;105:677–9.

[80] Sun Y, Zhang J, Lu L, et al. Aldosterone-induced inflammation in the rat heart: role of oxidative stress. Am J Pathol 2002;161:1773–81.

[81] Kuster GM, Kotlyar E, Rude MK, et al. Mineralocorticoid receptor inhibition ameliorates the transition to myocardial failure and decreases oxidative stress and inflammation in mice with chronic pressure overload. Circulation 2005;111:420–7.

[82] Funck RC, Wilke A, Rupp H, et al. Regulation and role of myocardial collagen matrix remodeling in hypertensive heart disease. Adv Exp Med Biol 1997; 432:35–44.

[83] De Angelis N, Fiordaliso F, Latini R, et al. Appraisal of the role of angiotensin II and aldosterone in ventricular myocyte apoptosis in adult normotensive rat. J Mol Cell Cardiol 2002;34:1655–65.

[84] Hein S, Arnon E, Kostin S, et al. Progression from compensated hypertrophy to failure in the pressure-overloaded human heart: structural deterioration and compensatory mechanisms. Circulation 2003;107: 984–91.

[85] Brilla CG, Janicki JS, Weber KT. Impaired diastolic function and coronary reserve in genetic hypertension. Role of interstitial fibrosis and medial thickening of intramyocardial coronary arteries. Circ Res 1991;69:107–15.

[86] Weber KT. Fibrosis and hypertensive heart disease. Curr Opin Cardiol 2000;15:264–72.

[87] Woodiwiss AJ, Tsotetsi OJ, Sprott S, et al. Reduction in myocardial collagen cross-linking parallels left ventricular dilatation in rat models of systolic chamber dysfunction. Circulation 2001;103:155–60.

[88] Sakata Y, Yamamoto K, Mano T, et al. Activation of matrix metalloproteinases precedes left ventricular remodeling in hypertensive heart failure rats: its inhibition as a primary effect of angiotensin-converting enzyme inhibitor. Circulation 2004;109:2143–9.

[89] Spieker LE, Noll G, Ruschitzka FT, et al. Working under pressure: the vascular endothelium in arterial hypertension. J Hum Hypertens 2000;14:617–30.

[90] Folkow B. Early structural changes in hypertension: pathophysiology and clinical consequences. J Cardiovasc Pharmacol 1993;22(Suppl 1):S1–6.

[91] Britton S, Di Salvo J. Effects of angiotensin I and angiotensin II on hindlimb and coronary vascular resistance. Am J Physiol 1973;225:1226–31.

[92] Frewin DB, Jellett LB, Whelan RF. Modification of the vasoconstrictor action of sympathomimetic agents by bretylium tosylate and tranylcypromine in man. Br J Pharmacol 1969;36(3):602–10.

[93] Prasad A, Halcox JP, Waclawiw MA, et al. Angiotensin type 1 receptor antagonism reverses abnormal coronary vasomotion in atherosclerosis. J Am Coll Cardiol 2001;38:1089–95.

[94] Takeishi Y, Minamihaba O, Yamauchi S, et al. Dynamic 123I-BMIPP single-photon emission computed tomography in patients with congestive heart failure: effect of angiotensin II type-1 receptor blockade. Clin Cardiol 2004;27:204–10.

[95] Flather MD, Yusuf S, Kober L, et al. Long-term ACE-inhibitor therapy in patients with heart failure or left-ventricular dysfunction: a systematic overview of data from individual patients. ACE-Inhibitor Myocardial Infarction Collaborative Group. Lancet 2000;355:1575–81.
[96] Weir MR, Gray JM, Paster R, et al. Differing mechanisms of action of angiotensin-converting enzyme inhibition in black and white hypertensive patients. Hypertension 1995;26:124–30.
[97] Exner D, Dries D, Domanski M, et al. Lesser response to angiotensin-converting enzyme inhibitor therapy in black as compared with white patients with left ventricular dysfunction. N Engl J Med 2001;344:1351–7.
[98] Shekelle PG, Rich MW, Morton SC, et al. Efficacy of angiotensin-converting enzyme inhibitors and beta-blockers in the management of left ventricular systolic dysfunction according to race, gender, and diabetic status: a meta-analysis of major clinical trials. J Am Coll Cardiol 2003;41:1529–38.
[99] Jorde U, Ennezat P, Lisker J, et al. Maximally recommended doses of angiotensin-converting enzyme (ACE) inhibitors do not completely prevent ACE-mediated formation of angiotensin II in chronic heart failure. Circulation 2000;101:844–6.
[100] Husain A, Li M, Graham R. Do studies with ACE N- and C-domain-selective inhibitors provide evidence for a non-ACE, non-chymase angiotensin II-forming pathway? Circ Res 2003;93:91–3.
[101] MacFayden RJ, Lee AFC, Morton JJ, et al. How often are angiotensin II and aldosterone concentrations raised during chronic ACE inhibitor treatment in cardiac failure? Heart 1999;82:57–61.
[102] Shirani J, Loredo ML, Dilsizian V. Evidence for disparate distribution of mast cell chymase and angiotensin converting enzyme in peri-infarct and non-infarct myocardium in ischemic cardiomyopathy. J Invest Med 2003;51(Supp 2):S366.
[103] Dilsizian V, Loredo ML, Jagoda EM, et al. Scintigraphic and immunohistochemical evidence for localization of angiotensin converting enzyme to myocytes in human ischemic cardiomyopathy. J Am Coll Cardiol 2003;41:427A.
[104] Benedict CR, Shelton B, Johnstone DE, et al. Prognostic significance of plasma norepinephrine in patients with asymptomatic left ventricular dysfunction. SOLVD Investigators. Circulation 1996;94(4):690–7.
[105] Rouleau JL, Packer M, Moye L, et al. Prognostic value of neurohumoral activation in patients with an acute myocardial infarction: effect of captopril. J Am Coll Cardiol 1994;24:583–91.
[106] van der Ent M, Remme WJ, Bartels GL, et al. Early administration of ramipril in acute myocardial infarction: neurohormonal and hemodynamic effects and tolerability. Cardiology 1997;88(6):548–55.
[107] Wilson Tang WH, Vagelos RH, Yee YG, et al. Neurohormonal and clinical responses to high- versus low-dose enalapril therapy in chronic heart failure. J Am Coll Cardiol 2002;39:70–8.
[108] Danser AHJ, Schalekamp MADH, et al. Angiotensin-converting enzyme in the human heart: effect of the deletion/insertion polymorphism. Circulation 1995;92:1387.
[109] Ueda S, Meredith PA, Morton JJ, et al. ACE (I/D) genotype as a predictor of the magnitude and duration of the response to an ACE inhibitor drug (enalaprilat) in humans. Circulation 1998;98:2148.
[110] Cicoira M, Zanolla L, Rossi A, et al. Failure of aldosterone suppression despite angiotensin-converting enzyme (ACE) inhibitor administration in chronic heart failure is associated with ACE DD genotype. J Am Coll Cardiol 2001;37:1808.
[111] Murphey LJ, Gainer JV, Vaughan DE, et al. Angiotensin-converting enzyme insertion/deletion polymorphism modulates the human in vivo metabolism of bradykinin. Circulation 2000;102:829–32.
[112] Hingorani AD, Jia H, Stevens PA, et al. Renin-angiotensin system gene polymorphisms influence blood pressure and the response to angiotensin-converting enzyme inhibition. J Hypertens 1995;13:1602–9.
[113] Watt GC, Harrap SB, Foy CJ, et al. Abnormalities of glucocorticoid metabolism and the renin-angiotensin system: a four-corner approach to the identification of genetic determinants of blood pressure. J Hypertens 1992;10:473–82.
[114] Hindorff LA, Heckbert SR, Tracy R, et al. Angiotensin II type I receptor polymorphisms in the cardiovascular health study: relation to blood pressure, ethnicity and cardiovascular events. Am J Hypertens 2002;15:1050–6.
[115] Gallinat S, Busche S, Raizada MK, et al. The angiotensin II type 2 receptor: an enigma with multiple variations. Am J Physiol Endocrinol Metab 2000;278:E357–74.
[116] Jaffer FA, Weissleder R. Seeing within: molecular imaging of the cardiovascular system. Circ Res 2004;94:433–45.
[117] Markham J, McCarthy TJ, Welch MJ, et al. In vivo measurements of pulmonary angiotensin-converting enzyme kinetics. I. Theory and error analysis. J Appl Physiol 1995;78:1158–68.
[118] Schuster DP, McCarthy TJ, Welch MJ, et al. In vivo measurements of pulmonary angiotensin-converting enzyme kinetics. II. Implementation and application. J Appl Physiol 1995;78:1169–78.
[119] Sun Y, Mendelsohn FAO. Angiotensin converting enzyme inhibitor in heart, kidney, and serum studied *ex vivo* after administration of zofenopril, captopril, and lisonopril. J Cardiovasc Pharamcol 1991;18:478–85.
[120] Cushman DW, Wang FL, Fung WC, et al. Differentiation of angiotensin-converting enzyme (ACE) inhibitors by their selective inhibition of ACE in physiologically important target organs. Am J Hypertens 1989;2:294–306.

[121] Hooper NM, Turner AJ. An ACE structure. Nat Struct Biol 2003;10:155–7.

[122] Moskowitz DW. From pharmacogenomics to improved patient outcomes: angiotensin I-converting enzyme as an example. Diabetes Technol Ther 2002; 4:519–32.

[123] Chai SY, Mendelsohn FA, Paxinos G. Angiotensin converting enzyme in rat brain visualized by quantitative in vitro autoradiography. Neuroscience 1987; 20:615–27.

[124] Lee YHC, Kiesewetter DO, Lang L, et al. Synthesis of 4-[^{18}F]fluorobenzoyllisinopril: a radioligand for angiotensin converting enzyme (ACE) imaging with positron emission tomography. J Labelled Comp Radiopharm 2001;44:S268–70.

[125] Dilsizian V, Shirani J, Lee YHC, et al. Specific binding of [^{18}F] fluorobenzoyl-lisinopril to angiotensin converting enzyme in human heart tissue of ischemic cardiomyopathy [abstract]. Circulation 2001; 104:II-694.

[126] Mathews WB, Burns HD, Dannals RF, et al. Carbon-11 labeling of the potent nonpeptide angiotensin-II antagonist MK-996. J Labelled Comp Radiopharm 1995;36:729–37.

[127] Hamill TG, Burns HD, Dannals RF, et al. Development of [11C] L-159,884: a radiolabelled, nonpeptide angiotensin II antagonist that is useful for angiotensin II, AT1 receptor imaging. Appl Radiat Isot 1996;47: 211–8.

[128] Szabo Z, Speth RC, Brown PR, et al. Use of positron emission tomography to study AT1 receptor regulation in vivo. J Am Soc Nephrol 2001;12: 1350–8.

[129] Lee SH, Jung YS, Lee BH, et al. Characterization of angiotensin II antagonism displayed by SK-1080, a novel nonpeptide AT1-receptor antagonist. J Cardiovasc Pharmacol 1999;33:367–74.

[130] Verjans J, Lovhaug D, Narula N, et al. Noninvasive imaging of myocardial angiotensin receptors in heart failure. 25th Annual Scientific Sessions, American Heart Association, Western States Affiliates. Irvine (CA), September 30, 2005.

[131] Hunt SA, Abraham T, Chin H, et al. ACC/AHA 2005 guideline update for the diagnosis and management of chronic heart failure in the adult: a report of the American College of Cardiology/American Heart Association Task Force on practice guidelines (writing committee to update the 2001 guidelines for the evaluation and management of heart failure): developed in collaboration with the American College of Chest Physicians and the International Society for Heart and Lung Transplantation: endorsed by the Heart Rhythm Society. Circulation 2005;112: e154–235.

ELSEVIER
SAUNDERS

Heart Failure Clin 2 (2006) 249–253

HEART
FAILURE
CLINICS

Index

Note: Page numbers of article titles are in **boldface** type.

doi:10.1016/S1551-7136(06)00046-8

D

E

F

G

H

I

L

M

N

P

R

S

Changing Your Address?

Make sure your subscription changes too! When you notify us of your new address, you can help make our job easier by including an exact copy of your Clinics label number with your old address (see illustration below.) This number identifies you to our computer system and will speed the processing of your address change. Please be sure this label number accompanies your old address and your corrected address—you can send an old Clinics label with your number on it or just copy it exactly and send it to the address listed below.

We appreciate your help in our attempt to give you continuous coverage. Thank you.

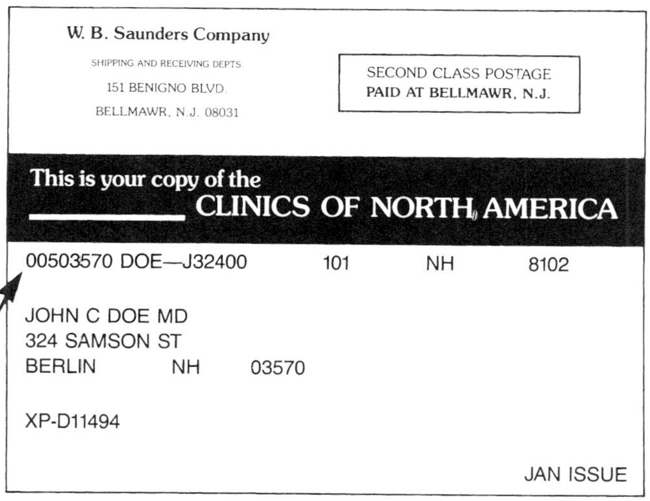

W. B. Saunders Company
SHIPPING AND RECEIVING DEPTS
151 BENIGNO BLVD.
BELLMAWR, N.J. 08031

SECOND CLASS POSTAGE
PAID AT BELLMAWR, N.J.

This is your copy of the
__________ CLINICS OF NORTH AMERICA

00503570 DOE—J32400   101   NH   8102

JOHN C DOE MD
324 SAMSON ST
BERLIN   NH   03570

XP-D11494

JAN ISSUE

Your Clinics Label Number

Copy it exactly or send your label
along with your address to:
W.B. Saunders Company, Customer Service
Orlando, FL 32887-4800
Call Toll Free 1-800-654-2452

Please allow four to six weeks for delivery of new subscriptions and for processing address changes.